7-05
P9-DBI-842
WITHDRAWN

The Chicken Health Handbook

Gail Damerow

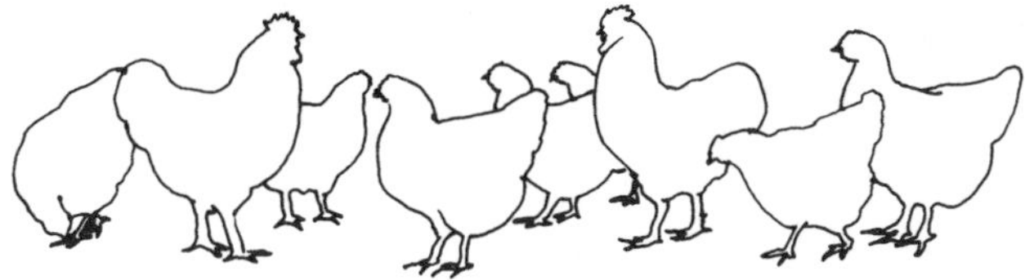

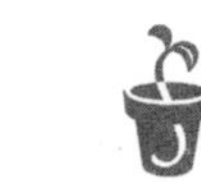

Storey Publishing

The mission of Storey Publishing is to serve our customers by publishing practical information that encourages personal independence in harmony with the environment.

Edited by Amanda R. Haar
Cover design by Meredith Maker
Text design and production by Cynthia McFarland
Cover photograph ©John Colwell from Grant Heilmann Photography
Line drawings by Elayne Sears except chapter opener line art and diagram art on pages 6 and 216 by Cynthia McFarland
Indexed by Gail Damerow

Copyright © 1994 by Gail Damerow

All rights reserved. No part of this book may be reproduced without written permission from the publisher, except by a reviewer who may quote brief passages or reproduce illustrations in a review with appropriate credits; nor may any part of this book be reproduced, stored in a retrieval system, or transmitted in any form or by any means — electronic, mechanical, photocopying, recording, or other — without written permission from the publisher.

The information in this book is true and complete to the best of our knowledge. All recommendations are made without guarantee on the part of the author or Storey Publishing. The author and publisher disclaim any liability in connection with the use of this information. For additional information, please contact Storey Publishing, 210 MASS MoCA Way, North Adams, MA 01247.

Storey books are available for special premium and promotional uses and for customized editions. For further information, please call 1-800-793-9396.

Printed in the United States by Versa Press
30 29 28 27 26 25 24 23 22 21 19 18

Library of Congress Cataloging-in-Publication Data

Damerow, Gail.
Chicken health handbook / Gail Damerow
p. cm.
Includes bibliographical references (p.) and index.
ISBN 0-88266-611-8 (pbk.)
1. Chickens — Diseases. 2. Chickens — Health. 3. Chickens — Parasites. I. Title.
SF995.D33 1994
636.5'089—dc20 93-33385
CIP

WITHDRAWN

Contents

Charts

Chapter 7 INFECTIOUS DISEASES

Chapter 8 ENVIRONMENT-RELATED PROBLEMS

Chapter 9 DIAGNOSTIC GUIDES

Chapter 10 POSTMORTEM EXAMINATION

Chapter 11 THERAPY

Chapter12 ENHANCING IMMUNITY

Chapter 13 INCUBATION AND BROODING

Chapter14 CHICKENS AND HUMAN HEALTH

Foreword

IN MY VETERINARY PRACTICE I work with many poultry fanciers and backyard poultry farmers. I am often asked what books I could recommend to help them learn better management and gain a better understanding of the diseases that may affect their birds. I have been unable to help them much with their requests, as most of the texts on avian diseases are written for veterinarians, of limited usefulness to the layperson. Very few books are available for the fancier, and those that I have seen are generally incomplete and not particularly accurate.

Therefore, I am delighted to see this publication being made available to the poultry fancier. Gail Damerow has covered the topic of small-flock poultry health management very completely and competently. The information is presented accurately and in enough detail to give the fancier a full understanding of the diseases, their prevention and treatments. Yet this is done in an easily understood manner through careful attention to definitions and explanations. It is not an easy task to convert scientific information that veterinarians study for years to understand into useful, management-bottom-line information for the average backyard poultry grower. I believe Ms. Damerow has accomplished this in her book.

Ms. Damerow has also presented her information in a quite accessible format for the fancier. She not only describes each disorder as a distinct entity, which can be looked up by the fancier who has just received a diagnosis and wants to learn more about the disease, but she also has provided a section arranged by clinical signs. The fancier, seeing certain clinical signs in the flock, can go to the book and look up what the possible causes are. Both of these approaches will have their usefulness for the fancier.

Prevention of disease through good management is essential when raising poultry, especially small flocks of poultry, which are often not vaccinated for many of the diseases that commercial poultry are, which often travel to and from shows, and which are maintained in multi-age facilities. Also, the generally low monetary value of individual birds makes costs of diagnosis and treatments impractical in many cases. Having a book such as this which outlines good disease prevention strategies, as well as disease management strategies should problems occur, is a valuable asset to the poultry fancier.

I believe the best use of this book is to read it through for the disease prevention management information whether you are having disease problems in your birds or not. Implement whatever management practices you are not already using. Then keep the book handy as a reference if you see a problem pop up in your flock.

Jeanne Smith, D.V.M.
Avian Health Services
3220 Quail Drive, Placerville, CA 95667

Introduction

THIS BOOK WAS BORN out of years of frustration in trying to deal with chicken diseases and not being able to find a clearly understandable, in-depth source of information. Books that are easy to understand are usually not complete — often failing to contain the very information needed most. On the other hand, comprehensive books rarely make sense to the non-specialist. Making matters worse, most printed information is geared toward operators of large commercial flocks, who deal with quite a different set of problems from those experienced by small-flock owners.

Since I couldn't find the book I needed, after years of experience raising chickens I decided to write it. I've tried to include all the information necessary to keep a small flock healthy, while avoiding technical details that have no practical application (do you *really* need to know which bacteria are gram-negative, polar-staining, and non-motile?).

I can't promise to have described every conceivable problem your chickens might experience, but I've covered all the common problems and many less common ones you'll likely never see but will surely be interested in, if one of them turns up in your flock.

Years ago, when I was secretary of the Pacific Poultry Breeders Association and was responsible for putting out the organization's newsletter, I was accused of placing too much emphasis on diseases. Complainers grumbled that chicken-keepers (especially novices) might get the idea that raising chickens involves a constant battle with diseases.

Those complaints haunted me as I wrote this book, so I wish to make clear that my aim is not to discourage you from keeping chickens. It is, rather, to help you fine tune your management practices so you can avoid diseases, and to increase your disease awareness so you can recognize any problem that might occur and take action before the problem gets out of hand.

How you approach injury or disease in your flock depends a great deal on your purpose in keeping chickens, whether it is to enjoy healthful meat and eggs, to have fun showing your birds, or to make money selling homegrown meat or eggs. This book provides information pertaining to all three situations. It is *not* for the commercial grower who takes an impersonal view of individual birds, who crowds them and thereby induces stress and disease, who medicates them to the max, and who breeds for ever-greater growth or production at the expense of disease resistance. (Diseases found primarily in commercial flocks are described here, however, so you can watch out for them if you live in a major poultry-producing area.)

I wish to thank Randy Holliman of Hoechst-Roussel Agri-Vet Company in Murfreesboro, Tennessee, for helping me learn how to do a home fecal test; L. Dwight Schwartz, D.V.M., avian health consultant with Avicon, Inc. in Okemos, Michigan, for reviewing my chapter on "Diseases and Disorders" and helping fill in the gaps; Arthur A. Bickford, D.V.M., of the California Veterinary Laboratory in Turlock for his thorough review and numerous helpful suggestions; and Jeanne Smith, D.V.M., of Avian Health Services in Placerville, California, for her technical review and wonderful insights into the problems of small-flock ownership.

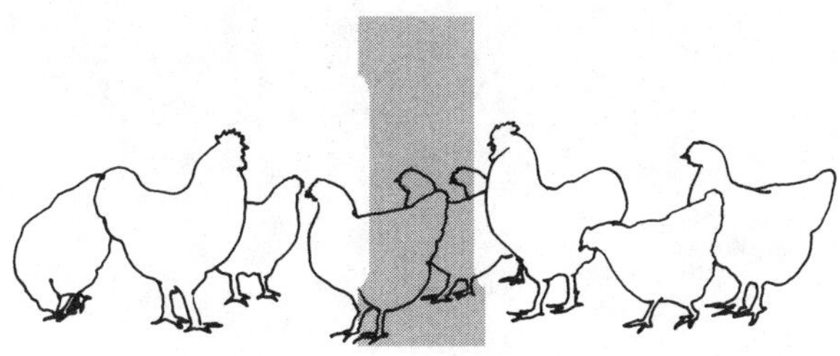

Chicken Health

DURING THE PAST CENTURY, most of the serious diseases that once plagued poultry keepers have been brought under control. It wasn't that long ago, for example, that we discovered viruses and invented vaccines against them, or that we first began to understand the life cycles of internal parasites and were finally able to control them.

While we have been busy learning to control old diseases, new ones have appeared. Some were always there, to be discovered as technology improved. Others have popped up out of the blue. Still others have been caused by the way modern poultry flocks are managed. So, while technology gives us new ways to fight diseases, it also gives us new diseases to fight.

What Is Disease?

Disease is defined as a departure from health and includes any condition that impairs normal body functions. Disease results from a combination of indirect causes (called "stress") that reduce resistance and direct causes that produce the disease.

Direct causes of disease can be divided into two categories: infectious and non-infectious. Infectious diseases result from invasion of the body by another living organism — bacteria, viruses, fungi, protozoa, and a variety of internal and external parasites. Non-infectious diseases are caused by nutritional problems (deficiency or excess), chemical poisons, traumatic injury, or even excessive stress.

ALLAN DAMEROW

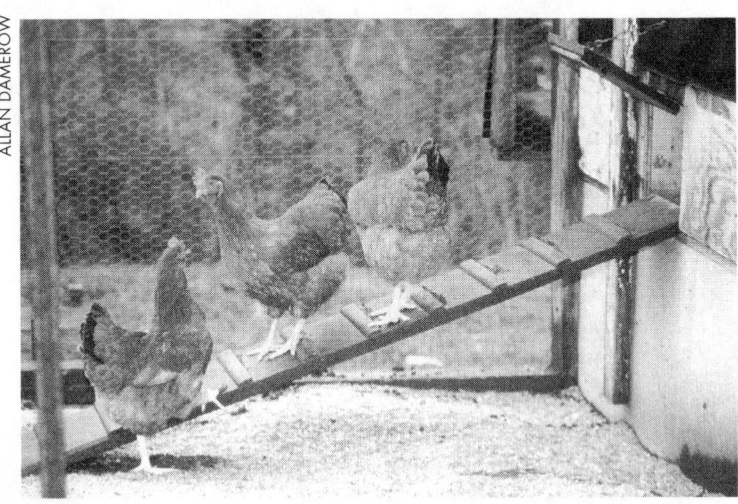

Fresh air and sunshine promote good health.

Technically speaking, all infectious diseases are parasitic, and all parasitic invasions are infectious. By convention, the word "parasite" is often used to identify infectious diseases caused by animal forms, most of which can be seen with the naked eye (worms, lice, mites, and the like).

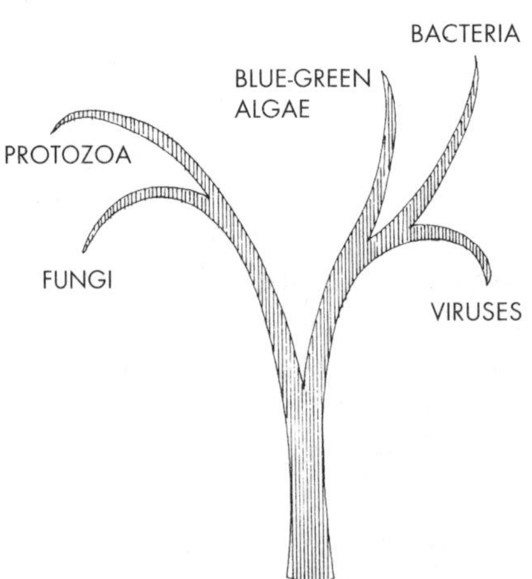

Microorganisms causing infectious disease

The word "infection" is generally reserved for invasion by other forms, which all happen to be microscopic (bacteria, virus, fungi, etc.). The distinction breaks down, however, in the case of protozoa, which are both animal forms and microscopic. (In this book, protozoa are grouped with the other animal forms.)

Regardless of a disease's cause, before you can effectively control it, you must know how diseases in general are introduced and how they spread.

Reservoirs of Infection

Diseases are introduced from reservoirs of infection, defined as any source or site where a disease-causing organism survives or multiplies and from which it can be transferred to a host — in this case, a chicken. A reservoir of infection may be animate or inanimate.

Animate or living reservoirs include:

- chickens and other domestic poultry
- exotic and cage birds
- wild birds
- wild animals (including rodents)
- livestock
- household pets
- humans
- earthworms, snails, and slugs
- arthropods (fleas, mites, ticks, lice, and mosquitoes that bite; sow bugs, crickets, and grasshoppers that chickens eat)

Some disease-causing organisms, such as the infectious bronchitis virus, are species specific for chickens, meaning they affect only chickens. Others are shared among different kinds of poultry, such as the avian reovirus, which infects both chickens and turkeys. Some microbes are harmless to one type of fowl but devastating to others, such as the Marek's disease virus that's common and harmless in turkeys but potentially deadly to chickens. Some microbes, including *Salmonella* bacteria, infect a wide variety of vertebrates including humans. A few infectious organisms spend part of their life cycles living in arthropods that parasitize chickens or that spread disease to chickens through their bites.

A chicken may serve as its own reservoir of infection, as occurs when a disease is caused by an organism the chicken normally carries on or in its body. Examples are streptococci and *Pasteurella* bacteria, both of which infect a bird after its resistance has been reduced by some other cause. Dead chickens, improperly disposed of, can also serve as reservoirs of infection, if their bodies are pecked by susceptible chickens.

Inanimate reservoirs of infection include:

- feed containing fungi or bacteria
- water, usually stagnant and rich in organic matter, in which bacteria, fungi, or protozoa thrive
- litter, soil, and dust harboring spore-bearing organisms that produce disease when they get into a chicken's tissue, often through a wound
- so-called "fomites" — articles that can be contaminated by disease-causing organisms. Examples of fomites include a crate used for carrying chickens, an incubator used for hatching chicks, or a brooder in which chicks are raised. A fomite can be either a reservoir of infection or merely a vehicle that serves as a means of spreading infectious organisms from one place to another.

How Diseases Spread

Once a disease has been introduced, it may spread from one chicken to another in two ways:

- vertically — from an infected hen to her chicks by means of hatching eggs (or, in the case of some viruses, from an infected cock through semen fertilizing the eggs);
- horizontally — from one bird to another through direct or indirect contact.

Direct contact occurs when an infected bird and a susceptible bird peck, preen, or mate one another. Diseases that spread through contact with the skin of an infected bird include pox and influenza (caused by viruses) and staphylococcal and streptococcal infections (caused by opportunistic bacteria). Staph and strep infections also spread through direct mucus-to-mucus contact during mating.

Indirect contact occurs by means of a vehicle (sometimes called a "mechanical vector"). A vehicle is anything, living or otherwise, capable of transporting disease-causing organisms from one place to another. Like reservoirs of infection, vehicles can be either animate or inanimate.

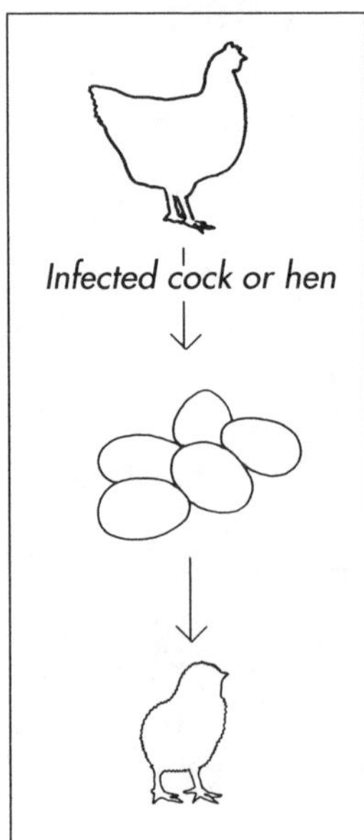

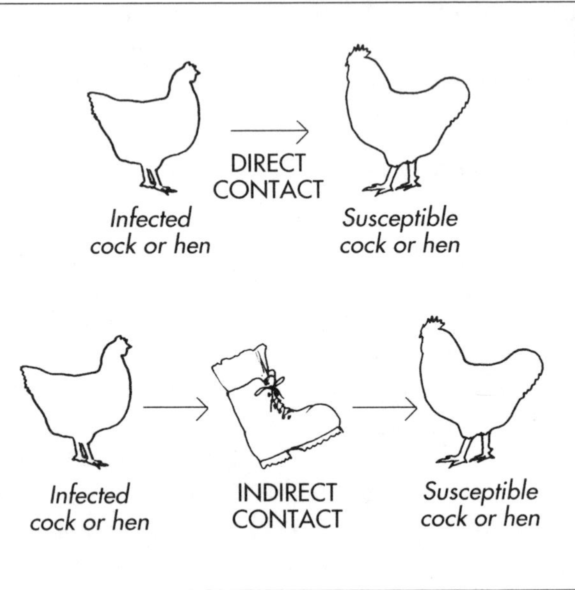

Animate vehicles include:

- wild birds, rodents, household pets, and other animals that carry infectious organisms on their feet, feathers, or fur (as distinct from diseased animals that spread infection through their saliva, droppings, or urine);
- flies and other arthropods that carry disease on their feet or bodies (as distinct from infected arthropods that spread disease by injecting contaminated saliva);
- humans who carry disease-causing organisms on their clothing, shoes, skin, or hair, including fanciers who visit one another, vaccination crews that travel from place to place, meter readers, electricians, plumbers, and feed delivery personnel.

Inanimate vehicles include:

- shed skin, feathers, droppings, broken eggs, and other debris from infected birds;
- feed and drinking water contaminated by body discharges from infected birds, including undrained puddles and streams that run past one flock and then another;
- air, which wafts dust, fluff, fine bits of dried droppings, and droplets of respiratory moisture expelled by breathing, sneezing, or coughing (most airborne infections do not spread far);
- needles that contaminate the blood of susceptible chickens during flockwide vaccination of infected and susceptible birds alike;
- used equipment, egg cartons, waterers, feeders, feed sacks, tires (of cars, trucks, or wheelbarrows), and other fomites to which body discharges containing disease-causing microbes may cling, to be transported for hundreds of miles.

Carriers

Many diseases are spread by carriers. A carrier is a bird that does not show symptoms of a disease, yet harbors the organism that causes the disease. Carriers may be active or passive. An active carrier once had symptoms of the disease but has since recovered. A passive carrier never developed symptoms. Whether active or passive, a carrier sheds and spreads disease-causing organisms.

Diseases that produce carriers usually are not worth curing. You can cure a bird of infectious coryza, for instance, but you have no way of knowing if the bird will become a carrier and spread the disease to susceptible birds in the future.

The older a bird is, the more exposure it has had to disease-causing organisms, and the more likely it is to be a carrier. Since growing and adult birds carry levels of microbes that chicks and young birds can't resist, birds of various ages should never be mixed together.

CHART 1-1

Diseases Spread by Carriers

Disease	*Cause*	*Incidence*
Air-sac disease	bacteria	common
Arizonosis	bacteria	rare
Blackhead	protozoa	rare
Bluecomb	unknown	rare
Campylobacteriosis	bacteria	common
Canker	protozoa	rare
Chlamydiosis	bacteria	rare
Cholera	bacteria	not common
Chronic respiratory disease	bacteria	common
Erysipelas	bacteria	rare
Infectious bronchitis	virus	common
Infectious coryza	bacteria	common
Infectious laryngotracheitis	virus	common
Infectious synovitis	bacteria	not common
Influenza	virus	rare
Leucocytozoonosis	protozoa	rare
Listeriosis	bacteria	rare
Lymphoid leukosis	virus	common
Marek's disease	virus	common
Newcastle	virus	common
Newcastle (exotic)	virus	rare
Parasites	worms	very common
Paratyphoid	bacteria	common
Pox	virus	common
Pullorum	bacteria	rare
Thrush	fungus	common
Typhoid	bacteria	rare
Ulcerative enteritis	bacteria	common

Biosecurity

"Biosecurity" is the latest buzzword in the world of poultry health. It means protecting your flock from infectious diseases and it encompasses any precaution you take to prevent diseases from entering or surviving in your yard.

Different sectors of the poultry industry place emphasis on different biosecurity measures. The USDA favors all-in, all-out management, which works fine for commercial broiler and layer operations, but not for an ongoing backyard flock. Manufacturers of pharmaceuticals promote the use of antibiotics and other drugs as a means of controlling disease, but the use of drugs for non-medical purposes has serious drawbacks in commercial and backyard flocks alike.

No single biosecurity measure provides the perfect answer to preventing disease. Instead, protect your flock with a well-thought-out program of interrelated precautions, thoroughly grounded in old-fashioned common sense.

As part of your common sense biosecurity program:

- keep a flock history
- start with good foundation stock
- maintain a closed flock
- breed for resistance
- medicate only as necessary
- provide a sound environment
- practice good sanitation
- minimize stress
- feed a balanced ration

Flock History

A flock history is basically a diary that includes anything and everything pertaining to your flock. Start it the moment you acquire your first birds, noting the date (or date of hatch — if you purchase by mail, it will be on the shipping carton), source, strain (if applicable), anything the seller tells you about the birds' past history, and any health certificates that come with the birds.

Document your feeding and management practices and any changes you make, including vaccinations you give and medications you use. Write things down as you go along. It may seem like a time-consuming chore, but it's a lot easier than trying to reconstruct events later if you need the information to help trace a health problem.

The "Flock History" chart on page 148 lists additional information to include in your flock history.

Foundation Stock

It's difficult to maintain a healthy flock unless you start out with healthy stock. The best way to make sure the birds are healthy is to purchase locally, so you can see whether or not they come from a healthful environment. You can then ask the seller, eye to eye, about the birds' ages and health history, and you can see for yourself if any of the seller's birds have symptoms of diseases that might be carried by the birds you plan to buy.

You'll have the least chance of getting diseased birds if you start with newly hatched chicks. The older the bird, the more disease problems it has been exposed to. If you do purchase older birds, take time to check their appearance. Make sure they have glossy plumage, look perky and active, and don't show any signs of stress behavior.

Flocks enrolled in the National Poultry Improvement Plan (NPIP) are certified to be free of pullorum and typhoid. Some are also free of mycoplasmosis. (Information on how to obtain the latest NPIP directory is offered in the appendix.) Unfortunately, you may not find an NPIP member who has the kind of birds you want.

Don't buy birds if you are not totally satisfied with their background in terms of genetics, management, sanitation, or health history. Above all, avoid birds from live-bird auctions, flea markets, wheeler-dealers, traders, uncertified hatcheries, and any other source where birds are brought together from far-flung flocks.

Closed Flock

Each flock is exposed to a unique set of disease-causing organisms, so that each develops its own distinct set of immunities. Birds from two healthy flocks can therefore give each other diseases for which the others have no defenses.

Once your flock is established, the best way to avoid diseases is to keep a closed flock. Keeping a closed flock means avoiding direct or indirect contact with other birds. Complete avoidance isn't always possible, but knowing the dangers helps keep them to a minimum.

Maintaining a closed flock means you don't:

- mix birds from various sources
- bring in new birds
- return a bird to your property once it's been elsewhere
- visit other flocks
- let owners of other flocks visit yours
- borrow or lend equipment

- hatch eggs from other flocks
- allow wild birds free access to your yard

Unfortunately for biosecurity, visiting other flocks is part of the fun of having chickens. If you do visit other flocks, slip plastic grocery bags over your shoes and tie the handles around your ankles. When the visit is over, seal the two bags in a third bag for disposal. If other flock owners visit you, ask them to do the same. You may feel foolish wearing plastic bags on your feet, but you'll feel even more foolish if you spread a disease to someone else's birds or bring a disease home to your flock.

Trading and showing birds are other fun activities that breach biosecurity. Although diseases are more likely to be spread by trading than by showing, occasionally a highly contagious disease (most often infectious laryngotracheitis) does make the show rounds. To be on the safe side, isolate any returning show bird or incoming new bird with two or three sacrificial culls from your flock. If your old chickens remain healthy after about a month, chances are good the incoming chicken is not a carrier.

Excluding Wild Birds

Wild birds are seriously endangered due to the cutting down of forests, draining of wetlands, and other disturbances to their natural environment. Instead of trapping or poisoning wild birds to keep them away from your flock, cover your run with wire or plastic mesh. If your chickens are range fed, so that an overhead cover is impractical, place their feeders indoors so spilled grain won't attract wild birds.

Breeding for Resistance

Old poultry books make frequent references to "constitutional vigor." The concept is quite simple: in every flock some individuals are less affected by diseases than others. Susceptible birds get sick or die when exposed to a disease. Resistant birds (those with "constitutional vigor") get mildly sick and recover quickly or don't get ill at all.

Developing your flock's genetic resistance means breeding only those birds that are less affected by disease, so you'll raise more like them. The remainder should be culled. In this context, cull means kill — it does not mean passing on your problem birds to someone else.

Some poultry specialists take the position that small-flock owners should purchase new stock each year and that raising chicks from your own breeder flock only promotes disease. Quite the contrary will be true, *if* you take care to cull sick birds so that your flock gradually develops genetic resistance. Fred P. Jeffrey (backyard fancier, retired professor of poultry science, and author of

Chicken Diseases) advocates the rigid culling of all snifflers, droopers, feather rufflers, poor eaters, and pale-headed birds to be sure they don't reproduce their kind.

Guidelines on Breeding for Resistance

- **Keep a minimum breeding flock of about fifty birds, so you'll have the leeway to cull vigorously and still maintain a viable flock.**
- **Use breeders that are at least two years old, which opposes the conventional wisdom that the older the bird, the more diseases it has been exposed to and the less healthy it is likely to be. Chicks hatched from survivors of disease exposure are particularly hearty and may carry maternal antibodies that give them further immunity. (Be sure that the disease cannot be egg-transmitted from survivor-carriers to their chicks.)**
- **"Progeny test" or evaluate your breeders based on the performance of their offspring. Progeny testing requires pedigreeing your birds; in other words, you must know exactly which cock and hen produced each chick (for ideas on how to keep track of chicks, see "Chick Identification," page 221). For progeny testing, Jeffrey suggests this criterion: if the majority of progeny from a particular mating live for 1½ years, keep the parents in your breeder flock; if the majority of progeny do not survive that long, cull the parents *and* the remaining progeny.**
- **Find indicators or factors known to be related to susceptibility or resistance to diseases prevalent in your area. Some indicators can be identified through blood typing, a potentially impractical, expensive, and time-consuming practice. Other indicators are more accessible to the owner of a small flock. For example, resistance to pullorum is associated with a higher than normal body temperature in chicks during their first six days of life.**
- **Give your flock a leg up on resistance by starting with a breed or strain that already has some natural resistance to the diseases and parasites they will encounter in your area. Leghorns and other light breeds, for example, are more resistant to pullorum than Rocks, Reds, and other heavy breeds; Rhode Island Reds are more resistant to worms than White Leghorns.**

Breeding for genetic resistance does have its down side: your birds can develop resistance only to diseases present in your yard. If a new disease is introduced, your chickens may have no defenses against it. Since no flock can be exposed to all possible diseases, no flock can be immune to all possible diseases. Even if you breed for genetic resistance, you must still take care not to introduce new diseases.

Another aspect to breeding for resistance is that disease-causing organisms are likely to evolve right along with your resistant strain of birds. These evolving new forms of bacteria and viruses make breeding for resistance a never-ending process.

Medication Schedule

Using drugs casually, rather than controlling disease through proper management, will only increase your problems and your costs. Instead, work out a disease prevention program based on the problems prevalent in your area. Vaccinate against serious diseases your flock is likely to be exposed to, especially epidemic tremor, infectious bronchitis, infectious bursal disease, and Marek's disease. Pay attention to your flock and know what to look for, so if a problem does occur you'll be ready to treat it properly and promptly.

Sound Environment

The way you house your chickens influences their state of health. Poultry housing falls into four basic categories:

- cage confinement — common for show birds, pedigreed breeders, and large, mechanized laying flocks
- confinement housing — common for broilers, breeder flocks, and floor-managed layers
- free range — favored for backyard laying flocks and range-fed or so-called "organic" meat birds
- yard and coop — preferred for backyard flocks in the suburbs and other areas where space is limited

Commercial flocks are confined indoors, in cages or on the floor, for several reasons: lighting can be strictly controlled, air can be filtered, and diseases that are spread by flying insects and wild birds can be excluded. While confined flocks are protected from some diseases, as a trade-off they incur other health problems due to lack of sunshine, fresh air, and activity. In addition, if a contagious disease does manage to get in, it spreads like wildfire.

No matter how you choose to house your chickens, they need protection from cold, heat, rain, and wind. A sound fence protects them from four-footed predators; a covered yard protects them from flying predators. The yard or pen should be free of junk and weeds to discourage mice and rats.

The single most important feature of any chicken house is ease of cleaning. If cleanup is a hassle, you won't do it as often as you ought. The tighter the construction, the easier cleaning is and the fewer cracks and crevices there will be where pathogens and parasites can hide.

Smooth surfaces are easier to clean than rough or porous surfaces. Old-time poultry keepers used to spray crankcase oil along the bottoms of walls and on wood and cement floors, to make these surfaces less penetrable and therefore easier to clean. The practice has the additional advantage of controlling roundworms, as well as common insects, but it has the disadvantage of creating a fire hazard in wood structures.

Floors. Flooring can be one of four basic types:

- A dirt floor is simple and cheap, and it keeps birds cool in warm weather. Its disadvantages are that it draws heat in cold weather, does not exclude burrowing rodents, and cannot be effectively cleaned.
- A wood floor invariably has cracks that get packed with filth, and most are built too close to the ground, providing a shallow air space that invites invasion by rodents.
- Droppings boards made of wood battens or welded wire have the advantage of allowing droppings to fall through where chickens can't pick in them. Like a wood floor, droppings boards must be placed high enough to discourage rodents.
- Concrete, if well finished, is the most expensive type of flooring, but requires minimal repair and upkeep, is easy to clean, and discourages rodents.

Floor Space. Crowded conditions get filthy fast, reduce the flow of fresh air, and cause stress — all inducements to disease. The minimum floor space requirements, including those listed in the accompanying chart, may need adjustment to suit your specific management practices.

To keep chickens evenly spread over the available space, use several feeders and waterers and spread them around in different locations. In extremely cold weather conditions, provide heat to prevent huddling.

Litter management. When chickens are kept on a flooring other than droppings boards, use litter to absorb droppings and moisture expelled by the flock. For chicks, use 3 inches (7.5 cm) or more of clean litter that's absorbent, non-toxic, free of mold, and has particles too large to be eaten. For adult birds, litter should be at least 8 inches (20 cm) deep. Dry pine shavings make

Roosts

Since droppings tend to accumulate where chickens perch at night, roosts should be placed over wooden battens or welded wire droppings boards. Allow at least 8 inches (20 cm) of roosting space per bird. Roosts should be approximately 2 inches (5 cm) in diameter (1 inch [2.5 cm] for bantams) and free of splinters and sharp edges that can cause foot injuries. To prevent breast blisters and bumblefoot in broilers and in cocks of the heavy breeds, do not allow these heavier birds to roost.

CHART 1-2

Minimum Space Requirements

Birds	*Age*	*Open Housing*		*ConfinedHousing*		*Caged*	
		sq ft/Bird	Birds/sq m	sq ft/Bird	Birds/sq m	sq in/Bird	sq cm/Bird
Heavy	1–7 days	-	-	0.5	20	(Do not house heavy breeds on wire)	
	1–8 weeks	1.0	10	2.5	4		
	9–15* weeks	2.0	5	5.0	2		
	15–20 weeks	3.0	4	7.5	1.5		
	21 weeks +	4.0	3	10.0	1		
Light	1 day–1 week	-	-	0.5	20	25	160
	1–11 weeks	1.0	10	2.5	4	45	290
	12–20 weeks	2.0	5	5.0	2	60	390
	21 weeks +	3.0	3	7.5	1.5	75	480
Bantams	1 day–1 week	-	-	0.3	30	20	130
	1–11 weeks	0.6	15	1.5	7	40	260
	12–20 weeks	1.5	7	3.5	3	55	360
	21 weeks +	2.0	5	5.0	2	70	450

*or age of slaughter

excellent litter. Hardwood shavings, on the other hand, should be avoided due to the danger of aspergillosis.

Remove and replace litter around feeders if it becomes thick with droppings. Remove and replace moist litter around waterers. Moist litter favors the growth of molds (such as those causing aspergillosis) and bacteria (that produce ammonia and other unpleasant gases), and aids the survival of viruses, protozoa (such as those causing coccidiosis), and nematodes (worms).

At least once a year, empty your coop, clean out and replace all the litter, and scrape manure from the walls and perches. Fall is the best time for this chore, since it puts your flock on clean litter at the start of winter, when bad weather keeps chickens indoors much of the time. Compost the used litter or spread it on a field where chickens will not range for at least one year.

If you use the built-up litter system of management (whereby litter is only infrequently removed and replaced), compost the litter if you plan to introduce a replacement flock. The heat produced during composting will destroy most pathogens and parasites.

Ventilation. Fresh air dilutes the population of microbes and reduces the buildup of airborne diseases. Good ventilation also keeps air in motion (without causing drafty conditions) and removes suspended dust and moisture. Moisture tends to be particularly high in a chicken house because chickens

ALLAN DAMEROW

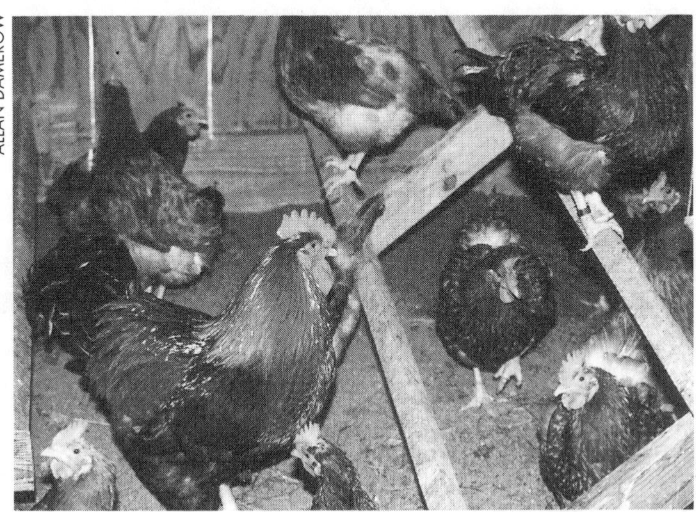

Pine shavings make excellent litter to absorb droppings and moisture.

breathe rapidly, thereby using more air in proportion to their size than any other animal. Another important benefit of good ventilation is preventing the buildup of ammonia fumes from accumulated droppings.

Providing an adequate flow of fresh air may require a fan to move out stale air and bring in fresh air. Fans are sold according to how many cubic feet of air they move per minute (cfm). A good rule of thumb is to get a fan that provides 5 cfm (.03 cubic meters per minute) per bird.

Ammonia Check

High levels of ammonia in the air can reduce feed consumption, affecting the growth rate of young birds and the production of laying hens. Ammonia gas dissolves in fluid around the eyes, causing irritation, inflammation, and blindness. Symptoms of ammonia-induced conjunctivitis are rubbing the eye with a wing and reluctance to move or go into sunlight. High levels of ammonia can also damage the mucous membranes of a bird's respiratory tract, allowing bacteria, dust, and viruses to travel down the tract to cause disease.

Ammonia that is concentrated enough to cause conjunctivitis or respiratory tract damage is concentrated enough to be detected by the human sense of smell. To check the ammonia level in your coop, squat or bend down until your head is 1 foot (30 cm) above the litter, or about the height of a chicken's head. Breathe normally for a moment or two. If your eyes, nose, or throat burn, the ammonia level is too high for your birds—decrease litter moisture and improve ventilation. Once the condition is corrected, a chicken's cells that were damaged by ammonia fumes should repair themselves within 2 weeks.

Sanitation

After a period of continuous use, chicken housing becomes contaminated with disease-causing organisms that may eventually reach infectious levels. Regular cleanup does not eliminate microorganisms, but it does keep them at bay. You can remove an estimated 95 percent of contamination with a thorough cleaning.

Dry cleaning is not nearly as effective as cleaning with water, and hot water cleans better than cold water. Detergent (or a 4 percent washing soda solution) added to the hot water reduces surface tension and helps the water penetrate organic matter. In addition, detergents are mildly germicidal.

During cleanup, wear a dust mask and avoid inhaling poultry dust, which can cause human respiratory problems. Methodically follow these steps:

- Choose a warm day so facilities will dry quickly.
- Suppress dust by lightly misting equipment and walls with water and a bit of detergent.
- Remove portable equipment, such as feeders, waterers, nests, and cages.
- Remove litter and droppings; compost them or spread them on land where your chickens will not range for at least a year.
- Use a broom, brush, or shop vac to remove dust and cobwebs from the ceiling and walls.
- Brush, blow, or vacuum dust from fans, vents, and any electrical equipment.
- Use a hoe or other scraper to remove manure and dirt clinging to the floor, walls, and perches; as long as you can see manure or dirt, keep scraping.
- Turn off electricity and protect electrical equipment and outlets with watertight covers or duct tape.
- Apply detergent or washing soda and hot water systematically to the ceiling, walls, floor, and washable equipment with a brush or fruit-tree sprayer that delivers 400 psi (pounds per square inch) or 28 kg per sq cm for good penetration.
- Open doors and windows, and turn on the ventilation fan, to air out and dry housing before letting the chickens back in.
- Finish the job by removing any debris that has accumulated around the yard since your last cleanup.

Disinfection

Thoroughly cleaning a chicken house is more important than disinfecting it, since many disease-causing organisms cannot survive long in an environ-

CHART 1-3

Survival Ability of Disease-Causing Organisms

Disease	*Cause*	*Survival off Birds*
Chlamydiosis	bacteria	hours to days
Cholera	bacteria	month or more
Coccidiosis	protozoa	months
Erysipelas	bacteria	years
Infectious bronchitis	virus	week or less
Infectious bursal disease	virus	months
Infectious coryza	bacteria	hours to days
Infectious laryngotracheitis	virus	days
Influenza	virus	days to weeks
Marek's disease	virus	years
Mycoplasmosis	bacteria	hours to days
Newcastle disease	virus	month or less
Pox	virus	months
Salmonellosis	bacteria	weeks to months
Tuberculosis	bacteria	months to years

ment away from birds or their debris. In addition, the microbes that cause some diseases — including infectious bursal disease, coccidiosis, and tuberculosis — resist disinfectants. Disinfection, in most cases, should be used only as a way to zap stragglers following cleanup.

Disinfection becomes a necessity if you acquire used equipment or your flock experiences an infection. Not all disinfectants work equally well against all disease-causing organisms. A veterinarian or poultry pathologist can help you select the appropriate disinfectant for your situation.

Check the date on any disinfectant to be sure it is not outdated. Store the disinfectant in a cool place. Some chemicals are quite toxic and should be stored away from children, pets, livestock, food, and feeds. To avoid a tragic error, keep disinfectants in their original containers with the labels intact.

Dilute a disinfectant according to either directions on the label or instructions provided by a vet or pathologist. Some disinfectants work best in hot water, but some evaporate too quickly in warm or hot water. Never mix different kinds of disinfectant, or you may render them all ineffective. Before mixing a disinfectant with detergent, lye, washing soda, or other cleaning product, check the label for information on compatibility.

Organic matter inhibits penetration by a disinfectant, and in some cases actually deactivates the disinfectant, so follow the above steps for thorough cleanup before applying a disinfectant. If surfaces cannot be scrubbed clean, use a disinfectant that is not readily deactivated by organic matter. Take care, though — such disinfectants are quite toxic and should never be applied with a spray.

Wear goggles to protect your eyes, and avoid inhaling disinfectant chemicals. After scraping and scrubbing housing clean, close doors and windows before applying the disinfectant. Work systematically, starting with the ceiling, then the walls, and finally the floor. Afterward, don't forget to disinfect your shovel, broom, rake, hoe, and other clean-up tools. Wait at least 20 minutes before rinsing equipment and tools to give the disinfectant time to do its job.

To protect your chickens from skin injury and from respiratory irritation due to inhaled chemicals, allow housing to dry thoroughly, and leave the facilities empty for as long as possible. The safe time between application and letting your chickens in varies from 4 hours to 2 days. Consult the label.

Chemical Disinfectants

Chemical disinfectants include:

Hypochlorites — chlorine-based disinfectants such as chlorine bleach (which contains 5 percent available chlorine) and swimming pool chlorine (which contains 15 percent). Common brand names are Clorox and Halazone. Chlorines work best in warm water but evaporate rapidly, so prepare a fresh solution right before use. Chlorine is destructive to fabric, leather, metal and some kinds of plastic.

Iodine, organic — mixture of iodine with some other chemical. Common brand names include Betadine and Isodyne. When the amber color fades, organic iodine is no longer effective.

Quat — quaternary ammonium compound (sometimes also referred to as QAC). Quats vary in composition and are widely available at drugstores, pet shops, feed stores, and poultry supply outlets. Common brand names include Germex and Zephiran. Quats have no strong odor, leave no stains, and are non-corrosive, non-irritating, and relatively non-toxic. They cannot be combined with soap or detergent and will not work on surfaces that are not completely free of soap or detergent.

Phenol — another name for carbolic acid, a coal tar derivative and the standard by which all other disinfectants are measured. Common brand names include Lysol and Orthophenylphenol. Most chicken keepers consider phenols too expensive for use in poultry houses.

Cresols — coal tar product related to phenol and similar in bactericidal properties, once found on every farm. Cresl-400 is one common brand name. Cresylic acid is cresol with soap added.

Quicklime — also called "slaked lime" is used primarily for damp yards where the sun does not shine (and where birds shouldn't be kept, anyway). Quicklime is highly caustic, so keep birds away until the area dries thoroughly.

CHART 1-4

Chemical Disinfectants

	Iodine	*Quat*	*Chlorine*	*Cresol*	*Phenol*
Used for:					
Eggs	yes	yes	yes	no	yes
Incubator	yes	yes	yes	no	yes
Housing	yes	yes	no	yes	yes
Equipment	yes	yes	yes	yes	yes
Troughs	yes	yes	yes	no	yes
Drinking Water	yes	no	yes	no	no
Bootbath	yes	yes	no	yes	yes
Effective against:					
Bacteria	yes	most	yes	yes	yes
Bacterial spores	some	no	some	no	no
Fungi	yes	some	yes	most	most
Viruses	some	some	some	some	some
Usage level (ppm):					
Disinfect	100	600	200	varies	varies
Sanitize	25	200	50	varies	500
Application:					
Water temperature	<110°F (43.5°C)	hot	<110°F (43.5°C)	hot	hot
Effective pH	acid	alkaline	acid	acid	acid
Deactivated by alkaline water	yes	no	yes	no	no
Deactivated by hard water	no	somewhat	no	no	no
Deactivated by organic matter	yes	somewhat	yes	no	no
Apply with brush	yes	yes	yes	yes	yes
Apply with spray	yes	yes	yes	no	no
Other Properties:					
Toxicity	low	low	low	high	high
Residual effect	no	yes	no	yes	yes
Odor	little	none	strong	strong	strong

Nonchemical Disinfectants

Not all disinfectants are chemicals. Here's the rundown on readily available nonchemical disinfectants:

Hot water increases the effectiveness of some chemical disinfectants, and boiling water and live steam are both effective disinfectants in their own right.

Sanitation Terminology

Products with names ending in "cide" kill the disease-causing agent named in the first part: a bactericide kills bacterial cells, a fungicide kills molds and fungi, a viricide kills or inactivates viruses, a germicide kills bacteria, but not necessarily their spores (most germicides are also viricides).

Products ending in "stat" retard the growth of the organism named in the first part: a bacteriostat slows the growth of bacteria, a fungistat slows the growth of molds or fungi, and so forth.

Antiseptic — destroys or retards the growth of microorganisms
Detergent — improves the cleaning action of water, acts as a wetting agent or surfactant to help water penetrate the surface of organic matter, and is mildly germicidal
Disinfectant — inactivates or kills microorganisms, but not necessarily their spores
Sanitizer — reduces microbial contamination to a level considered safe
Sterilizer — destroys all microbes, including bacteria, spores, fungi, and viruses

Resting housing by keeping chickens out for 2 to 4 weeks after cleanup helps reduce the microorganism population, since many cannot live long in the absence of chickens.

Drying also reduces the population of microorganisms, but killing a significant number of microbes by drying takes a long time.

Sunlight speeds up drying of portable equipment (such as feeders, waterers, cages, and nests) and housing that can be readily opened up to direct rays. Sunlight does not penetrate deeply, but will destroy microbes on the surface. Sunlight and normal soil activity will effectively disinfect a yard or run from which surface organic wastes have been removed.

Heat produced by composting will destroy most of the bacteria, viruses, coccidial oocysts, and worm eggs present in litter. Heap the litter into a pile (but not on a wood floor, or you could start a fire). If the litter is dry, dampen it a little to start fermentation. Let the pile heat up to at least 125°F (52°C), leave it for 24 hours, then turn it so the outside is on the inside. Let it heat for another 24 hours before spreading the litter back out. Composting litter to destroy its microbes is a good idea, whether the litter will be reused for chickens or used to fertilize a garden or field.

Flame is an effective disinfectant, but a hazardous one, especially around wood structures. It is best reserved to disinfect concrete pads and to sear away feathers stuck to wire cages, but take care: if you hold a torch to galvanized wire long enough for the wire to get hot, the galvanizing will be damaged.

Stress Management

Stress encompasses anything that reduces resistance to disease. Some microbes are so strong (or "virulent") that they readily overcome a bird's normal resistance. Many microbes, on the other hand, cause no illness or only mild illness, unless stress lowers the bird's resistance.

Some diseases are themselves stress factors — they are not serious, but they lower a bird's resistance to a more serious infection. Internal parasites (worms) are a prime example of a mild infection that can open the door to something more serious or that can become serious in combination with other stress factors.

No matter how much natural resistance a chicken has, its resistance will be reduced to some extent by stress. Stress cannot be avoided. It is normal in every chicken's life. Most chickens are able to adapt, even to times of peak stress: hatching, reaching maturity, and molting. Additional stresses are caused by the environment (such as chilling, heating, and excessive humidity) and by routine management procedures (debeaking, vaccinating, and any procedure in which birds are handled or herded).

Stress management involves providing clean, dry litter and range, adequate protection from the elements, good ventilation without draftiness, contamination-free feed and water, adequate feed and water space, proper nutrition, and freedom from crowding. Avoidance of crowding is especially important for chicks, since they grow fast and can quickly outgrow their living quarters. As birds grow, they develop immunities through gradual exposure to disease-causing microbes. Stress due to crowding can cause disease instead of immunity.

Stress reduction also involves avoiding the indiscriminate or improper use of medications, as well as avoiding handling birds at critical times, including when pullets are just starting to lay, when a flock has recently been moved or vaccinated, and when the weather is extremely hot or cold.

Gentle handling as a stress-reduction measure is more important to chicken health than fancy housing, according to a study by W. B. Gross at Virginia Tech. Gently treated birds are easier to handle and experience less stress during procedures that require handling. Compared to birds that are ignored or are treated roughly, birds that are handled gently grow to a more uniform size and are more resistant to infections.

Preconditioning is another stress-reduction technique. Whenever you make a management change, precondition your birds by making the change gradually so that each step is relatively minor. If, for example, you plan to cage your pullets for laying, move them at least a week before you expect them to start production. If you plan to move or separate breeders, give them plenty of time to adjust to their new surroundings before the start of breeding season.

Showing and Stress

Showing causes stress by exposing a bird to unfamiliar and confusing surroundings, strange people, different-tasting water, and any number of new and potentially frightening experiences. Excessive showing can be so stressful that it affects the fertility and hatchability of eggs. Hens are more easily stressed by showing than cocks.

If you show your chickens, precondition them by coop training them prior to the show so they'll get used to being caged alone and handled frequently. At show time, bring along your own feed and water — if your chickens don't like the feed or water at the show, they won't eat or drink well, their stress level will go up, and they'll be more susceptible to diseases. Some exhibitors add antibiotics or electrolytes to water during a show, but if a bird doesn't like the taste it won't drink, increasing its stress level.

Stress Behavior

If you're familiar with the way your chickens normally act, you can readily notice changes caused by stress and can take appropriate action. You may be able to alleviate the stress behavior through a simple management change. Continuing stress that causes long-term behavioral changes seriously reduces a chicken's resistance to disease. Sometimes the stress behavior itself is a first sign of disease.

Stress behavior falls into three basic categories:

- diarrhea
- labored breathing
- changes in normal behavior or activity patterns

Diarrhea becomes evident as a stress sign when you grab a bird suddenly and it reacts by pooping on you. Diarrhea can also be a sign that there's something wrong with the feed or water or that your birds are suffering from a digestive disorder. Labored breathing can be caused by crowding, panic, high temperatures, and respiratory distress. Changes in normal behavior or activity can be triggered by any number of factors including boredom, fear, crowding, constant introduction of new birds, frequent showing, insufficient or unpalatable water, uncomfortable temperatures, and disease.

The study of animal behavior and its relationship to health is called "veterinary ethology." For observation purposes, ethologists divide the behavior of chickens into eleven distinct areas:

Reflex behavior involves any automatic reaction, such as flinching or shying away from sudden movement. A frightened chicken, for example, might shake its head from side to side. A sick chicken reacts more slowly than usual to perceived danger.

Feeding behavior includes both the frequency of visiting feed or water troughs and the amount ingested. Under normal circumstances, a chicken visits feed and water stations often and eats or drinks a little at a time. Stress usually makes a bird eat and drink less, although some diseases increase thirst. Anomalous feeding behaviors that call for management action include feather picking, cannibalism, drinking excessive amounts of water, eating litter or soil, and eating eggs.

Rest patterns, including sleep, are easily disturbed during times of stress. A classic example is restlessness at roosting time, caused by anticipation of being bitten by external parasites that feed on birds at night.

Exploratory behavior satisfies the need to investigate new things in the environment, including new birds. Excess stress can be induced by the sudden introduction of something a bird can't see or doesn't understand (such as the loud noise of machinery operating nearby). Excessive stress leads to overreaction, often in the form of flightiness (the "Chicken Little syndrome"). Flightiness is relative, however, since some breeds naturally tend to be more flighty than others. Anomalous behavior that may be an early sign of disease is loss of interest by a bird in its surroundings.

Body activity relates to motion, including moving from place to place or wing flapping for the sheer joy of it. A stressed-out chicken may pace up and down, indicating either frustration (as in the case of one cock trying to get away from another) or boredom (in the case of a caged chicken).

Grooming activities include head scratching, preening, mutual grooming, and dust bathing. If you're not familiar with dust-bath behavior, the first time you see your chickens laid out in the dirt, you'll surely think they died a sudden death. Loss of interest in grooming behavior, so that birds take on a scruffy look, is a common early sign of disease.

Sexual behavior on the part of a cock involves courtship (pecking the ground, waltzing, and wing fluttering) and crowing (to establish location and warn off competitors — a behavior that's territorial as well as sexual). Sexual behavior on the part of a hen largely involves crouching when a cock puts his foot on her back in preparation for mating. Hens that are low in the pecking order will crouch as the rooster nears and will be mated more often than other hens. You can readily identify these subordinate hens by the broken or missing feathers on their backs or sometimes by wounds inflicted by the mounting cock. Such wounds may be serious enough to require isolation and treatment.

Parental behavior refers to the relationship between a hen and her chicks, since a cock develops no special relationship with his offspring. A hen protects her chicks, leads them to feed and water, and communicates with them (and they with her) through a series of vocalizations that each have a specific meaning. Anomalous parental behavior includes leaving the nest before the eggs hatch (perhaps because the hen was bothered by mites), attacking chicks when they hatch, or abandoning chicks. Some breeds, particularly those best known for their laying abilities, have been selectively bred not to have the brooding instinct.

Territorialism involves aggressive behavior used in an effort to maintain personal and territorial space. Crowding increases aggression, which increases stress. Stress behavior in the form of so-called "displacement" activity commonly occurs when one cock of a sparring pair suddenly starts preening or pecking the ground. Anomalous territorial behavior includes attacking intruders, other chickens, or humans and refusing (or being unable) to move due to fear.

Social relations in a flock of chickens boil down to the peck order. Birds that are low in peck order get chased away from feeders, don't get enough to eat, and don't grow as well or lay as many eggs as others. The more birds you have, the more important it is to have several feeders and waterers, and to spread them around. Stress goes up when the peck order is disrupted for any reason, such as sickness or the removal or addition of birds. As a result, birds eat less, grow slowly or lose weight, and lay fewer eggs.

Relationship to man starts with imprinting, a phenomenon occurring in chicks during their first day of life. By the time a chick is 3 days old, it starts experiencing fear, which is why you'll never develop the same friendly relationship with mail-order chicks that you can have with chicks hatched in your incubator. Whether or not your chickens are imprinted on you, minimize stress by talking or singing softly when you work among them, and by moving calmly and avoiding abrupt movements.

Balanced Rations

The best way to ensure that your chickens are getting a balanced ration is to purchase commercially prepared feed designed to suit your flock's stage of maturity: chick starter for young and growing birds, layer ration for table-egg production, and breeder (or gamebird) ration for hatching-egg production. The relationship between health and nutrition is covered in the next chapter.

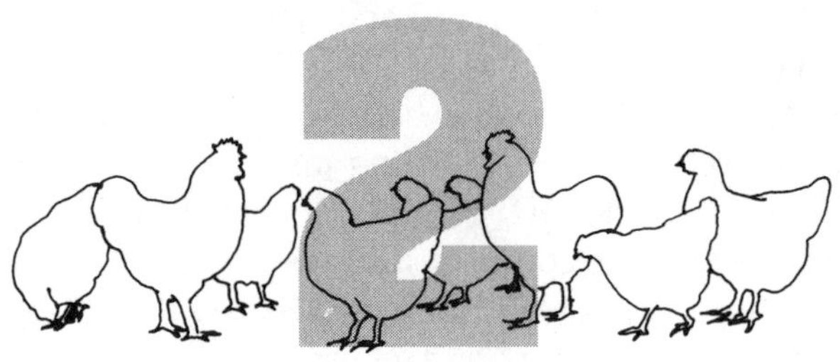

Health and Nutrition

HEALTH AND NUTRITION INTERACT in many ways. Disease isn't always caused by bacteria, viruses, or other parasites. Disease can also be caused by a nutritional deficiency. The nutritional deficiency may, in turn, inhibit the body's immune response, opening the door to infection.

Conversely, an infectious disease may reduce a bird's appetite or inhibit absorption of nutrients from its digestive system. The resulting nutritional deficiencies may either delay recovery or further reduce the bird's resistance, increasing its susceptibility to secondary infection.

Nutrients

Free-ranged flocks are able to forage for natural sources of the nutrients their bodies need. Other nutrients are manufactured within their bodies, aided by sunlight. Some nutritional deficiencies occur only in chickens confined indoors, away from sunlight. Others occur due to incorrect formulation or improper storage of prepared feeds.

More than thirty-six nutrients have been identified as being essential to chickens. Since no single ingredient contains all the necessary nutrients, the best ration includes a combination of ingredients that together satisfy a chicken's requirements.

Nutritional problems don't always result from deficiencies, but can be caused by excess. Too much of any nutrient, or a lack of balance between nu-

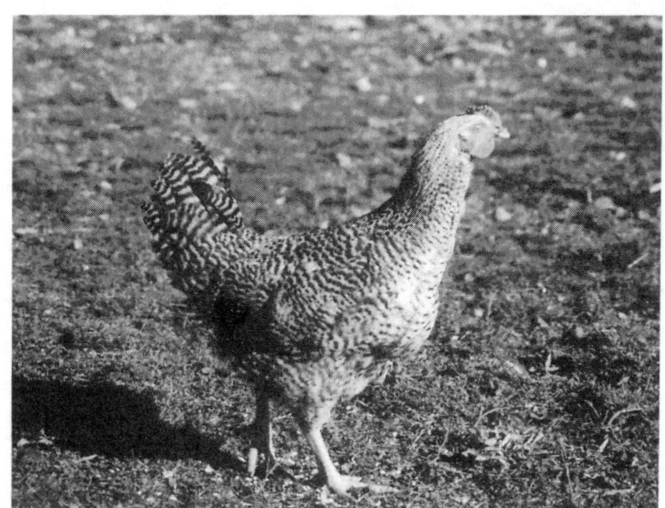

Free-ranged chickens forage for natural sources of nutrients.

trients, can be just as devastating as a deficiency, so don't be too quick to pump your birds full of nutritional supplements.

Protein

A chicken's body uses protein to produce antibodies that fight disease. During infection, a bird rapidly loses its protein stores, causing its protein requirement to go up. If the bird cannot obtain additional protein, its resistance level drops.

Feathers are 85 percent protein. Protein requirements therefore increase during the annual molt, when all of a bird's feathers are replaced with new ones. When your flock is about to molt — as indicated by plumage taking on a dull look — begin tossing a handful of dry cat food into the yard every other day, and continue until the molt is over. Use cat food, rather than dog food, because cat food contains animal protein (which is rich in amino acids), while most brands of dog food are top-heavy with grains.

A hard molt — where feathers fall rapidly but grow back slowly — may indicate animal protein deficiency. Another indicator is feathers that become brittle and break easily. If the deficiency is unlikely to be caused by a dietary problem, look for a disease (recent or current) that may be inhibiting protein absorption.

General symptoms of protein deficiency are similar to general symptoms of infection: decreased appetite, slow growth in chicks or weight loss in mature birds, decreased laying, and smaller egg size.

Excess protein in a chicken's diet is converted to uric acid and deposited as crystals in joints, causing gout. The excess use of meat scraps as a source of protein can also result in an imbalance of phosphorus (described later in this chapter).

Vitamins

Vitamins are divided into two groups: fat soluble and water soluble. The fat soluble vitamins (A, D, E, and K) are retained in body fat and used as they are needed. The water soluble vitamins (C and the B complex) are not stored by the body, which uses only what it immediately needs and expels any excess in droppings. Water-soluble vitamins must therefore be replenished more often than fat-soluble vitamins.

Every known vitamin is needed by chickens in some amount. A flock's vitamin requirements are interrelated with and must be balanced against other nutritional components — protein, minerals, and energy. Of all the nutrients, chickens are most likely to be deficient in vitamins A, D, and B2 (riboflavin).

Caged birds are more prone to vitamin deficiencies than floor-raised birds, since the latter pick up some of the vitamins they need from litter. Similarly, housed chickens are more prone to deficiencies than free-ranged flocks, since the latter enjoy a more diverse diet.

Stress, including disease-induced stress, increases the effects of a vitamin deficiency. Heat stress causes birds to eat less and worsens a deficiency. A vitamin supplement will give your chickens' immune systems a boost during times of stress, such as when their bodies are battling a disease, when the weather is unpleasant, during a move, before and after a show, and during breeding season. Chicks will get off to a good start if you give them a vitamin supplement during their first 3 weeks of life.

Fat-Soluble Vitamins

Vitamin A is needed for vision, growth, and bone development. It is called the "anti-infection" vitamin because it helps maintain the immune system. It also aids disease resistance by playing a role in maintaining the linings of the digestive, reproductive, and respiratory tracts.

Vitamin A deficiency is unlikely to result from improper diet, but may be caused by a health condition that interferes with nutrient absorption, such as coccidiosis or worm infestation.

If a chicken misses the mark when pecking, suspect poor eyesight due to vitamin A deficiency. An increase in blood spots in eggs may be another sign, since the amount of vitamin A needed to minimize blood spots is higher than the amount needed to keep a laying hen healthy.

Vitamin A deficiency can cause nutritional roup which produces respiratory symptoms similar to those of infectious bronchitis or infectious coryza; it can also cause the upper digestive tract to develop blisters resembling those of fowl pox. The damage caused to linings of the upper digestive and respiratory tracts can open the door to bacterial or viral invasion. Deficiency increases the severity of respiratory infections such as bronchitis and chronic respiratory disease, and increases a chicken's susceptibility to parasites such as coccidia.

Cod liver oil mixed into mash at the rate of 2 percent is a good source of vitamin A. Take care not to go overboard — too much vitamin A is toxic to chickens.

Vitamin D is necessary for the absorption of calcium to make strong bones, beaks, claws, and eggshells. A bird's body synthesizes vitamin D from sunshine, making deficiency more likely in caged or housed chickens than in penned or range-fed flocks. Deficiency can also occur in chickens fed rations intended for other livestock, since chickens need vitamin D3 while most other stock require vitamin D2.

A typical sign of vitamin D deficiency is a continuing cycle of normal egg production followed by the appearance of thin- and soft-shelled eggs followed by a drop in production followed by a return to normal production. A deficient hen may have weak legs right before she lays an egg, causing her to squat in a penguin-like stance. If the deficiency is not corrected, her beak, claws, and keel will become soft and her eggs will be small with reduced hatchability. Deficiency can be easily corrected by adding cod liver oil to mash at the rate of 2 percent or by adding vitamin AD&E powder to drinking water three times a week.

A chicken's need for vitamin D is intimately tied with its needs for the minerals calcium and phosphorus. A deficiency in any of these three nutrients can result in rickets (in young birds) or cage fatigue (in older birds). A deficiency may also cause egg eating.

Excess vitamin D causes kidney damage. One sign of too much vitamin D in a hen's diet is calcium "pimples" on eggshells that, when scraped off, leave little holes in the shell.

Vitamin E is necessary for normal reproduction and for resistance to *Escherichia coli* infection (colibacillosis). Wheat germ oil is a good source if used fresh — vitamin E in fortified rations degenerates rapidly, especially when temperature and humidity are high. Deficiency is most likely to occur in confined young birds fed a diet that's high in soy bean oil or cod liver oil and in birds fed rations containing rancid fats. Deficiency in chicks can result in encephalomalacia, exudative diathesis, or white muscle disease. Deficiency in cocks can cause loss of fertility.

Vitamin K is necessary for normal blood clotting. Signs of deficiency are profuse bleeding from slight wounds and internal bleeding (under the skin or into the body cavity). Vitamin K may trigger infectious anemia, especially in chicks treated for extended periods with the coccidiostat sulfaquinoxaline. Alfalfa leaves are a good source of vitamin K.

Water-Soluble Vitamins

Vitamin B is actually a whole group of unrelated substances whose names change so often it's hard to keep up. Vitamin B deficiency was not an issue in the days when chickens roamed pastures, freely picking in cow patties and horse apples. Health problems occurred when breeders started to specialize and began penning their chickens. In those early days, poultry keepers kept their flocks healthy by tossing them fresh horse or cow manure, but no one knew why it worked until 1948, when researchers discovered that manure contains vitamin B12. This B vitamin is unique among nutrients in being found almost exclusively in animal products.

Today, deficiency is not a problem where poultry keepers have returned to the practice of letting chickens run with other livestock. Chickens raised on

CHART 2-1

Vitamin Benefits and Sources

Vitamin	*Source*	*Benefit*
A	cod liver oil AD&E powder	vision, growth, bone development, resistance to diseases & parasites
B complex		growth & hatchability (all B complex vitamins)
thiamin (B1)	whole cereal grains	
riboflavin (B2)	leafy greens, grass, milk, yeast	
pyridoxine (B6)	many sources	
nicotinic acid (niacin)	meat protein, whole grain	
pantothenic acid	many sources	
biotin (H)	brewer's yeast, leafy greens, molasses	
inositol	many sources	
para-amino-benzoic acid	yeast, many sources	
choline	many sources	
folic acid (folacin)	green leaves	
B12	meat protein	
C	ascorbic acid	stress reduction
D	cod liver oil AD&E powder	strong bones, beaks, claws, & eggshells; hatchability
E	wheat germ oil AD&E powder	fertility, resistance to colibacillosis
K	alfalfa leaves	normal blood clotting

built-up floor litter get enough vitamin B12 by picking in the litter. Deficiency can occur in housed flocks, especially those fed soymeal as the sole or main source of protein.

Curled-toe paralysis in chicks is a sign of riboflavin (vitamin B2) deficiency, occurring when penned breeder hens are fed unsupplemented lay ration. Greens, including young grass, are good sources of riboflavin. Milk, whey, and other dairy products are also good sources, but too much can cause diarrhea.

All the B vitamins, along with other vitamins, are added to commercial rations and are otherwise so readily available in a wide variety of feedstuffs that, in a properly managed flock, deficiency is unlikely.

Vitamin C helps prevent diseases by reducing the harmful effects of stress. Chickens make their own vitamin C and do not need a supplement except when the absorption of vitamin C and other nutrients is inhibited by stress, such as might be induced by high environmental temperatures.

Minerals

While vitamins have their origins in organic plant or animal matter, minerals are inorganic elements. They give bones rigidity and strength, and they interact with other nutrients to keep the body healthy. Just as caged birds are more prone to vitamin deficiencies than floor-raised birds, they're also more prone to mineral deficiencies. But, unlike vitamins, minerals do not go stale. Most commercial feeds contain adequate amounts, with the possible exception of calcium.

Calcium and phosphorus are needed by chicks for bone formation and by hens for eggshell formation. Calcium and phosphorus are interrelated, and both require the presence of vitamin D to be metabolized. A deficiency in vitamin D can cause a deficiency of calcium and/or phosphorus.

Regardless of the cause, a deficiency of calcium and phosphorus increases a chicken's susceptibility to parasitic infection. Beetles and other hard-shelled bugs contain lots of calcium and phosphorus; ironically, they may also be a source of parasitic infection. A good supplemental source of calcium is ground oyster shells or limestone (but *not* "dolomitic" limestone, which can inhibit egg production).

Older hens need more calcium than younger hens, and all hens need more calcium in warm weather. Rough eggshells are a sign that a hen is getting too much calcium.

Magnesium is needed for bone formation, eggshell formation, and the metabolism of carbohydrates. A chicken's diet is more likely to have too much magnesium than too little, leading to diarrhea and smaller eggs with thin shells.

Salt in the form of sodium and chlorine can be deficient in a flock's diet, causing chicks to grow slowly and hens to abruptly lay fewer, smaller-sized eggs, lose weight, and become cannibalistic. But chickens are more likely to get too much salt than too little. The result is increased thirst, inability to stand, weak muscles, convulsions, and death. A lethal dose of salt is 0.06 ounce per pound (4g/kg) of body weight.

Chicks are more susceptible to salt poisoning than adults. Salt poisoning can occur when a flock's sole source of drinking water is saline water, although chickens can tolerate salt in water up to 0.25 percent. Poisoning can also occur when chickens pick in rock salt used for de-icing sidewalks and driveways.

Salt poisoning can be caused by a normal amount of salt in rations during summer, if chickens run out of water, and during winter, if drinking water freezes. Obviously, the way to avoid salt poisoning is to be sure your chickens have fresh, clean water at all times.

Potassium deficiency can occur during times of heat or other stress, resulting in decreased egg production, thin shells, and general weakness.

Manganese is needed for normal bones, for good eggshell quality, and to prevent slipped tendon. Coccidiosis interferes with its metabolism.

Copper deficiency can cause a loss of feather color in New Hampshires and Rhode Island Reds. As with manganese, the metabolism of copper is affected by coccidiosis.

Selenium deficiency is associated with white muscle disease; an excess of selenium increases susceptibility to salmonellosis. Corn and other grains may be low in selenium if they are grown east of the Mississippi River and in the Pacific Northwest, where the soil is selenium deficient. Grains may be especially high in selenium if they are grown in the Great Plains or parts of Canada where soils contain an excess of selenium.

Energy

A chicken's protein requirement goes up during the annual molt, its vitamin and mineral needs remain fairly constant year around, and its energy requirements fluctuate with outside temperature. Where the temperature range is extreme, energy must be adjusted seasonally — upward during cold months, downward during warm months. Energy can be lowered by adding wheat bran (but too much affects laying). Energy can be increased by increasing protein or carbohydrates.

Although protein contains a certain amount of energy, the cheapest form of energy is carbohydrates found in cereal grains. Grains are also the most caloric form of energy, so they must be used judiciously. Since a chicken eats to satisfy its energy needs, if its ration is too high in carbohydrates, the bird gets fat; if too low, the bird becomes underweight. In both cases, the bird is more susceptible to disease.

CHART 2-2

Nutritional Diseases and Disorders

Disease caused by:	*Deficiency of:*	*Excess of:*
Cage fatigue	calcium/phosphorus	
Curled-toe paralysis	riboflavin (vitamin B2)	
Egg binding	calcium/phosphorus	
Encephalomalacia	vitamin E	
Exudative diathesis	vitamin E	
Fatty liver syndrome		carbohydrate
Gout	water	protein
Infectious anemia	vitamin K	
Prolapsed oviduct	calcium/phosphorus	
Rickets	vitamin D	
Roup (nutritional)	vitamin A	
Slipped tendon	calcium/phosphorus manganese vitamins	
White muscle disease	vitamin D vitamin E/selenium	

Nutritional Diseases

Nutritional research has traditionally focused on broiler chicks and laying hens. More is therefore known about the requirements for rapid early growth in heavy breeds and about the maintenance needs of light laying breeds than about the requirements of breeder flocks, especially in the heavy breeds. Commercial feeds designed for mature birds are formulated for maintenance, ensuring that hens lay well but not necessarily providing sufficient nutrition for the eggs to develop into strong viable chicks. (See chapter 13 for more about the influence of nutrition on the hatchability of eggs and viability of chicks.)

Chickens, like humans, depend for good health on the existence of beneficial bacteria and other microorganisms living in their digestive tracts. A bird's nutritional requirements go up when the delicate balance of these microflora is upset by illness, drugs, stress, or an abrupt change in feed.

A bird's nutritional requirements can also be increased by any condition that causes nutrients to be destroyed before they can be absorbed or that inhibits the chicken's ability to absorb them. Interference with the absorption of nutrients, called "malabsorption," can be caused by parasite loads including worms or coccidia, infection, drug use, and environmental stress due to low humidity or temperature extremes. Any of these conditions can make even the most perfectly formulated rations insufficient to prevent a deficiency.

Deficiency Symptoms

A nutritional deficiency may be:

- borderline — resulting in slow growth, poor or rough feathering, lack of energy, lack of appetite, a slight drop in egg production, and slightly reduced hatchability;
- serious — birds become crippled, hens stop laying;
- extreme — ending in death.

Nutritional diseases tend to be quite similar to one another, making it hard to tell specifically which nutrient is lacking. In addition, deficiencies are rarely simple (having a single cause) but are more likely to be multiple (caused by the lack of more than one nutrient). Symptoms of a simple deficiency are determined by deliberately putting chickens on a deficient diet and observing the results. In a real-life multiple deficiency, symptoms combine to complicate the diagnosis.

Chart 2-3

Nutritional Symptoms

Body Part	*Disease/Condition*	*Deficiency*	*Excess*
Beak	soft	vitamin D	
Blood	excessive bleeding	vitamin K	
Bones	brittle	calcium	
		vitamin D	
	soft	calcium	
		phosphorus	
		vitamin D	
Brain	greenish yellow	vitamin E	
Claws	soft	vitamin D	
Droppings	loose & runny		salt
			magnesium
Eggs	blood spots	vitamin A	
	small		magnesium
			protein
	pale yolk		vitamin A
	calcium pimples		vitamin D
	low fertility	vitamin E	
	low hatchability*	calcium	
		magnesium	
		vitamin A	
	low production	potassium	
		protein	
			vitamin A

Body Part	*Disease/Condition*	*Deficiency*	*Excess*
Eggs (cont.)	no production	calcium	
	soft shell	calcium/vitamin D	
	thin shell		magnesium
		potassium	
		vitamin D	
	no shell	vitamin D	
	eating of	calcium	
		vitamin D	
Eyes	pale	vitamin A	
	poor vision	vitamin A	
	watery	vitamin A	
Feathers	black, in ermine pattern	vitamin D	
	brittle	protein	
	curled	protein	
	hard molt	protein	
	missing	protein	
	pale, in black & red breeds	copper	
	ruffled	vitamin A	
Keel	deformed	vitamin D	
Legs	stiff walk	biotin	
	penguin squat	vitamin D	
	weak or bowed	vitamin D	
Mouth	whitish sores	vitamin A	
Muscle	swollen joints	vitamin D	
	weak muscles	vitamin E	
			salt
Respiratory	general symptoms	vitamin A	
Ribs	collapsed (adult)	vitamin D	
	beaded (chick)	vitamin D	
Skin	inflamed	biotin	pantothenic acid
Susceptibility	general	vitamin A	
	colibacillosis	vitamin E	
	parasites	calcium & phosphorus	
	salmonellosis		selenium
	slipped tendon	manganese	
Weight	emaciation	vitamin A	
	fat		carbohydrate
	slow growth	protein	
		vitamin A	
		vitamin D	
	weight loss	carbohydrate	
		protein	

*See "Nutrition-Related Hatching Problems," p. 217.

Feeds

Certain feedstuffs themselves affect digestion and nutrient absorption. The growth rate of chicks, for example, is retarded by uncooked soybeans and soymeal. Deficiencies sometimes occur when commercial feeds are manufactured under new technologies. When processors switched from the expeller method to the solvent method of extracting soybean meal, feeds were deficient in folic acid and had to be reformulated to include an increased amount of that B vitamin. Even feedstuffs that are high in nutrients may contain them in "bound" form, meaning the nutrients are unavailable to or poorly utilized by chickens.

If you stockpile feed or continuously buy from the same stockpiled source, diagnosis of a nutritional deficiency may involve analyzing your feed. For most small flocks, though, feed is bought in small batches, and one batch is not likely to be around long enough to cause a serious deficiency, let alone be analyzed for its nutritional content.

A good rule of thumb is to buy only as much feed as you can use within 6 weeks of manufacture. Store the feed in such a way that it won't go rancid, moldy, or stale. Mold and other spoilage organisms destroy nutrients, and even the best commercial rations lose nutritional value during prolonged storage at a warehouse or on your back porch. Despite the inclusion of antioxidants to retard deterioration, nutrients are destroyed over time by heat, sunlight, and oxygen.

CHART 2-4

Feeding Schedule

Flock Type	*Age*	*Feed**
Broilers	1 day–5 weeks	starter
	5–7 weeks	finisher
	or 1 day–7 weeks	starter/grower
Roasters and Capons	7 weeks–slaughter	finisher + corn
Layers and Breeders	1 day–6 weeks	starter
	6–13 weeks	grower
	13–20 weeks	pullet developer
	or 1 day–20 weeks	starter/grower
	20 weeks	lay ration + oyster shell *or* limestone grit

*In many areas, the only feeds readily available for small flocks are starter/grower and lay ration. **Gradually make any feed change by adding progressively more of the new ration until the changeover is complete.**

Nutritional content holds up best in feed stored in a cool, dry, place, away from direct sunlight. Once you open a bag, transfer its contents to a sealed container such as a clean plastic garbage can with a tight-fitting lid; don't store feeds in metal cans, which sweat in warm weather, causing the feed to go moldy. Never feed chickens moldy rations, whether the mold developed in a storage container or in a sack that got wet.

Avoid cheap feeds that don't contain animal protein or high-fiber ingredients such as alfalfa or wheat products. Such feeds start out missing nutrients and go downhill from there. Also avoid the temptation to save money by feeding your flock copious amounts of scratch grains or stale bakery products, both of which will upset the nutritional balance of even the best feeding program. Corn and other treats should never make up more than 5 percent of a flock's total diet.

Feeders

CHART 2-5

Feeder Space

Age	*Space per Bird*	
Layers:		
0–6 weeks	1.0"	2.5 cm
7–18 weeks	2.0"	5.0 cm
19 weeks and up	3.0"	7.5 cm
Broilers:		
1 day–1 week	1.0"	2.5 cm
1–4 weeks	2.0"	5.0 cm
4–8 weeks	2.5"	5.0 cm
8–20 weeks	4.0"	10.0 cm
21 weeks and up	5.0"	12.5 cm

Feeder design can affect health by allowing droppings to accumulate in the feed. Droppings can be excluded by hanging feeders from the rafters or by fitting them with perch guards that rotate and dump any bird trying to roost on them.

Feeder design can also affect health by allowing feed to be scattered on the ground, where it not only attracts rodents but combines with manure and moisture to provide a good environment for disease-causing organisms. Billing out (the bad habit chickens have of using their beaks to toss feed out of a trough) can be prevented by using a feeder with an inwardly rolled lip and by positioning the feeder so the hopper is approximately the height of the birds' backs. Here, again, a hanging feeder is ideal because its height can easily be adjusted as birds grow.

Feed Amount

How much chickens eat varies with the ration's palatability, texture, energy, and protein content, as well as with the chickens' breed and strain, degree of activity, and condition of health. How much a chicken eats also varies with environmental temperature. Chickens subjected to cold winter temperatures need more feed than chickens raised in a warm climate or in a controlled environment. Hot weather causes a chicken to eat less; the ration's nutritional value must therefore be increased to meet the bird's needs.

Depending on their breed and purpose, chickens may be either fed free choice (given a constantly ready suppy) or placed on a restricted feeding schedule. Broilers and roasters should be fed free choice, since the idea is to get them to butchering age as quickly as possible. Pullets of the lightweight laying breeds may also be fed free choice, since they have been bred for efficient feed utilization.

Older lightweight hens, as well as breeders in the dual-purpose or meat categories, should be kept on a restricted diet. Restricting the feed intake of pullets past the age of 4 weeks slows their growth and delays the onset of laying, causing them to do better when they become layers and/or breeders. Restricting the intake of mature breeders keeps them from getting unhealthily fat and developing fatty liver syndrome.

CHART 2-6

Restricted Feeding Schedule for Pullets

*Age**	*Body Weight***		*Feed per Bird*	
weeks	pounds	grams	pounds	grams
Laying Breeds:				
4	0.59	270	0.06	28
6	0.88	400	0.07	36
8	1.32	600	0.08	39
10	1.60	730	0.09	42
12	1.87	850	0.09	45
14	2.09	950	0.10	49
16	2.55	1160	0.11	53
18	2.72	1240	0.14	64
20	3.03	1380	0.14	79
Meat Breeds:				
4	1.16	530	0.19	90
6	1.68	765	0.22	100
8	2.01	915	0.23	105
10	2.34	1065	0.25	115
12	2.67	1215	0.27	125
14	3.17	1445	0.29	135
16	3.72	1695	0.33	150
18	4.30	1955	0.37	170
20	4.89	2225	0.41	190

*To age 4 weeks, each layer pullet averages 1.47 pounds (672 grams) of feed, each broiler pullet averages 1.09 pounds (954 grams).

**Average expected body weight under restricted feeding program.

Rations-Related Problems

Starvation occurs when newly hatched chicks do not learn to eat quickly enough, causing them to lose energy rapidly until they can no longer actively seek food. In older birds, starvation occurs when rations are too high in fiber (common in cheap feeds). Starvation may also be related to climate: during cold weather, chickens may not get enough to eat to keep warm; during extremely dry weather, vegetation may be scarce for free-ranged chickens.

Obesity is most likely to occur in chickens kept as pets and in caged birds that are inactive and therefore eat more energy-rich feed than they need. Some breeds, especially New Hampshires and other dual-purpose breeds, have a natural tendency to put on fat. Fat hens do not lay well and are prone to heat stroke, reproductive problems, and fatty liver syndrome.

Xanthomatosis, a condition in which thick yellow or orange patches appear on the skin, is apparently caused by toxic fats in rations.

Water

A chicken's body is 50 percent water and an egg is 65 percent water, making water the most important nutrient in a chicken's diet. Water serves many func-

CHART 2-7

Diseases Affecting Water Consumption

Increase Consumption	*Decrease Consumption*
Blackhead	Infectious coryza
Cholera	Omphalitis
Enteritis	
Typhoid	
Infectious bursal disease	
Leucocytozoonosis	
Newcastle disease	
Salmonellosis	
Spirochetosis	

CHART 2-8

Diseases Related to Drinking Water

*Disease**	*Cause*
Algae poisoning	algae toxins in surface water
Bluecomb	stress triggered by lack of water
Botulism	rotting organic matter in water
Gout	insufficient drinking water
Salt poisoning	insufficient or saline drinking water
Thrush	water contaminated with fungus

*Numerous bacteria, protozoa, and viruses are spread by means of drinking water contaminated with droppings or mucus from infected birds.

CHART 2-9

Environmental Temperature and Water Consumption

Temperature		*Ratio of Water to One Part Feed*
60°F	16°C	1.8 parts
70	21	2.0
80	27	2.8
90	32	4.9
100	38	8.4

tions; among them is to transport other nutrients throughout the body and to keep the body cool through evaporation.

An old saying points out the perversity of chickens: "A flock's water supply is no better than the poorest drinking water available." You can bring your flock the purest, freshest water, yet your birds will persist in drinking from filthy puddles. Good yard drainage prevents stagnant puddles in which disease-causing microbes and parasite-carrying insects thrive. If your soil is neither sandy nor gravelly, enhance drainage by locating your coop on a slight slope. Many microbes and parasites can't survive long in the absence of moisture.

Provide your flock with water from a clean, reliable source. Avoid surface tanks, ponds, or streams, all of which are easily contaminated. Chickens prefer drinking water with a temperature of about 55°F (13°C), and will drink less if water is much above or below that.

The average chicken drinks between 1 and 2 cups (237 to 474 ml) of water per day, depending on numerous factors including its size, the environmental temperature, water palatability, feed intake, feed composition, condition of health, and whether or not the bird is laying.

The average layer drinks twice as much as the average non-layer. Some disease conditions cause chickens to drink more, as do rations that are high in protein or salt. Chickens drink less if the water contains medication or an excessive amount of dissolved minerals that the birds find unpalatable. Chickens that don't drink enough because water is unpalatable, dirty, or warm (or there simply isn't enough) can die from kidney failure.

Under normal conditions, a chicken will drink approximately twice as much as it eats, by weight. A layer, for example, may eat ½ pound (224 g) of feed and drink 2 cups (474 ml) of water per day. As the temperature goes up, the ratio of water to feed also goes up, as high temperatures cause a chicken to eat less and drink more.

Dehydration

A chicken can survive longer without feed than without water. Chickens drink only a little at a time, so they must drink often. Insufficient water slows growth in chicks and reduces egg production in hens.

Water deprivation can occur at any age and for a variety of reasons. Water may be available to chicks, but perhaps they are too small to reach it. Chickens of any age will be deprived of water if the water quality is poor or they simply don't like the taste of it. Diarrhea causes dehydration by passing water through the body too quickly to be absorbed. Hens may have plenty of water in winter, but if the water freezes, egg production will drop. In warm weather, water deprivation occurs when a flock's water needs go up but the supply remains the same.

If a laying hen goes without water for as little as 24 hours, she may take as long as 24 days to recover. If she goes without water for 36 hours, she may go into a molt, followed by a lengthy period of poor laying from which she may never recover.

CHART 2-10

Signs of Water Deprivation

Body Part	*Change*
Comb and wattles	shrunken and bluish
Tendons on backs of legs	stand out prominently
Droppings	off color

CHART 2-11

Watering

Waterer Space

Age	*Trough/Bird*		*Birds/Fount*	*Caged Birds/Cup*	*Nipple*
Layers:					
0–6 weeks	1.0"	2.5 cm	100	25	15
7–18 weeks	1.0"	2.5 cm	50	12	8
19 weeks and up	2.0"	5.0 cm	30	12	8

			Founts or Cups/100 Birds
Broilers:			
1 day–1 week	1.0"	2.5 cm	1
1–8 weeks	1.0"	2.5 cm	2
8 weeks and up	1.0"	2.5 cm	2
Breeders:	1.0"	2.5 cm	2*

Minimum Water Needs

Age	*Water Per Dozen Birds*	
1 day–1 week	1 quart	1 liter
1–4 weeks	2 quarts	2 liters
4–12 weeks	1 gallon	4 liters
12 weeks and up	1.5 gallons	6 liters

*Double in hot weather

Waterers

A good waterer is designed so chickens can't step in the water or roost over it, and it holds enough to last until it can conveniently be refilled. Automatic watering is, of course, ideal, provided you check it daily to make sure the system is functioning properly. Once a week, add 1 tablespoon of sodium bicarbonate (baking soda) per gallon to the automatic watering tank to keep slime from forming in the pipes, valves, and drinkers. Diseases can be spread through drinking water, so clean and disinfect all waterers regularly.

In winter, coils or a heating pan will keep water from freezing. In summer, place waterers in a shady place where the water won't be warmed by the sun. A gravel or sand bed beneath the waterer, topped with droppings boards, will keep chickens from drinking spills and picking in moist, filthy soil that invariably surrounds a waterer.

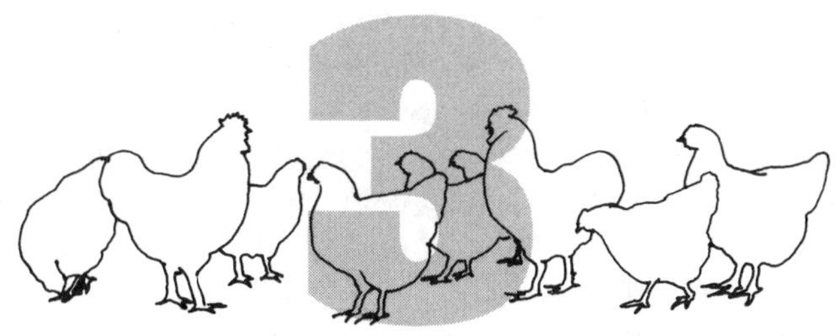

Anatomy of a Chicken

DIFFERENT DISEASES AFFECT DIFFERENT PARTS of a chicken's body in different ways. When a bird gets sick, knowing what part of its body is affected may help you determine what disease the bird has.

If your flock keeps getting diseases that always affect the same body system, some management change may be in order. Frequent bouts with digestive disorders, for example, may indicate a need for improved sanitation, while repeated respiratory problems may signal a need for improved ventilation.

Vital Statistics

Maximum Life Span: 30–35 years
Maximum Productive Life: 12–15 years

Body Temperature		
	adult	**103°F (39.5°C)**
	chick	**106.7°F (41.5°C)**
Respiratory Rate		
	cock	**12–20 breaths per minute**
	hen	**20–36 breaths per minute**
Heart Rate*		
	adult	**250–350 beats per minute**
	chick	**350–450 beats per minute**

*Heart rate varies with breed and sex; a mature New Hampshire cock has a heart rate of 250 beats per minute, a mature Leghorn hen 350 beats per minute.

Immune System

A chicken's first defense against disease is its skin, the largest organ and the main one by which a bird comes into contact with its environment. The majority of disease-causing organisms can enter a chicken's body only through the skin protecting the outside of its body or the mucous membranes lining the openings on the inside of its body.

On the skin live certain microbes that, through competition, keep other microorganisms away. If the skin is broken, even these "good" microbes may get into the body and cause disease. Microbes have an easier time getting through mucous membranes than through the skin. They are kept out by moving fluids (mucus and tears) and by enzymes that destroy invaders.

If a microorganism manages to break through the defenses of the skin or mucous membranes, the bird's lymphatic system takes up the battle. All body tissues are lubricated by watery fluid, called "lymph," that's derived from the bloodstream and that accumulates in the spaces between tissue cells. The lymphatic system drains lymph from all over the body and returns it to the bloodstream, after passing it through lymph glands (or lymph nodes) that filter out microbes and other foreign bodies.

Lymph contains specialized white blood cells of several kinds, technically called "lymphocytes" but popularly known by such names as "engulfing"

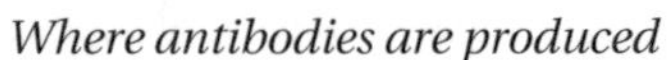
Where antibodies are produced

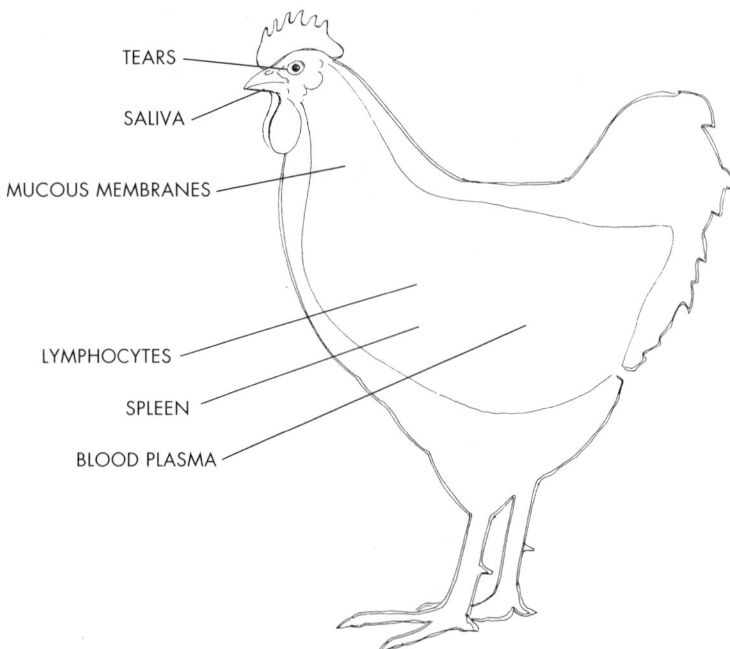

cells and "killer" cells. Lymphocytes neutralize or destroy invading microbes, which they recognize as antigens. An antigen is, quite simply, a protein that differs from any natural protein in the body.

When lymphocytes detect an antigen, they respond by producing substances to fight the invader. These substances are called "antibodies" or "immunoglobulins." No one knows exactly how antibodies are produced. What is known is that antibodies attach themselves to antigens, making it easier for engulfing cells, killer cells, and other lymphocytes to destroy the antigens.

CHART 3-1

Diseases Involving the Cloacal Bursa

Disease	*Effect*
Infectious anemia	atrophy
Infectious bursal disease	atrophy
Lymphoid leucosis	tumor
Marek's disease	tumor
Runting syndrome	atrophy

Antibodies are also produced by the spleen (the additional function of which is to remove and destroy worn-out blood cells). Many diseases affect the spleen, causing it to swell (paratyphoid), turn mushy (histoplasmosis), or atrophy (infectious anemia). The spleen is not a vital organ, however, and if it ceases to function, other parts of the body take over its job.

Immunity is controlled and antibody production is activated in chicks by a rose-shaped organ behind the cloaca, called the "cloacal bursa" (or "bursa of Fabricius"). Some viral diseases damage the cloacal bursa, permanently compromising the bird's immune system. Infectious bursal disease, the most common cause of immunosuppression, is a fairly common infection of chicks 3 to 6 weeks old that attacks lymph tissue and destroys the cloacal bursa. Marek's disease, a common tumor disease of birds 3 to 6 months old, may also damage the cloacal bursa.

Location of cloacal bursa, organ responsible for antibody production

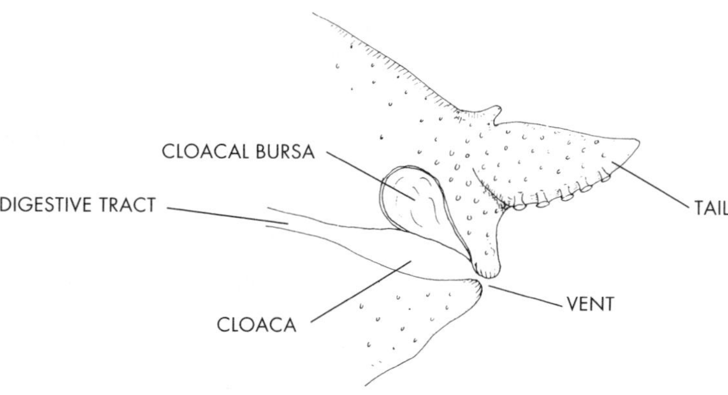

Digestive System

A chicken has no teeth. Saliva starts breaking down feed as soon as it enters the bird's mouth. Its tongue pushes the feed toward the back of its mouth. The feed then slides down the esophagus, a tube leading to the crop where the feed is temporarily stored. You can sometimes see a full crop bulging at the base of a bird's neck.

Occasionally the crop becomes impacted (see "Crop Impaction," page 264). Crop impaction may occur when feed is withheld preparatory to worming, causing chickens to eat too much at once afterward. Crops may also get packed when birds are free ranged where little is available to eat but tough, fibrous vegetation. Even if the bird continues to eat, nutrition cannot get through. The swollen crop may cut off the windpipe, suffocating the bird. Crop impaction is not likely to occur in properly fed birds.

Digestive System

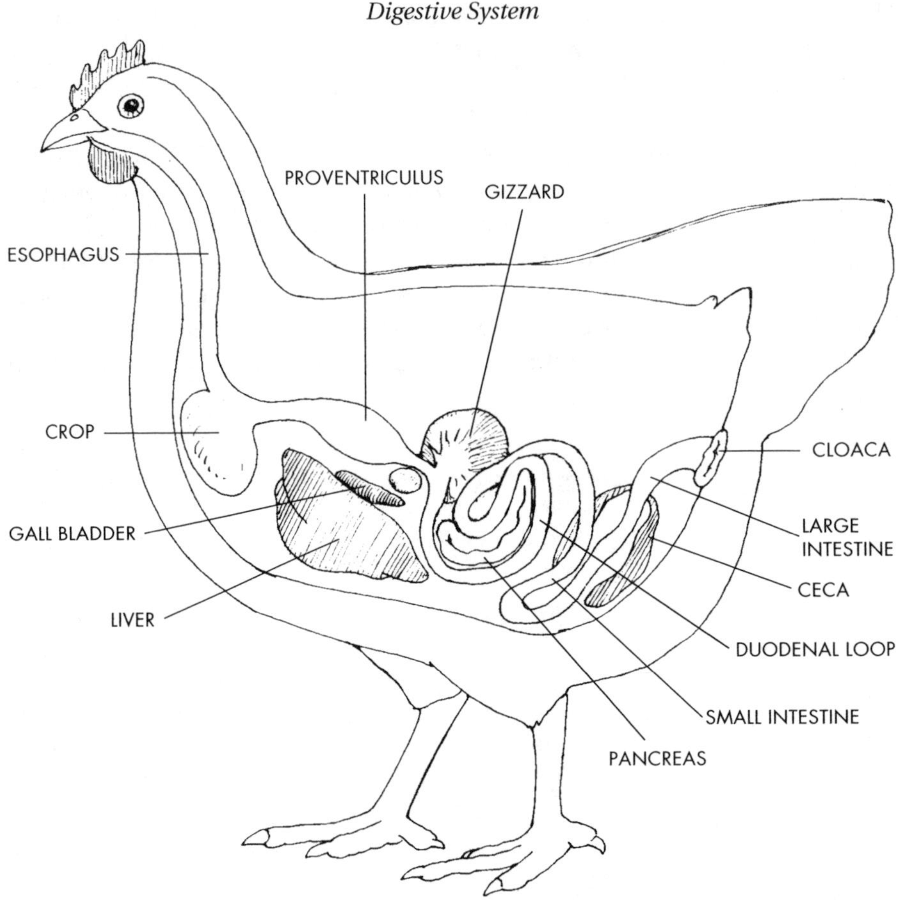

From the crop, feed is moved to the proventriculus or true stomach, where enzymes break it down further. It is then passed along to the gizzard, or mechanical stomach, an organ with strong muscles, a tough lining, and a collection of small stones or grit for grinding up grains.

A chicken fed only commercially prepared mash or pellets does not need grit. Its digestive efficiency will be impaired, however, if it eats grains without having access to grit for its gizzard. If a bird eats a small, sharp object such as a tack or staple, the object is likely to lodge in its gizzard and, due to the strong grinding motion of the gizzard muscles, may eventually pierce the gizzard wall. As a result, the bird will grow thin and eventually die — a good reason to keep the yard free of nails, glass shards, bits of wire, and the like.

From the gizzard, feed passes into the small intestine for absorption. The upper portion of the small intestine, called the "duodenum," forms a loop. Enclosed by the duodenal loop is the pancreas, which secretes enzymes to aid digestion, bicarbonate to neutralize acids, and hormones to regulate blood sugar.

Between the duodenal loop and the lower small intestine is connected the liver, an organ that secretes green bile (or gall) to aid in the absorption of fats in the intestine. Attached to the liver is a transparent pouch, the gall bladder, where bile is stored until it is needed.

Branching off between the small and large intestine are two blind pouches, called the "ceca" (one is a "cecum"), that have no known function. The ceca empty their contents two or three times a day, producing pasty droppings that often smell worse than regular droppings.

The last portion of the intestine, the large intestine or "rectum," is relatively short. It absorbs water from feedstuffs as they pass through.

Both the small and large intestine are normally populated by beneficial bacteria, referred to as "microflora" (*micro* meaning very small and *flora* meaning plants). Microflora aid digestion and enhance immunity by guarding their territory against invading microbes. An intestinal disease occurs when the balance of microflora is upset or the normal microflora are overrun by too many foreign organisms (usually eaten in contaminated feed or water). The result is enteritis or inflammation of the intestines; symptoms include diarrhea, increased thirst, dehydration, loss of appetite, weakness, and weight loss or slow growth.

Enteric diseases tend to be complex. Combinations of and interactions between various organisms — worms, bacteria, protozoa, viruses, and natural microflora — determine the severity of the disease. Successfully treating enteritis requires knowing what organism, or combination of organisms, is causing the illness.

The large intestine ends at the cloaca, where the digestive, reproductive, and excretory tracts meet. The cloaca has three chambers:

- the fecal chamber, at the end of the rectum
- the urogenital chamber, where the excretory and reproductive systems come together
- the vestibule, into which the cloacal bursa empties

In the fecal chamber, a final bit of moisture is absorbed from feedstuffs leaving the body, which are then expelled through the vent in the form of droppings. In a healthy chicken, feed passes through the entire digestive system in 3 to 4 hours.

Excretory System

The excretory system consists basically of the kidneys (lying along the chicken's back) connected to the cloaca's urogenital chamber by means of tubes called "ureters." The kidneys are responsible for filtering and removing wastes from the blood. In humans, these waste products are expelled in urine. A healthy chicken does not excrete urine, but expels blood-wastes in the form of semi-solid uric acid, called "urine salts" or "urates," that appear as white, pasty caps on droppings.

Urates may be improperly metabolized due to water deprivation, excess dietary protein or calcium, or certain diseases. Droppings may then contain more than the usual amount of urates (as occurs in spirochetosis), or urates may accumulate as pasty deposits in the joints (articular gout) or collect as crystals that block the ureters (as in the case of infectious bronchitis).

Respiratory System

The function of the respiratory system is to circulate oxygen throughout the body and to aid in temperature regulation. Parts of the respiratory system include the nose, throat, trachea or windpipe, lungs, air sacs, and certain bones.

Chickens, like other birds, are peculiar in having an extensive system of air sacs, or thin-walled pockets, that circulate air from the lungs into other parts of the body. The system of air sacs extends around the internal organs and into

CHART 3-2

Air Sacs

Number	*Name*	*Location*
2	abdominal	surrounding intestine
1	cervical	neck, above esophagus
2	interclavicular	shoulder
2	thoracic, anterior	beneath lung
2	thoracic, posterior	behind lung

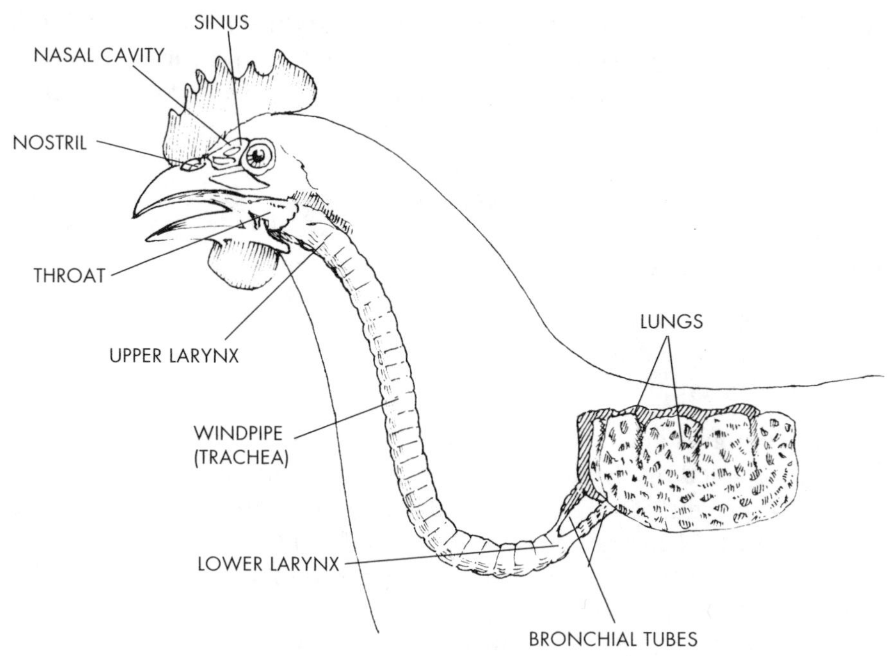

Respiratory System

some bones, called "pneumatic" bones, that are hollow. While the lungs are rigid, air sacs are flexible. All but one come in pairs. The largest pair is in the abdomen, surrounding the intestine.

Respiratory Disease

Respiratory disease has always been a problem in poultry. At one time, all respiratory diseases were lumped together as "colds" or "roup." During the middle part of the 20th century, they were recognized as a group of separate, sometimes unrelated, infections with common characteristics similar to a human cold: labored breathing, coughing, sneezing, sniffling, gasping, runny eyes and nose.

In these modern times, respiratory diseases are classified according to their cause, whether nutritional, parasitic, bacterial, fungal, viral, or environmental. Most serious respiratory diseases are caused by viruses, for which there is no cure and which are easily spread in moisture expelled by a sick bird that coughs, sneezes, or simply breathes. Respiratory distress can also occur as a reaction to vaccination, especially against Newcastle disease or infectious bronchitis.

Respiratory diseases often occur in combination, so that a flock cured of one disease may continue to have symptoms produced by a second disease. The best defense against respiratory illness is to develop your flock's genetic resistance. The best management practices are to provide good ventilation and avoid introducing carriers into your flock.

Skeletal System

The skeletal system of a chicken has three functions:

- to support the bird
- to transport calcium
- to aid respiration

Respiration is aided by a system of hollow pneumatic bones. Calcium transport is aided by a system of so-called "medullary" bones, from which a hen gets 47 percent of the calcium used in eggshell formation.

Skeletal problems can be caused by insufficient calcium, either because the diet is deficient or because a disease or other condition keeps calcium from being properly metabolized. Common problems include crooked or humped back, crooked keel, and wry tail (that flops to one side).

By far the most common problem is weak legs, which may be related to genetics, nutrition, infection, or some combination thereof. In hens, the problem is usually the result of mineral imbalance. Leg weakness is more likely to occur in heavy breeds than in light breeds. Guard against it by keeping young birds off slippery surfaces, by feeding a balanced diet, and by not breeding lame or deformed birds. Be aware that lameness is not always a skeletal disorder, but may result from nerve or muscle damage.

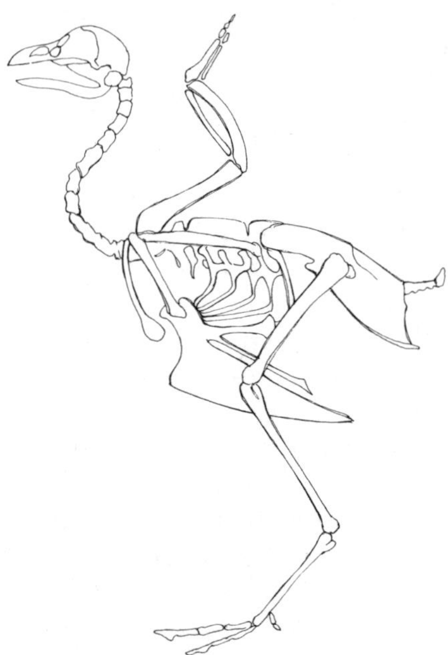

Skeletal System

Another common skeletal problem is inflammation of the joints and synovial membranes — thin membranes lining joint cavities and tendon sheaths. The synovial membranes secrete synovia, a fluid resembling thin egg white that lubricates joints. Inflammation of the synovial membranes, called "synovitis," causes excess synovia to be secreted, making the joint swell and become warm and painful. The most likely joint affected is the hock. Non-infectious synovitis may be caused by injury or nutritional problems. Infectious synovitis may be caused by bacteria, staphylococci, or viruses.

Near the joints, at places where a tendon or muscle crosses a bone or muscle, are small, fluid-filled sacs, called "bursa," that cushion pressure points. Inflammation of the bursa (bursitis) can be caused by pressure, friction, or injury to the membrane surrounding the joint. If the bird is not reinjured or does not become infected, after a time the excess fluid is reabsorbed by the bloodstream. The most common form of bursitis is keel bursitis, popularly known as "breast blister." Breast blister is caused by pressure against the keel, usually in a bird with weak legs (so it cannot keep its weight off the keel while resting) and/or poor feathering (that offers little protection to the keel).

Reproductive System

A cock's reproductive system consists of two sperm-producing testes and the accompanying equipment necessary to get the sperm into a hen. A hen's reproductive system consists of one ovary and a passageway or oviduct that's slightly more than 2-feet long.

A female chick embryo actually starts out with two ovaries, but the right one atrophies. Only the left one continues to develop and become functional. For some unknown reason, occasionally the right oviduct develops partially and becomes cystic, eventually growing so large it presses against other internal organs and causes death.

The functioning left ovary consists of a clump of undeveloped yolks or ova (one is an "ovum") located just beneath the hen's backbone, approximately halfway between the neck and tail. As each ovum develops and matures, it is released into the oviduct, usually about an hour after the previous egg was laid. Double-yolked eggs, laid most often by pullets and by heavy-breed hens, occur when two yolks are released within 3 hours of each other.

During a yolk's journey through the oviduct, it is fertilized (if sperm are present), encased in albumen or egg white, wrapped in a membrane, and sealed in a shell. The whole process takes about 25 hours, causing a hen to lay her egg a little later each day. Since a hen rarely lays in the evening, as the cycle progresses she'll eventually skip a day and start a new cycle the following morning. A group of eggs laid within one cycle is called a "clutch." A hen with a longer cycle (say, 28 hours) lays fewer eggs per clutch than a hen with a shorter cycle.

Any interruption in normal cycling can result in abnormal shell patterns. Abnormal patterns also occur when yolks are released less than 25 hours apart, causing two eggs to move through the oviduct close to each other. The second

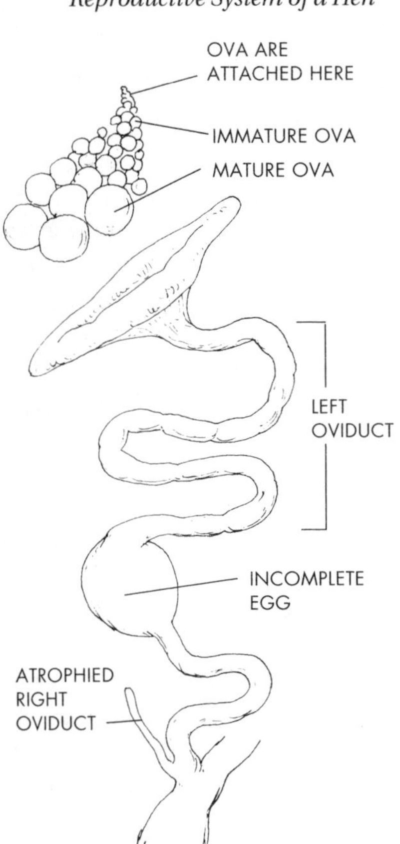

Reproductive System of a Hen

egg will have a thin, wrinkled shell that's flattened toward the pointy end. If it bumps against the first egg, the shell may crack.

Egg shape is inherited, so you can expect to see family similarities. Occasional variations are normal, and so are seasonal variations. Shells will be thicker and stronger in winter, but will get thinner in warm weather due to a reduction in calcium mobilization. Soft-shelled eggs are common when production peaks in spring.

A hen lays best during her first and second year. Thereafter, as long as she is healthy she will continue to lay, but not efficiently enough for commercial production. Regardless of a hen's age, the number of eggs she lays, their size, shape, and internal quality, and shell color, texture, and strength can be affected by a variety of things including environmental stress, improper nutrition, medications, vaccinations, parasites, and disease.

Reproductive Disorders

Soft-shelled, thin-shelled, or misshapen eggs, ruptured yolks within eggs, reduced production, and prolapse may be the result of either poor nutrition or infection. Watery whites and weak or misshapen shells with altered texture and strength can be caused by a viral respiratory disease, such as infectious bronchitis or Newcastle, or sometimes by vaccination. A coccidiostat in a hen's rations may alter egg size, color, and shell texture.

Tumors occur in the reproductive organs of hens more often than in any other animal and are a common cause of poor laying. Some tumors have known causes — notably lymphoid leukosis and Marek's disease — others do not. Slow-growing tumors occuring in older hens are understood least of all, since only young hens are kept in commercial flocks that sponsor most of the research.

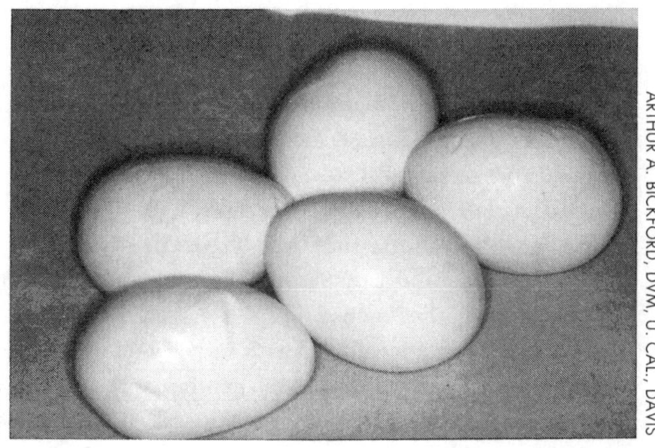

ARTHUR A. BICKFORD, DVM, U. CAL., DAVIS

Wrinkled and misshapen eggs

Prolapsed oviduct, also called "blowout" or "pickout," is a condition in which the lower part of a hen's oviduct turns inside out and protrudes through the vent. Prolapse occurs most often when a hen starts laying at too young an age, is too fat, or lays unusually large eggs. Caught in time, the prolapse can sometimes be reversed by applying a hemorrhoidal cream (such as Preparation H) and isolating the hen until she improves. Otherwise, the other chickens will pick at her vent, eventually pulling out her oviduct and intestines and causing the hen to die from hemorrhage and shock. Not all vent picking is due to prolapse, but instead may result from faulty management — feeders, waterers, and roosts may be positioned in such a way that birds below can pick at the vents of birds above.

A false layer is a hen whose egg-laying mechanism malfunctions due to damage in chickhood, usually by infectious bronchitis. The hen acts normal, visits the nest regularly, but leaves no egg. Instead, yolks drop into the hen's abdominal cavity and are partially reabsorbed by the hen's body. A postmortem examination (see Chapter 10) of a false layer will reveal large quantities of orange fat in the body and coagulated, cooked-looking yolk in the abdominal cavity. The latter is called "yolk peritonitis" and can be caused, as well, by a variety of bacterial infections.

An internal layer is a hen with partially or fully formed eggs in her abdominal cavity, caused by reverse peristaltic action (the rhythmic, wavelike motion that moves an egg through the oviduct). No one knows what causes peristaltic action to reverse, and no treatment is known. An internal layer is easily recognized by her lowered rear end, causing her to stand like a penguin.

Salpingitis, or inflammation of the oviduct, derives its name from the Greek word "Salpinx," meaning trumpet — the shape of the oviduct. Salpingitis is the most common cause of death in layers. It usually results from a respiratory infection, in which bacteria invade the oviduct via one of the ab-

Egg Binding

An egg travels down the oviduct pointed end first. When it gets to the urogenital chamber of the cloaca, it turns end for end so it will come out large end first. Sometimes an egg gets stuck. The egg may be too large (for example, if a pullet lays unusually large eggs), or a disease may cause the oviduct to swell or its muscles to become partially paralyzed. The stuck egg then causes future eggs to accumulate behind it, distending the hen's abdomen. Unless you can get things moving again, the hen will die.

Lubricate a forefinger with mineral oil or KY Jelly and insert it into the vent. With your other hand, push gently against the hen's abdomen to force the egg toward the vent. If you can see the egg, but it is too big to pass through the vent, puncture the shell and remove it in pieces (with great care not to let a sharp shard injure the hen). Rinse the cloaca with hydrogen peroxide.

If the egg was stuck in the cloaca too long, cloacal tissue may protrude through the vent. In that case, protect the hen from cannibalism by isolating her until her muscle tone is back to normal.

dominal air sacs. Most hens die within 6 months of becoming infected; survivors do not lay. If you conduct a postmortem on such a hen, you will find a cheesy mass in the oviduct. The longer the infection has gone on, the bigger the mass will be.

Atrophy of the ovary can occur due to disease or to severe stress caused by lack of feed or water. Symptoms, in addition to cessation of laying, are emaciation and dehydration accompanied by a neck or body molt.

Spontaneous sex change is a phenomenon whereby an old hen develops the characteristics of a cock, perhaps because an infected ovary has caused hormonal changes. The hen's comb grows larger, she molts into male plumage, and she may crow or mount other hens. If the infection is successfully treated, the "cock" will revert back to a hen at the next molt. If the infection is cured before the next molt, the "cock" will lay eggs. This phenomenon was once considered witchcraft, the most famous case being a "cock" named Basel who was burned at the stake in 1474 for laying eggs.

Nervous System

The nervous system is the network coordinating all the other systems. It consists of two parts:

- the central nervous system, responsible for voluntary movements (like eating)

- the peripheral nervous system, responsible for involuntary body functions (like breathing)

The nervous system can be disrupted by poisoning (as in the case of botulism), by a virus (such as the herpes virus causing Marek's disease), or by a hereditary defect (such as the recessive genetic trait that causes congenital tremor). Typical symptoms of a nervous disorder are incoordination, trembling, twitching, staggering, circling, neck twisting, convulsions, and paralysis of a wing, leg, or the entire body.

Circulatory System

Blood type influences a chicken's resistance to disease, a hen's egg production and vigor, and the hatchability of her eggs. A chicken may have one of twelve blood types: A, B, C, D, E, H, I, J, K, L, P, and R, which explains why certain breeds and strains are more vigorous and less susceptible to disease than others. The resistance factor B21, for example, is found in birds that are immune to Marek's disease.

Blood is part of the circulatory system, which includes the heart and a network of blood vessels. The heart is a pump that keeps blood circulating through the vessels. The function of the circulatory system is to transport oxygen, hormones, and nutrients throughout the body, but it can also transport disease-causing microbes.

The blood may be invaded by bacteria, viruses, fungi, protozoa, and other parasites that get into the blood through mucous membranes or through the skin, introduced by wounds or insect bites. Some species of parasitic worms temporarily travel through the blood stream on their way to the organ or tissue in which they will grow to maturity.

Septicemia occurs when any infectious organism enters the bloodstream and becomes "generalized" or "systemic" by invading the whole body. Typical symptoms that a disease has gone septicemic are weakness, listlessness, lack of appetite, chills, fever, and prostration. In acute septicemia, chickens that are in good flesh and appear healthy die suddenly. Sudden death with a full crop is a good indication of acute septicemia, since any other fatal condition is likely to cause loss of appetite.

Anemia, or "going light," is a condition in which the blood is deficient in quantity (blood loss) or quality (low hemoglobin, red blood cell count, or both). Anemia may be caused by dietary iron deficiency, worms, bloodsucking parasites (mites and lice), coccidiosis, and some infectious diseases — notably infectious anemia, caused by a virus known as "chicken anemia agent." Signs of anemia include pale skin and mucous membranes, loss of energy, loss of weight, and death.

CHART 3-3

Disorders by the Body System They Affect

Skin
Breast blister
Bumblefoot
Favus
Flukes
Lice
Mites
Necrotic dermatitis
Pox (dry)

Digestive
Arizonosis
Blackhead
Bluecomb
Campylobacteriosis
Canker
Cholera
Coccidiosis
Colibacillosis
Crop impaction
Necrotic enteritis
Newcastle (exotic)
Paratyphoid
Pasted Vent
Pullorum
Rotaviral enteritis
Roundworms
Infectious stunting syndrome
Tapeworms
Thrush
Typhoid
Ulcerative enteritis

Reproductive
Egg drop syndrome
Flukes
Fusariotoxicosis

Joint and Bone
Arthritis
Cage fatigue
Gout (articular)
Infectious synovitis
Kinky back
Osteopetrosis
Rickets
Slipped tendon
Twisted leg

Respiratory
Air-sac disease
Aspergillosis
Chlamydiosis
Cholera
Chronic respiratory disease
Cryptosporidiosis
Emphysema
Flukes
Gapeworms
Infectious bronchitis
Infectious laryngotracheitis
Infectious synovitis
Influenza
Newcastle disease
Pox (wet)
Roup (nutritional)
Swollen head syndrome

Blood and Cardiovascular
Ergotism
Infectious anemia
Leucocytozoonosis
Malaria

Nervous
Algae poisoning
Botulism
Congenital tremor
Epidemic tremor
Ergotism
Marek's disease
Newcastle disease
Toxoplasmosis

Generalized (Entire Body)
Aflatoxicosis
Arizonosis
Blackhead
Campylobacteriosis
Chlamydiosis
Cholera
Chronic respiratory disease
Colibacillosis
Erysipelas
Histoplasmosis
Infectious bursal disease
Infectious stunting syndrome
Listeriosis
Lymphoid leukosis
Marek's disease
Newcastle disease
Paratyphoid
Pseudomonas
Pullorum
Runting syndrome
Spirochetosis
Staphylococcosis
Streptococcosis
Toxoplasmosis
Tuberculosis
Typhoid

Temperature Control

A second function of the circulatory system is to aid in regulating body temperature. The normal body functions of a chicken depend on a relatively steady temperature of just under 107°F (42°C).

A chicken's temperature normally decreases slightly at night and during cool weather. Heat is lost through droppings, evaporation (primarily from the lungs), conduction (sitting on a cool surface), and radiation (heat lost to surrounding air that is appreciably cooler than the bird). In an infection that causes fever, a drop in body temperature to below normal means death is near.

Body heat normally increases slightly during the day and in warm weather. A rise in body heat also occurs naturally during physical activity and digestion. Fever is a symptom of certain infections, including influenza, infectious bursal disease, and spirochetosis, and any infection that becomes septicemic.

General Symptoms of Systems Diseases

Enteritis: **diarrhea, increased thirst, dehydration, loss of appetite, weakness, weight loss or slow growth**

Nervous Disorder: **incoordination, trembling, twitching, staggering, circling, neck twisting, convulsions, paralysis**

Respiratory Disease: **labored breathing, coughing, sneezing, sniffling, gasping, runny eyes and nose**

Septicemia: **weakness, listlessness, lack of appetite, chills, fever, prostration**

Acute Septicemia: **sudden death in an apparently healthy bird in good flesh with a full crop**

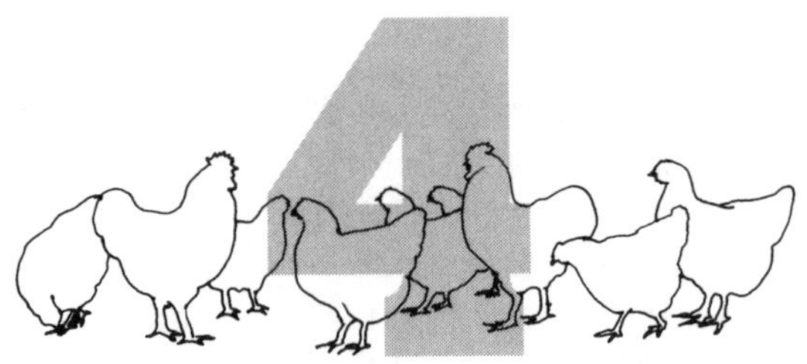

External Parasites

A PARASITE IS A LIVING ORGANISM that invades the body of another living organism and survives without providing benefit. Any living thing that invades a chicken's body and produces an infectious disease is, by definition, a parasite. Those organisms commonly called parasites, however, have certain characteristics that set them apart from other infectious agents.

- They are animals, while other infectious agents are primitive plant forms.
- They primarily cause mechanical damage to the body, rather then poisoning the body with toxins, as do other infectious agents.
- They normally cause a long-term decline in health, rather than the usual brief life-or-death struggle triggered by other infectious agents.

Parasites are divided into two groups: internal parasites that invade the internal organs (discussed in the next two chapters), and external parasites that generally stay on the outside of a chicken's body.

External parasites, in turn, are divided into two groups: insects (bugs, fleas, flies, lice) and mites (chiggers, mites, ticks). Most external parasites produce similar results: weight loss or slow growth, reduced egg production, and aesthetic damage to meat birds. Serious infestations may cause death, particularly to young birds. Some parasites carry diseases from one bird to another.

Chart 4-1

Diseases Spread by External Parasites

Disease	*Transmitted by*	*Disease*	*Transmitted by*
Chlamydiosis	shaft louse	Marek's disease	darkling beetle
Cholera	fowl ticks	Pox	mosquitoes
Epidemic tremor	fowl ticks	Spirochetosis	fowl ticks
Leucocytozoonosis	blackflies	Variety of bacterial diseases	flies
Malaria	mosquitoes		

Insects

Bugs, fleas, flies, and lice all belong to class Insecta. They all have three-part bodies and three pairs of legs attached to the middle part. They develop to maturity in stages, and young insects do not look like mature ones.

Most insects spend at least part of their lives off the bird's body, making it possible to control them by eliminating their favorite hiding places and breeding grounds — cracks and crevices inside buildings, junk piles outside.

Bugs

Bugs are flat-bodied insects belonging to the family Cimicidae, order Hemiptera. They all bite to get a blood meal. In doing so, they inject saliva that causes itching and swelling.

The poultry bug *(Haematosiphon modoru)* — also called "adobe bug," "curuco," or "Mexican chicken bug" — occurs in southern and western states. It attacks humans as well as chickens.

The swallow bug *(Oeciacus vicarius)* is spread to poultry flocks by barn swallows. It has a fierce bite and, like the poultry bug, attacks humans.

The cone-nose assassin bug *(Triatoma sanguisuga* in California, Florida, Maryland, and Texas, *T. protrata* in California and Utah) bothers chickens but is a relatively minor pest.

Bedbug

The most common bug that affects chickens is the bedbug *(Cimex lectularius* in temperate areas, *C. boueti* and *C. hemipterus* in the tropics and subtropics). This bloodsucking parasite is so well-known for attacking humans that it is mentioned in an old nursery rhyme ending with the line, "Don't let the bedbugs bite."

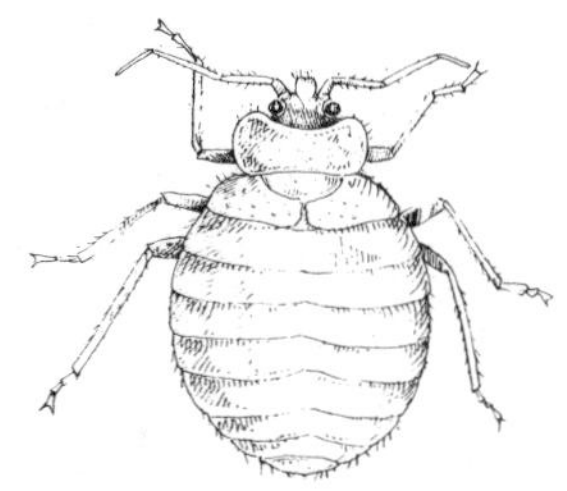
Bedbug
(Cimex lectularius)

The bedbug infests cracks, crevices, and litter, where it can survive for as long as a year without a blood meal. It feeds at night, for about 10 minutes at a time, and is rarely seen on birds during the day. Evidence of bedbug infestation is black fecal spots deposited on eggs and in cracks, and the characteristic unpleasant odor created by the bugs' stink glands.

Adult bedbugs are up to ¼ inch (0.5 cm) long. The female lays several eggs per day until she has produced between 70 and 200 eggs. Depending on the temperature, the eggs hatch in 6 to 17 days. In 1 to 3 months, again depending on temperature, young bedbugs go through several stages to reach maturity and begin reproducing. Control includes removing infested litter, cleaning out housing, and dusting cracks and crevices with an insecticide approved for poultry.

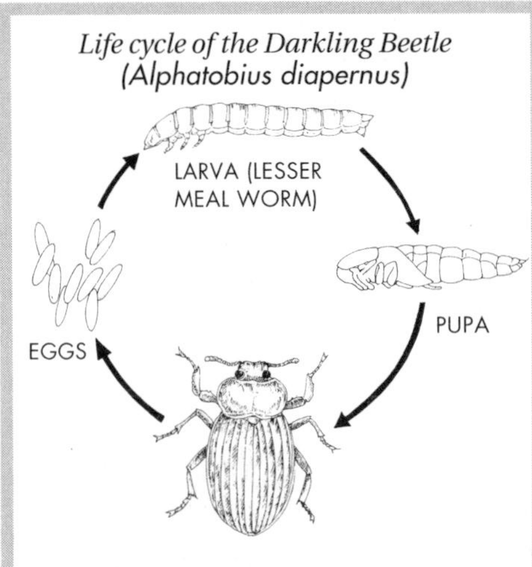

Darkling Beetle

The darkling beetle *(Alphatobius diaperinus)* and its larvae, the lesser mealworm, are not, strictly speaking, parasites of chickens, but they're often found in and around poultry houses. This beetle is about ¼ inch (0.5 cm) long and likes to hide in corners and under feeders. It is difficult to control unless you can take advantage of its extreme sensitivity to low temperatures: if the temperature falls below 40°F (8°C), thoroughly clean out the coop and open it up to the chill.

Fleas

Fleas are insects (order Siphonaptera) with an enlarged third pair of legs that allow them to jump. They spend most of their lives off their host, usually in bedding or grass. They live for weeks off the host, but survive for up to a year if they temporarily return for a blood feeding. Females lay several eggs per day, which hatch in bedding, litter, or grass.

Most fleas are brown and are large enough to see with the naked eye. They are particularly abundant in temperate and warm climates. Of the six species that attack poultry, three are important in North America.

The European chick flea *(Ceratophyllus gallinae)* is most likely to be found in northeastern areas. It lives in nests and litter, and stays on birds only long enough for a blood meal.

The western hen flea *(C. niger)* is common along the Pacific Coast and northward into Alberta. It is similar to the European chick flea, but occurs in a different geographical area. It breeds in poultry droppings and only occasionally returns to birds for feeding.

Sticktight Fleas

The sticktight flea *(Echidnophaga gallinacea)* — also called "southern chicken flea" or "tropical hen flea" — is quite common all across the southern United States and as far north as New York. It is particularly prevalent in sandy areas.

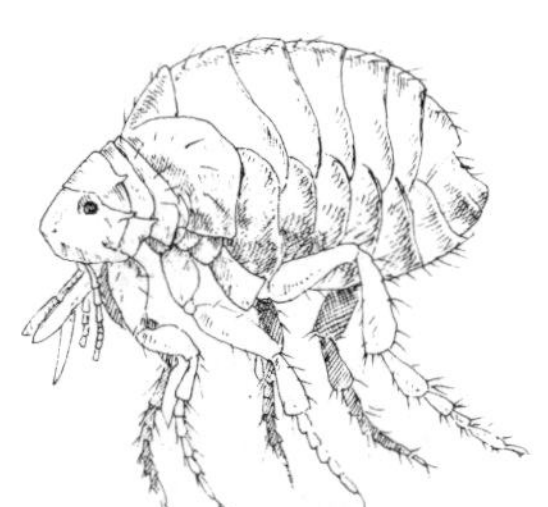

Sticktight Flea *(Echidnophaga gallinacea)*

The tiny, reddish brown fleas measuring 6⁄100 of an inch (1.5 mm) attack humans and other mammals as well as chickens. They attach themselves in clusters of 100 or more to the skin of a chicken's head, where they remain for weeks. Sometimes they imbed their mouths permanently into the skin to suck the chicken's blood. The resulting blood loss may cause death, especially to young birds.

Sticktight fleas are easy to control on birds using a flea salve or poultry-approved insecticide. Unfortunately, they are difficult to remove from housing, due to the female's habit of forcefully ejecting eggs so they will lodge and hatch in sand or litter. Control involves removing infested litter and heavily dusting the floor with an approved insecticide. Repeat the application two or three times at 10- to 14-day intervals to kill fleas that hatch in the meantime.

Sunlight, heat, excessive moisture, and freezing all inhibit sticktight and other fleas. Moisture may be used to control fleas when housing is empty between flocks. Sunlight, heat, or cold may be used effectively in a clean coop that can be opened up for complete exposure.

Flies

Flies are insects of the order Diptera, meaning "two-winged." One pair of wings is for flying, the other is for balance. Flies that bother chickens fall into two categories: biting flies and filth flies. Both kinds spread diseases and parasitic infections.

Biting Flies

Biting flies are found primarily around bodies of water. The two main kinds that bother chickens are black flies and biting gnats.

Blackflies *(Simulium* spp) — also called "buffalo gnats" or "turkey gnats" — are found at the edge of flowing water. They are approximately the same size as mosquitoes, but are chunkier and have rounded or humped backs. They transmit leucocytozoonosis and sometimes attack in swarms large enough to

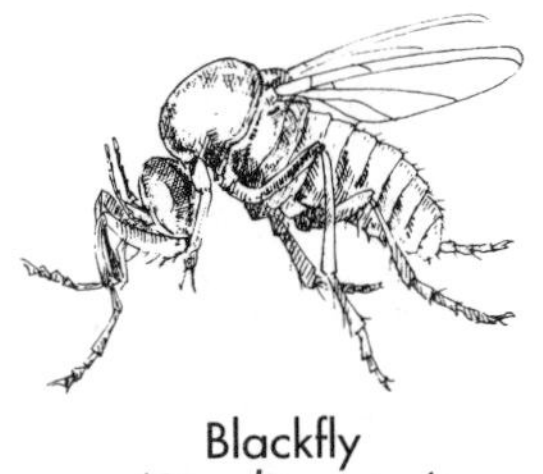
Blackfly
(Simulium spp)

cause anemia and death.

Blackflies are difficult to control. Your best bet is to control larvae in spring (using an insecticide locally approved for the purpose), before adults emerge. Chickens kept in strict confinement may be protected from blackflies by windows fitted with fine-mesh screens.

Biting gnats *(Culicoides* spp) — also called "midges," "no-see-ums," "punkies," or "sandflies" — are found in swampy areas. Attacks irritate chickens, causing them to become restless and to eat less. Like blackflies, biting gnats are difficult to control. A good start is to eliminate sources of stagnant water.

Filth Flies

The common house fly *(Musca domestica)* and other filth-breeding flies don't bite, but they irritate birds, transmit tapeworm (by ingesting tapeworm eggs that infect a chicken when it eats the fly), and spread bacterial diseases. Flies also leave annoying specks on eggs, and they bother neighbors, sometimes leading to nuisance-abatement lawsuits.

Fly problems are a direct result of housing a flock in an artificial environment without providing proper management. Flies breed in damp litter and manure. An important fly-control measure is keeping litter dry by guarding against leaky waterers, leaky roofs, and run-off seepage due to improper grading outside.

Good ventilation also helps dry out manure and litter. Since flies don't like moving air, a ceiling fan not only improves ventilation on hot days, but keeps

Life cycle of House Fly
(Musca domestica)

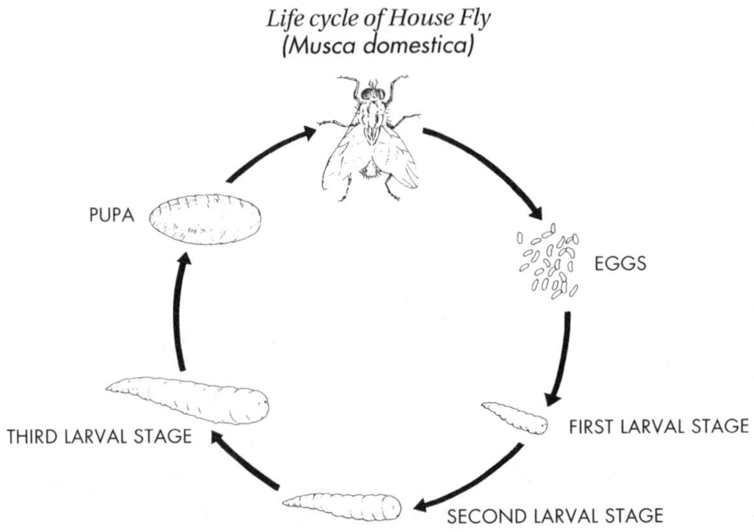

flies from bothering chickens.

A common mistake that can lead to a warm-weather population explosion of flies is to remove litter without thoroughly cleaning the coop. When manure accumulates and dries out, it attracts fly parasites and predators that naturally control flies. If you remove litter and manure, you also remove the natural fly predators.

Letting manure accumulate during warm weather, and making sure it stays dry, is a good fly-control method. Another is cleaning out litter and manure at least once a week. The cleaning must be absolutely thorough — one small clump of manure contains enough fly eggs to produce hundreds of flies. Dispose of the litter by composting it, burying it, or spreading it on a field where chickens won't roam within the next year.

If flies get out of hand, avoid using insecticides or you'll run the risk of breeding a resistant fly population. One alternative is to introduce fly predators, purchased from one of several mail-order sources. Another alternative is to buy or make fly traps.

Homemade Fly Trap

How many traps you need depends on how big your chicken house is and on how bad the fly problem is. For each trap, you'll need a milk jug or similar container. Cut four 3-inch (6 cm) diameter holes into the upper one-third of the jug, one hole in each face. In the bottom of the jug, place 2 tablespoons of commercial fly bait granules containing the fly sex pheromone (common brand names include Muscalure and Tricolure). Hang the jug close to the ceiling. Flies will enter the jug to feed on the bait and die before they can leave. As dead flies accumulate, replace the jug with a new one.

Mosquitoes

The occasional mosquito does not seriously bother a chicken, but a mass attack lowers egg production and can cause death. Several mosquito species *(Aedes* and *Culex* spp) transmit poultry diseases, including malaria and pox. Such diseases are most likely to occur in late summer and early fall, when cool nights attract mosquitoes to the warmth and lights of a poultry house.

Control mosquitoes by eliminating their principal breeding grounds — stagnant water in persistent puddles, old tires, and swampy areas. Where mosquitoes are dense, vaccinate against pox.

Lice

Lice come in two varieties: blood-sucking and chewing. Bloodsucking lice attack only mammals. Chewing or biting lice (order Mallophaga) attack both mammals and birds. Several species infest chickens, and a bird may be infected by more than one species at a time.

Lice are species specific, meaning a louse that prefers chickens doesn't like any other kind of bird or animal. How seriously chickens become louse-infested, or lousy, depends in part on their strain — some strains are more resistant than others. Debeaked birds, because they can't groom properly, are more likely to become seriously infested than other chickens.

An infested bird becomes so irritated from being chewed on that it doesn't eat or sleep well. Egg production may drop as much as 15 percent, and fertility may also drop. Chickens get restless and injure themselves by scratching and pecking their own bodies. In the process, feathers get damaged — an important consideration if the birds are raised for show. In a serious infestation, especially in chicks, birds die.

Louse infestation (technically called "pediculosis") often accompanies poor management and associated problems such as malnourishment, internal parasites, and other infections. Whether louse infestation causes these problems, or these other problems make chickens more susceptible to lice, is arguable but entirely academic.

Lice Species

Lice species vary in shape and size, ranging in length from 1⁄25 to 1⁄4 inch (1 to 5 mm) — big enough to see with the naked eye. Most lice are yellow or straw-colored, making them difficult to see on white chickens, but easy to spot on dark-feathered varieties.

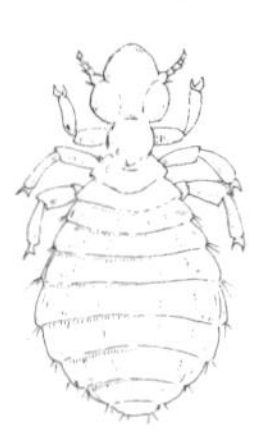

Head Louse *(Cuclotogaster heterographa)*

Among the different species that attack chickens, each has a preference for feeding on certain parts of the body, resulting in descriptive common names such as wing louse, head louse, and fluff louse. Most lice eat feathers, skin scales, and other organic matter on the skin. An exception is the body louse, which chews through skin and punctures growing quills to get blood. Body and head lice are the two most serious louse pests of poultry.

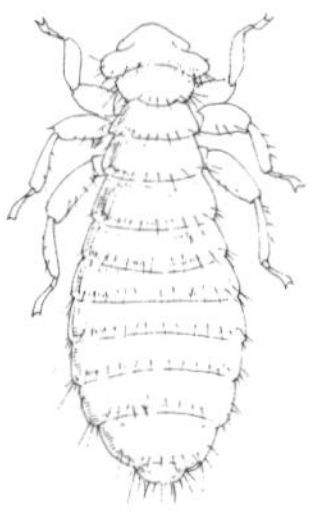

Body Louse *(Menacanthus stramineus)*

In a heavy infestation of body lice *(Menacanthus stramineus)*, you'll find numerous scabs on the bird's skin and pearl-colored egg masses at the base of feathers. Body lice move fast — when you part a bird's feathers, take a quick look before the lice scurry into hiding.

The head louse *(Cuclotogaster heterographus)* is the most serious louse pest of young birds, particularly in heavily feathered breeds like Polish and Cochin. It spreads from a hen to her chicks, causing the little guys to become

Chart 4-2

Lice

Common Name Scientific Name	*Body Part Affected*	*Where Found*	*Appearance of Louse*	*Appearance of Egg*	*Common in North America*
head louse *Cuclotogaster heterographus*	head and neck	base of feathers	oblong, grayish, 0.1" (2.5 mm) long	white, attached to down or feather base	very
small body louse *Menacanthus cornutus*	vent, breast, head, under wings	close to skin	like body louse, but smaller	like body louse eggs, but smaller	no
body louse *M. stramineus*	vent, breast, head, under wings	close to skin in sparsely feathered areas	straw-colored, moves	in clusters near feather base	very
small body louse *M. pallidulus*	vent, breast, head, under wings	close to skin	like body louse, but smaller	like body louse eggs, but smaller	no
shaft louse *Menopon gallinae*	feather shafts	body feathers	like body louse, but smaller and paler	in strings on feathers	yes
wing louse *Lipeurus caponis*	feather barbules	wing, tail, back, and neck feathers	slender, gray, moves slowly	in clusters near feather base	yes
fluff louse *Goniocotes gallinae*	body feather fluff	back and vent	small, broad, yellow, slow	in clusters near feather base	no
large chicken louse *Goniodes gigas*	body and feathers	body feathers	dark, smokey gray 0.25" (5 mm) long	in clusters near feather base	no
brown chicken louse *G. dissimilis*	feathers	body feathers	large, reddish brown	in clusters near feather base	no

droopy and weak. Seriously infested chicks may die before they reach 1 month of age.

The shaft louse *(Menopon gallinae)*, which does not infest young birds until they become well feathered, is a possible transmitter of chlamydiosis. It punctures soft feather quills near the base and leaves strings of light-colored eggs on feathers. It likes to rest on feather shafts, but scurries toward the bird's skin when you part the feathers.

The fluff louse *(Goniocotes gallinae)* is fairly common. It stays mainly on fluff and is relatively inactive, so it causes little irritation or injury. Similarly, the brown chicken louse *(Goniodes dissimilis)* which occurs primarily in the South, lives on body feathers. Two species of small body lice *(Menacanthus cornutus* and *M. pallidulus)* are similar to each other, and both are often mistaken for immature body lice. These and other lice species are not particularly common in North America.

Life Cycle and Treatment

A louse lives for several months, going through its entire life cycle on a bird's body. It can survive less than a week off the body. The female louse lays her eggs, called "nits," on a chicken's feathers and makes sure they stay there by sticking them down with glue.

Nits hatch in 4 to 7 days. Young lice, called "nymphs," are unlike other insects in that they look like adults, only they're smaller and nearly transparent. They go through several molts and develop color as they grow.

When a louse matures, it mates on the bird and starts laying nits. One female may lay as many as 300 nits in her lifetime. Since lice go through one generation in about 3 weeks, in just a few months one pair explodes into 120,000.

Lice usually travel to chickens by way of wild birds or used equipment. They spread by crawling from bird to bird or through contact with infested feathers, especially during a molt.

Lousiness is usually worse in fall and winter. Suspect lice if your chickens are restless and constantly scratch and pick themselves. Look for moving lice on feathers and skin, and for white or grayish egg clusters at the base of feathers. If you see lice on one bird, chances are good the whole flock has them, or soon will.

Inspect your birds at least once a month. As soon as you spot lice, treat the flock by spraying or dusting with an insecticide approved for poultry. Spray caged birds from the bottom as well as from the sides and top. Treat litter-reared birds by sprinkling powder on the litter and in preferred dusting areas. Treat individual birds by placing a pinch of powder beneath each wing and in the vent area. For head lice, mix insecticide powder with Vaseline and rub it on each bird's head and neck. Since no insecticide kills nits, repeat the treatment twice at 7-day intervals.

Mites

Mites belong to the tribe Arthropoda, characterized by exterior skeletons and jointed limbs. They are members of the class Arachnida, a group of spider-like creatures with single-segmented bodies and four pairs of legs.

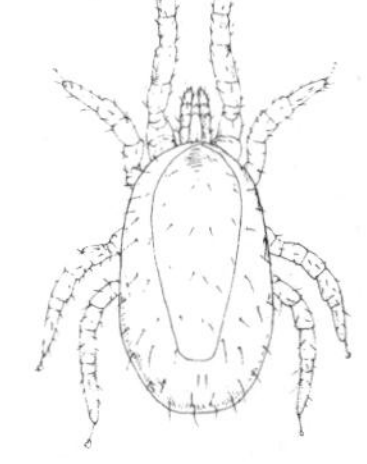

Red Mite *(Dermanyssus gallinae)*

Mites are quite small, usually under 1⁄25 inch (1 mm) in length; some are microscopic. All have mouths designed for piercing or chewing. Depending on the species, they live on blood, tissue cells, or feathers.

Most mites spend a lot of time off the bird and are spread by contaminated equipment, shoes, or clothing. They are also spread by infested birds, including wild ones.

Some mites remain on a chicken's skin. Others hide in feather parts, burrow under the skin, or make their way deep within the body to live in the lungs, liver, or other organs. Mite infestation (technically called "acariasis") causes irritation, low vitality, plumage damage, increased appetite accompanied by low egg production, reduced fertility, retarded growth in young birds, and sometimes anemia and death.

Red Mites

The red mite *(Dermanyssus gallinae)* — also called "chicken mite," "poultry mite," or "roost mite" — is the most common mite found in warm climates and is a bigger problem in summer than in winter, since it becomes inactive when the temperature drops. The red mite is more likely to be found on litter-raised birds than on those kept in cages.

Red mites are grey until they suck a chicken's blood and turn red. They live and lay their eggs in cracks near roosts or nests. They survive for up to 6 months off chickens, so housing may remain infested long after chickens have been removed.

The red mite population increases rapidly in hot weather; one female lays as many as 120,000 eggs. The mites feed at night. In a heavy infestation, some mites may stay on birds during the day and can kill chicks and setting hens. In a particularly severe infestation, red mites invade the roof of a bird's mouth, causing serious anemia. Red mites, when abundant, will also attack humans.

Check birds at night, when mites are on the prowl. You'll see little specks crawling on the roost or on the birds themselves. Red mites can be controlled solely by cleaning up the birds' environment — no need to treat individual

CHART 4-3

Mites

Suborder	*Family*	*Species*	*Common name*	*Where found*	*Common in North America*
Sarcoptiformes	Sarcoptidae	*Knemidocoptes mutans*	scaly-leg mite	unfeathered part of legs	yes
		K. gallinae	depluming mite	in skin at base of feathers	no
	Epidermoptidae	*Epidermoptes bilobatus*	scaly-skin mite	body and upper legs on birds	no
		Rivoltasia bifurcata	feather-eating mite		
	Cytoditidae	*Cytodites nudus*	air-sac mite	respiratory system	unknown
	Laminosioptidae	*Laminioptes cysticola*	cyst mite	under skin	unknown
	Analdesidae	*Megninia gallinulae*	feather mite	legs and head	no
		M. cubitalis	feather mite	on birds	
	Pterolichidae	*Dermogylphus minor*	quill mite	inside quills	no
		D. elongatus	quill mite	inside quills	
		Pterolichus obtuses	feather mite	on flight and tail feathers	
Trombidiformes	Trombiculidae	*Acomatacarus galli*	chigger	hedgerows and dense brush	southern states
		Neoschongasti a. americana	chicken chigger		
		Trombicula alfreddugesi	chigger		
		T. batatas	chigger		
		T. splendens	red bug		
	Myobiidae	*Syringophilus bipectinatus*	quill mite	inside quills	no
Megostigmata	Dermanyssidae	*Dermanyssus gallinae*	red mite	at night in nests and cracks; during day on birds	very
		Ornithonyssus sylviarum	northern fowl mite	on birds	northern states
		O. bursa	tropical fowl mite	on birds	warm regions
Ixodoidea	Argasidae	*Argas* spp.	fowl tick	wood litter, cracks	yes
	Ixodidae	*Amblyomma americanum*	lone star tick	wood litter, cracks	southern states
	Ixodidae	*A. maculatum*	Gulf Coast tick	wood litter, cracks	southern states

birds. Clean facilities thoroughly and dust with a pesticide powder approved for poultry, with particular attention to cracks and crevices. Repeat the dusting in 5 to 7 days.

Fowl Mites

The Northern fowl mite *(Ornithonyssus sylviarum)* is the most serious external parasite of chickens and the most common one found in cooler climates. It completes its entire life cycle in less than a week, so an infestation worsens rapidly. In contrast to red mites, Northern fowl mites increase more rapidly in cold weather.

Northern Fowl Mite *(Ornithonyssus sylviarum)* found in cool climates

This mite differs from the red mite in another way — it survives only about a month off the bird. It lives its entire life on the bird and therefore does more damage than the red mite.

Evidence that northern fowl mites are present includes mites crawling on eggs in nests, large numbers of mites on the skin of birds during the day, darkened vent feathers, and blackened, scabby skin around the vent. This mite moves quickly and will crawl up your arms when you handle your chickens. Control involves dusting individual birds with a pesticide approved for poultry. Repeat the dusting again in 5 to 7 days.

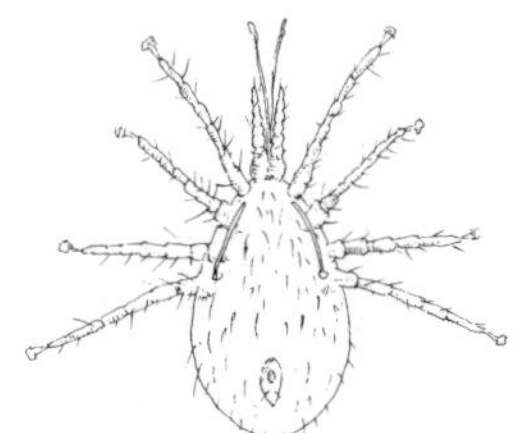

Nearly identical Tropical Fowl Mite *(Ornithonyssus bursa)* found in warmer areas

The tropical fowl mite *(Ornithonyssus bursa)* resembles the northern fowl mite and seems to replace it in warm areas. Like the northern fowl mite, the tropical mite lives its entire life on the bird, but by contrast is more likely to lay eggs in poultry nests. Control involves dusting nests as well as individual birds.

Skin Mites

The scaly-leg mite *(Knemidocoptes mutans)* is a pale gray, round, tiny creature, only about 1/100 of an inch (0.5 mm) in diameter. It is more likely to attack older birds, but also affects young birds kept with old birds. It burrows into the unfeathered portion of the skin on a chicken's shanks, raising the scales by generating debris that accumulates beneath them. As a result, the legs thicken and crust over. In severe infestations, this mite attacks combs and wattles as well as legs.

The scaly-leg mite spends its entire life on the chicken. Once it invades,

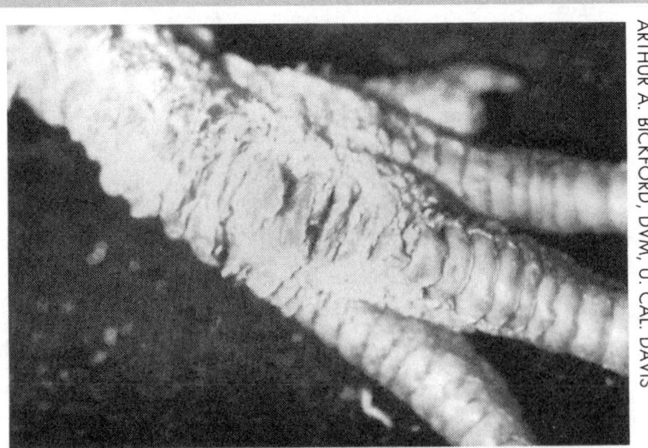

ARTHUR A. BICKFORD, DVM, U. CAL. DAVIS

Controlling Scaly-Leg Mites

Scaly-leg mites spread slowly by traveling from bird to bird. They can be controlled by brushing perches and chickens' legs once a month with a mixture of one part kerosene to two parts linseed oil (not motor oil).

Scaly-leg and other burrowing mites can be controlled in exhibition birds with ivermectin (trade name Ivomec), an over-the-counter cattle wormer sold at most feed stores. Give a bantam 5 to 7 drops by mouth; give a larger bird ¼ cc by mouth. Since the withdrawal time is not known, ivermectin should not be used on birds kept for meat or eggs.

you'll have a hard time getting rid of it. The best approach is to cull affected birds. Treatment involves smothering the mites by applying a kerosene-linseed oil mixture (see box) to the chicken's legs every 10 days until the problem clears up. Coat the legs with mineral oil or warmed petroleum jelly (Vaseline) to loosen old, crusty scales, but don't expect raised scales to return to normal.

Scaly-skin mite *(Epidermoptes bilobatus)* is a relatively rare parasite that causes avian scabies. The mite burrows into the skin of a chicken's body and thighs, causing inflammation and itchiness. The skin thickens with brownish-yellow scabs that may become infected with fungus. A serious infestation causes emaciation and death. The scaly-skin mite is difficult to control. Keep it from spreading by isolating or culling infested birds.

Feather Mites

Feather mites live on and eat plumage, ruining feathers by chewing stripes across them or by damaging the feather base. Luckily, these mites are not common in North America.

Perhaps the most common among them is the depluming mite

(Knemidocoptes gallinae), a tiny creature that is barely visible to the naked eye. It burrows into the skin at the base of feathers, causing the chicken to scratch and pull out its feathers in an effort to reduce the irritation. The problem increases in warm weather. This mite is difficult to control; cull birds to avoid its spread. Treatment involves dipping individual birds in a solution made up of 1 ounce (30 grams) soap, 2 ounces (60 grams) sulfur, and 1 gallon (4 liters) warm water.

The quill mite *(Syringophilus bipectinatus)* inhabits a feather quill, resulting in partial or total loss of the feather. Evidence of its presence is the powdery residue it leaves in the quill stump. Since these mites hide inside feathers, the only known way to control them is to dispose of affected birds and thoroughly clean their housing. Quill mites occur in the eastern states, but are quite rare.

Also rare are:

- the feather-eating mite *(Rivoltasia bifurcata)*, which does little damage
- the Canadian feather mite *(Megninia gallinulae)*, which causes crusty heads and the loss of leg scales
- the southern feather mite *(M. cubitalis)*, which is similar to the Canadian feather mite but occurs primarily in the southern United States.

Internal Mites

Although mites are basically external parasites, they sometimes invade the inside of a chicken's body, either by burrowing under the skin or by invading internal organs. No one knows how common they are. Since they do not cause serious health problems, few people look for them. As a result, little is known about them.

The cyst mite *(Laminosioptes cysticola)*— also called "flesh mite" or "subcutaneous mite" — is a tiny creature visible only under a microscope. It burrows into a chicken's skin, where it does little damage until it dies. Then it becomes encased in a yellowish nodule (somewhat resembling a nodule caused by tuberculosis). The main problem cyst mites cause is destroying the aesthetic appeal of meat birds. The only known way to get rid of them is to destroy infected birds.

The air-sac mite *(Cytodites nudus)* invades a chicken's respiratory system, where it seems to do little damage unless it becomes abundant. A serious infestation produces symptoms that resemble avian tuberculosis: emaciation, anemia, and death. During postmortem examination (see chapter 10), you can see the mites as slow-moving white dots on the air-sac surfaces. The only known method of control is to cull affected birds. Unlike other mites, which hatch from eggs and molt several times to reach maturity, air-sac mites are born live and spend their entire life cycles in a chicken's windpipe, lungs, air sacs, and bone cavities.

Chigger Mites

Chigger mites — also called "jiggers," "harvest mites," and "red bugs" — infest the skin of birds, humans, and other animals. Of the 700 known species, only 4 are common in the United States and Canada. Chiggers are most prevalent east of the Rockies, although some species occur in Arizona and California. The adult, identified by its red, figure-eight shaped body, feeds on plants. Only the larval stage is parasitic. In southern states chiggers go through several generations per year; in the north, they go through only two or three generations.

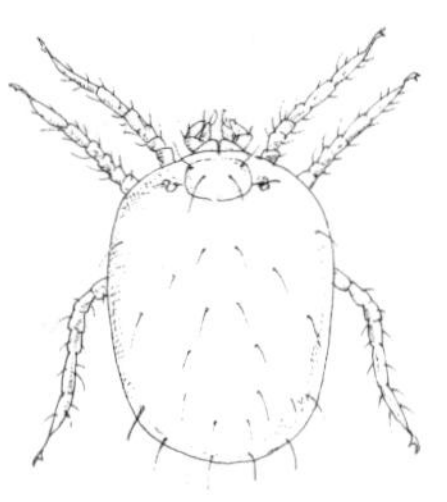
Chigger Mite Larvae *(Trombicula alfreddugesi)*

Chigger larvae have three pairs of legs, instead of the usual four of other mite forms. They are about 1⁄150 inch (0.17 mm) long — so small they can barely be seen with the naked eye. They are straw-colored, making them even more difficult to see until after they feed, when they look like red dots.

Chiggers are fond of attacking a chicken's neck, breast, and wings. They pierce the skin with their mouths, inject poisonous saliva that liquifies the skin, and feed on liquified skin for up to 6 days before dropping off. The bite causes itching, swelling, and irritating scabs that may last for weeks. Young birds become droopy, stop eating and drinking, and sometimes die.

Since chiggers prefer tall weeds, they can be a problem for free-ranged chickens. The best method of control is to keep weeds mowed around your coop. Where chiggers are especially numerous, repel them by dusting or spraying with sulfur.

Chart 4-4

Chiggers

Species	*Distribution*	*Habitat*
Acomatacarus galli	southern U.S.	grassy meadows, dense brush
Neoschongastia a. americana	southern U.S.	dry soil and rocks
Trombicula alfreddugesi	widespread	dry, brushy areas
T. batatas	tropical areas	sunlit, grassy meadows
T. splendens	eastern U.S.	swamps, bogs, rotten logs

Scavenger Mites

Scavenger mites (family Uropodidae) live in poultry litter and feed on fungi. They are especially numerous where new pine shavings are thrown on top of old litter. Discovering an infestation of scavenger mites can be alarming, but don't worry — these mites do not attack chickens.

Ticks

Ticks are really nothing more than big mites. They are divided into three families, two of which are parasitic — Argasidae or soft ticks and Ixodidae or hard ticks.

Soft Ticks

Of several species of soft ticks, *Argas persicus* is the most prevalent in the United States. It is commonly known as the "fowl tick," "adobe tick," "blue bug," "chicken tick," or "tampan." It mainly occurs in the southwestern states and along the Gulf Coast.

Fowl ticks are leathery, egg-shaped, flattish and up to ½-inch (12 mm) long. They feed only on blood and can survive as long as 4 years between feedings. They are tan or reddish-brown until they feed, then they turn bluish.

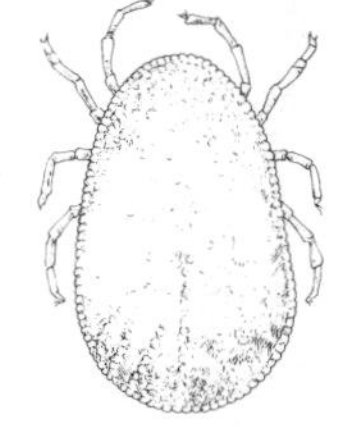

Fowl Tick
(Argas persicus)

A female tick lays as many as seven batches of eggs containing up to 150 eggs each. She deposits her eggs under tree bark and in coop walls. In warm weather, the eggs hatch in about 10 days; in cool weather, they take up to 3 months. Tick larvae crawl around until they find a host, attach themselves, and feed for about a week. They leave the bird to molt, then return for another blood meal.

Ticks are particularly active during dry, warm weather. They hide in cracks and crevices during the day and come out at night to feed. Feeding takes 15 to 30 minutes and leaves red spots on the bird's skin. Chickens that expect to be bitten become restless at roosting time.

Other signs of infestation are ruffled feathers, weakness, depressed appetite, weight loss, a drop in laying, and sometimes diarrhea. The bite wound may become infected with bacteria. In a growing or mature hen, toxins released from the ticks' saliva can cause transient paralysis that is sometimes mistaken for botulism or Marek's disease. Soft ticks also spread a number of diseases, including cholera, epidemic tremor, and spirochetosis. A large infestation causes anemia, emaciation, and death.

Control includes housing chickens in a metal building (to eliminate hiding places), and installing suspended roosts or keeping birds in cages (so ticks can't easily climb onto them). Eradicating ticks is difficult. It involves thoroughly cleaning housing and spraying with a pesticide labeled for ticks that is approved for use with poultry. Use a high-pressure sprayer and pay special attention to cracks and crevices. If birds must be individually treated for larval ticks, dipping is more effective than spraying.

Since ticks molt several times before reaching adulthood, and the entire process takes about 8 weeks (longer, in winter), spray every week for at least 8 weeks to destroy all stages in the life cycle, then spray once a month thereafter. Alternate the type of insecticide you use so the ticks don't become resistant to one type.

A serious tick infestation involving the transmission of a disease may require such drastic measures as cutting down and burning nearby trees in which chickens roost and/or burning down infested housing. Moving tick-infested chickens to new housing will, however, only move the problem to a new location.

Hard Ticks

Hard ticks are most likely to be found on free-ranged chickens in temperate and tropical climates. Two kinds affect chickens in North America.

The lone star tick *(Amblyomma americanum)* occurs from southern Iowa eastward to the Atlantic Coast and southward into Mexico. It is found in woodland and brushy areas, and attacks dogs and humans as well as chickens. Since it transmits human diseases, you don't want one of these to bite you.

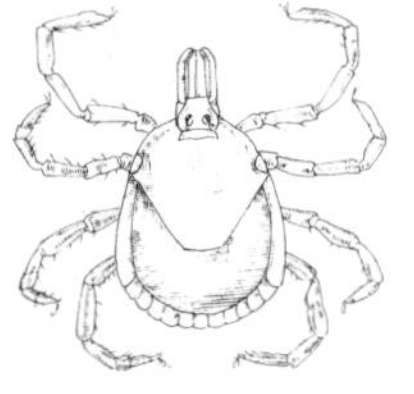

Lone Star Tick *(Amblyomma americanum)*

The adult female lone star tick is pear-shaped and chestnut-brown with a pale spot on her back. She'll lay between 5,000 and 7,000 eggs, which take 32 days to hatch. The larvae, called "seed ticks," are straw-colored and crawl around in bunches. Nymphs are light to dark tan and are smaller than adults. The lone star tick has a 1-year life cycle, during which it feeds three times on three different hosts.

The Gulf Coast tick *(Amblyomma maculatum)* is chestnut-brown with colorful patterns on its back. It occurs along the Atlantic Coast from Virginia southward into Florida and westward along the Gulf Coast into Texas, decreasing in numbers as it moves inland. Although it attacks chickens, it prefers humans, dogs, and other large animals. Each female lays 15,000 to 19,000 eggs, which take 19 to 28 days to hatch. Larvae usually attach themselves to the neck area and feed in groups.

Parasite Control

Not all external parasites are equally common in all areas of the country. Your state Extension poultry specialist can tell you which parasites are most likely to be found in your area and can advise you on currently approved methods for their control.

Many parasites can be controlled through good management, including giving housing a periodic thorough cleaning. Once parasites invade a coop, sometimes the only way to get rid of them is to use a pesticide.

Methods for applying pesticides to birds can be divided into two categories: individual treatment and flock treatment. Individual treatment is more effective, but flock treatment is more practical for a large flock.

No pesticide destroys parasite eggs. To avoid reinfestation when eggs hatch, a repeat application is necessary, timed to coincide with the hatching cycle of the parasite involved.

Pesticide Use

The list of pesticides recommended for poultry is fairly short and changes often due to two things: continuing development of resistant strains of parasites and new knowledge about the dangers of various products. Even approved pesticides are toxic and should be handled with care. Always read the label and follow all precautions.

Before applying any pesticide, remove or cover feeders and waterers and gather eggs. Wear gloves and a face mask, and avoid inhaling sprays or dusts. If you spill any on yourself, wash your skin and launder your clothing. After applying a pesticide, wash your clothing separately.

Store pesticides away from children, pets, livestock, foods, and feeds. Keep them in their original containers with their labels intact. Puncture empty containers so they can't be reused. Due to laws regarding toxic wastes, getting rid of empty containers can be difficult. Check with your local waste-disposal agency.

Some pesticides approved for poultry are restricted, meaning you must obtain a permit to use them. Contact your county Extension office or state poultry specialist for details. Obviously, your best bet is to avoid using toxic chemicals by managing your flock so you don't need them.

Pyrethrum. One fairly safe natural pesticide is pyrethrum, a plant extract that's relatively non-toxic to humans and birds but is highly toxic to insects. Put into a squeeze bottle and puffed into cracks and crevices, or powdered onto vent fluff and beneath wings, it wards off body parasites and flies.

Dust baths. Old-time poultry keepers controlled external parasites by providing their flocks with bins of fine road dust or ashes, sometimes adding sulfur or lime-and-sulfur garden dust to enhance the beneficial effects of the dust bath. Chickens instinctively dust themselves to keep clean and rid themselves of external parasites, which they dislodge by pulling feathers through their beaks while grooming. But dusting in ashes, sulfur, or other chemicals involves a trade-off — chickens are highly susceptible to respiratory problems, and inhaling exotic materials makes matters worse.

Nicotine sulfate. Another old-time treatment that works wonderfully well is the gardening pesticide nicotine sulfate (sold as a 40 percent solution under the trade name Black Leaf-40). It works by evaporating when it is warmed by a bird's body heat. It's painted on roosts just before nightfall or dabbed on vent fluff. As a 2 percent dust it's puffed into vent feathers. The use of nicotine sulfate on poultry has been banned in some states because it is highly toxic if spilled on the skin of chickens (or humans). Old-timers could sometimes revive a poisoned bird by tossing it into the air, causing the bird to flap its wings and inhale oxygen by reflex, but the trick didn't always work and the bird often died.

Petroleum oil. A safer old-time method that's messy but effective against parasites living off a bird's body is to paint petroleum oil onto roosts and nests and into cracks and crevices. It works by coating and smothering lice and mites, but can create a fire hazard in a wooden building.

Dog dip/shampoo. Two other products that work quite well for chickens are flea dips and flea-tick-louse shampoo for dogs. Shampooing is ideal if you wash your birds for exhibition anyway. On a warm, sunny day, wash each bird in warm water, soaking the bird thoroughly and working a good lather among the feathers. Rinse the bird at least twice in warm water. Pat the feathers dry with towels. Let the bird dry in a warm area, away from drafts, or hasten drying with a blow dryer.

Systemic inhibitors. A fairly new idea being developed for chickens is the use of systemic inhibitors that minimize infestation by making a chicken's body unpleasant to parasites. Commonly used systemic inhibitors include brewer's yeast fed to cats to ward off fleas, and vitamin B taken by humans to keep mosquitoes away. Some drugs, including the coccidiostat sulfaquinoxaline and the cattle wormer ivermectin, work similarly.

Precaution

Despite the success of extra-label uses such as those suggested above, it isn't a good idea to experiment with products that are not specifically intended for poultry unless: a) you do not plan to eat meat or eggs from your flock in the near future, and b) you're prepared to lose birds treated with inappropriate products.

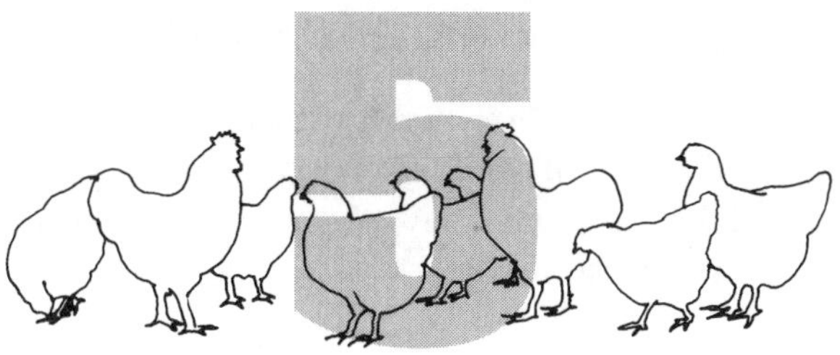

Internal Parasites: Worms

INTERNAL PARASITES ARE DIVIDED into two major categories — protozoa (discussed in the next chapter) and the group commonly known as worms. Worms can become a problem in ground-reared flocks, particularly where chickens are kept in the same place year after year. Most infestations develop rather slowly.

Under good management, worms and chickens become balanced in peaceful co-existence. Through gradual exposure, birds can develop resistance to most parasites. An overload is usually caused by disease or stress.

If the scale tips in favor of the worms, the chickens may gradually lose weight as the worms interfere with food absorption and other digestive processes. Some worms, instead of invading the digestive tract, invade the respiratory system, causing breathing difficulties and gradual blockage of airways. Less common worms invade other parts of the body.

Worms are divided into two main groups, according to the shapes of their bodies. Roundworms or Nemathelminthes have cylindrical bodies; flatworms or Platyhelminthes have flattish bodies. In turn, roundworms, are divided into two groups, nematodes (also called "roundworms") and acanthocephalans (thorny-headed worms). Flatworms are also divided into two groups, cestodes (tapeworms) and trematodes (flukes).

Intermediate Host

Some worms have direct life cycles whereby female worms living in a chicken's body shed eggs that pass out of the chicken in droppings and are eaten by the same or another chicken to begin a new life cycle. Other worms have an indirect cycle that requires an intermediate host. A host is any living thing in which

Direct Life Cycle of Roundworm

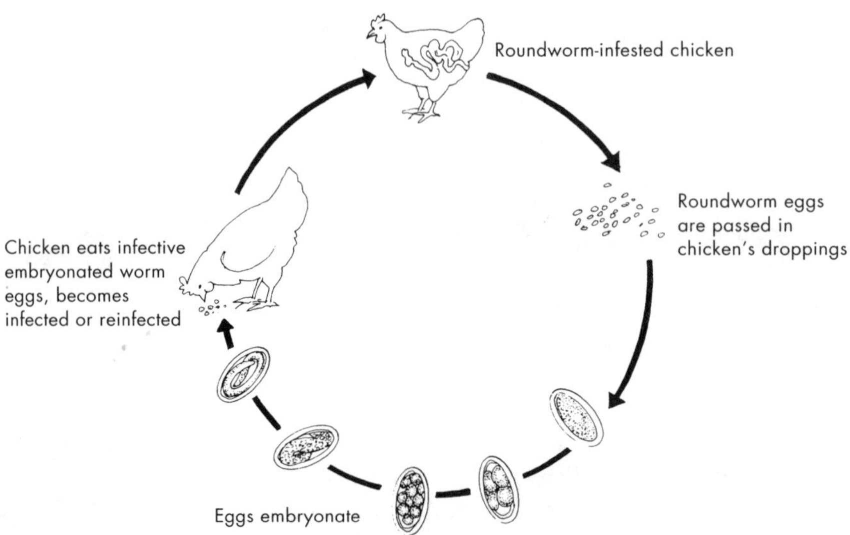

Indirect Life Cycle of Roundworm or Tapeworm

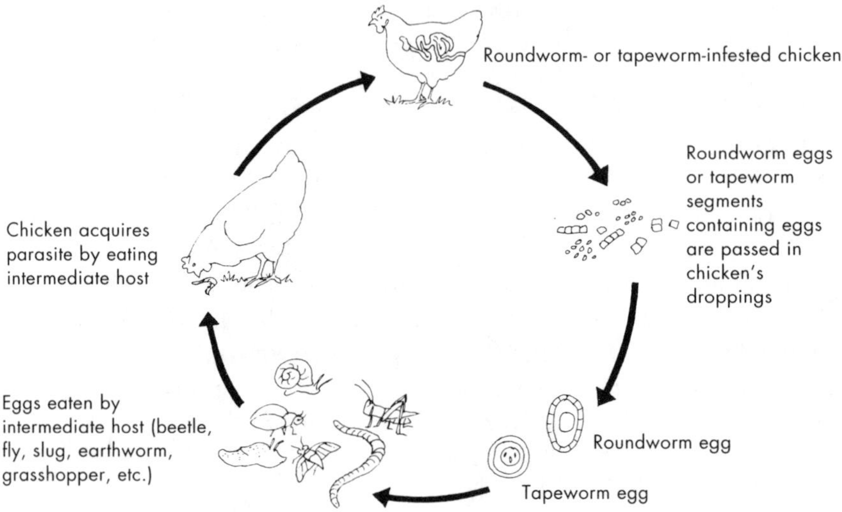

a parasite resides. In an indirect cycle, worm eggs expelled by a chicken are eaten by a grasshopper, earthworm, or other intermediate host. A chicken becomes infected or reinfected by eating the intermediate host (or being bitten by the intermediate host, which releases parasite larvae in its saliva).

More than half the nematodes and all the tapeworms that invade chickens require an intermediate host. These indirect-cycle parasites create greater problems in late summer, when beetles, grasshoppers, and other intermediate hosts proliferate. Knowing which parasites have indirect life cycles, and which intermediate hosts are involved, is an important part of any parasite control program.

Parasitic Worms of Chickens

Nemathelminthes (roundworms)
- Nematodes (roundworms)
- Acanthocephalans (thorny-headed worms)

Platyhelminthes (flatworms)
- Cestodes (tapeworms)
- Trematodes (flukes)

Controlling Worms

Controlling parasitic worms requires good management rather than constant medication. Not only can parasites become resistant to medication, but worming becomes an expensive and never-ending cycle unless you eliminate the source of infection.

Reducing the need for worming medications includes providing a proper diet; a diet that's high in vitamins A and B and animal protein enhances immunity to roundworms. Good management involves these sensible parasite-control measures:

- practice good sanitation
- eliminate intermediate hosts
- rotate the range of free-ranged birds
- avoid mixing chickens of different ages
- don't raise turkeys with chickens

Most worms spend part of their life cycles away from the bird's body, offering a good handle on parasite prevention and control. To avoid direct-cycle parasites, design housing

General Symptoms of Worm Infestation

Usual Symptoms

Pale head (anemia)
Droopiness/depression
Reduced laying
Gradual weight loss

Ocassional Symptoms

Foamy diarrhea
Death

so chickens can't pick in their own droppings. To avoid indirect-cycle parasites, keep intermediate hosts away from the coop. Take care when using insecticides, though, since chickens can be poisoned from eating poisoned insects. When possible, use an insecticide only in an unoccupied house, then thoroughly clean up before introducing a flock.

Wormers

A healthy chicken can tolerate a certain amount of parasitic invasion. Avoid using a wormer unless parasites cause your chickens to look scrawny and scruffy, lose weight, and lay fewer eggs. If worms get out of control and reach the point where they begin to affect the chicken's health, you may have no choice but to use a wormer. Wormers are more properly called

Wormers

Different brands of the following anthelmintics come in varying strengths. Dosages vary accordingly. Always follow label directions.

***Coumaphos* (Meldane) is a feed additive approved for large roundworms, capillary worms, and cecal worms. It is not readily available for small-scale use. For replacement pullets, 10 to 14 days before laying starts coumaphos is added to mash at the rate of 0.004 percent. For hens that are already laying, the rate is 0.003 percent for 14 days. Since coumaphos has cumulative toxic effects, it should not be used within 3 weeks of a previous worming. The withdrawal period is 7 days.**

***Hygromycin B* is a feed additive approved for large roundworms, capillary worms, and cecal worms. It is not readily available for small-scale use. Minute amounts are added to mash at a continuous rate of 0.00088–0.00132 percent. The withdrawal period is 7 days.**

***Piperazine* is a readily available wormer approved for large roundworms. Despite its wide safety margin, it is currently under FDA scrutiny and may one day be withdrawn for use in chickens. Piperazine is rapidly absorbed and rapidly excreted. It acts as a narcotic, weakening and paralyzing adult worms and causing them to be expelled from the chicken, live, with a bird's digestive wastes, but requires a high concentration to be effective. Piperazine works best as a one-time oral dose of 50 to 100 mg per bird. The next most effective method, and one that's more practical for large flocks, is to add piperazine water-wormer to the birds' sole source of drinking water at the rate of 0.1 to 0.2 percent (3 ml per gallon) for 4 hours. Repeat the dosage in 7 to 10 days. The withdrawal period is 7 days.**

***Phenothiazine* is approved for cecal worms. It works only against cecal worms and has a narrow margin of safety, so take care not to exceed the recommended**

"anthelmintics" (from the Greek words *anti* meaning "against" and *helmins* meaning "worms").

How often your chickens need worming, if they need it at all, depends in part on the way your flock is managed. Chickens on open range may need worming more often than confined chickens. Caged chickens need worming least often of all. Flocks in warm, humid climates, where intermediate hosts are prevalent year-around, are more likely to need worming than flocks in cold climates, where intermediate hosts are dormant part of the year.

To ensure a wormer's effectiveness (especially if you're battling tapeworm), withhold feed from the flock for 18 hours before worming. About an hour after worming, feed a moist mash, which causes hungry chickens to eat slowly.

After you've used one wormer for a time, parasites will become resistant to

dosage of 0.05 grams per bird for 1 day only. The withdrawal period is 7 days.

Drugs not approved for poultry use (withdrawal periods are therefore not made public):

***Levamisole,* the active ingredient in tetramisole, is effective against a wide variety of nematodes. It acts on a worm's nervous system, paralyzing the worm and causing it to be expelled, live, with digestive wastes. Levamisole drench (for oral use) is added to water at the rate of 0.03 to 0.06 percent (10 ml per gallon) for one day only. Levamisole injectable is injected subcutaneously (beneath the skin) one time only at the rate of 25 mg per 2 pounds of body weight (25 mg/kg). Levamisole's therapeutic effect in treating a variety of infectious diseases is under investigation.**

***Thiabendazole* is a rapidly absorbed, rapidly metabolized, rapidly excreted wormer used to kill gapeworm and common roundworm. It is less potent than more slowly absorbed and excreted products, making a divided dose (administered over a period of time) more effective than a single dose. The dosage rate in feed is 0.5 percent for 14 days; individual treatment calls for 75 mg for each 2 pounds of a bird's weight (75 mg/kg). Due to its extended treatment period, thiabendazole is effective against emerging worm larvae as well as adult parasites. Since thiabendazole moves through a chicken quickly, the withdrawal time is relatively short.**

***Mebendazole* is based on thiabendazole and is used for spiral stomach worm, common roundworm, and thorny-headed worm. The dosage rate is 10 mg for each 2 pounds of body weight (10 mg/kg) for 3 days.**

***Ivermectin* is effective against a wide variety of internal and external parasites (excluding flukes and tapeworm). It can be toxic to chickens in relatively small amounts. Given orally, ¼ cc is enough to worm a large chicken; up to 7 drops will worm a bantam.**

it. Resistance takes between eight and ten generations. To minimize the development of resistant strains, avoid always using the same anthelmintic. Don't alternate too quickly, though, or the parasites may become resistant to *all* the wormers you use. For maximum benefit, rotate wormers annually.

In the old days, anthelmintics worked against a narrow range of parasites. Today's more potent wormers work against a wider variety of parasites. They work in two ways: by interfering with the parasite's feeding pattern (in other words, by starving it), or by paralyzing the parasite so it is expelled live in the chicken's body wastes.

A wormer may be administered to chickens in one of two ways:

- orally (added to feed, water, or given directly by mouth), to be absorbed through the digestive tract;
- injected, to be absorbed from tissue under a chicken's skin.

Either way, the wormer is transported throughout the chicken's body, metabolized, and eventually excreted.

Withdrawal Period

Different wormers require different amounts of time before they disappear entirely from a bird's body. Each drug approved for use in poultry has an established "withdrawal period" — the amount of time it takes before the drug no longer shows up in the bird's meat or eggs. The withdrawal period for most wormers is 1 week.

Because an approved drug against a particular parasite isn't always available, many flock owners use drugs that are not approved. Such use is considered "experimental" (a designation that allows the drug to be used by qualified researchers) or "extra label" (a designation that allows veterinarians to prescribe the drug as needed). Since no withdrawal period has been established for them, drugs that are not approved should not be used on chickens kept for meat or eggs. (Chickens raised for meat reach butchering age so quickly that worming them shouldn't actually be necessary.)

Drug approval keeps changing, so what was "in" today is "out" tomorrow, and vice versa. Check with your state poultry specialist, veterinarian, or veterinary products supplier regarding the latest regulations. Carefully follow the label directions of any drug you use.

Roundworms

In the number of species involved and the damage they do to chickens, roundworms are the most significant parasitic worm. They belong to the phylum Nemathelminthes (*nema* means "thread" and *helmins* means "worm" in Greek). Most nematodes are long and thin, appearing somewhat threadlike.

Nematodes are less common in caged layers than in floor-reared birds. Direct-cycle nematodes and those requiring an indoor-living intermediate host (such as cockroaches or beetles) are more of a problem in penned birds; indirect-cycle nematodes requiring an outdoor-living intermediate host (such as grasshoppers and earthworms) are more of a problem in free-ranged flocks.

Embryonation

Not all nematode eggs are infective when they are expelled from a chicken. Some require development or "embryonation" to become infective. Some eggs embryonate in as little as 3 days, others require 30 days or more.

In order to embryonate, nematode eggs must encounter just the right conditions of temperature and humidity. In less than favorable conditions, embryonation may take longer or may not occur at all. In general, eggs embryonate more quickly under fairly warm, humid conditions. Minimizing moisture inhibits embryonation and slows the buildup of parasite loads.

Large Roundworm

The large roundworm *(Ascaridia galli)* is one of the most common poultry parasites. Roundworm or ascarid infestation is called "ascaridiasis." The large roundworm is approximately the same thickness as pencil lead and grows as long as 4½ inches (9 cm) — big enough to be seen without a magnifying glass.

Adult large roundworms roam a chicken's small intestine. Occasionally one will migrate from the intestine up the cloaca and get trapped inside a newly forming egg — a decidedly unappetizing occurrence. Such a roundworm can easily be detected during candling.

One female roundworm lays up to 5,000 eggs, which take 10 days or more to embryonate. Embryonated eggs survive in the soil for a year or longer. Roundworms are spread by direct cycle — embryonated eggs are picked up by a chicken from droppings, soil, feed, and water.

Birds that are over 3 months old are more resistant to ascaridiasis than younger birds. Heavier breeds such as Rhode Island Red and Plymouth Rock are more resistant than lighter breeds such as Leghorn and Minorca. Chickens that eat primarily animal protein are more resistant than chickens that eat primarily plant protein.

Signs of ascaridiasis are pale head, droopiness, weight loss or slow growth, emaciation, and diarrhea. In a severe infestation, the intestines become plugged with worms, causing death. Even a somewhat mild infestation may be devastating when combined with some other disease, particularly coccidiosis or infectious bronchitis. In addition, ascarids have been implicated in the spread of avian reoviruses (see "Viral Diseases," page 119).

Of the drugs approved for ascarids in chickens, only piperazine is readily available to owners of small-scale flocks, although levamisole is often used for backyard flocks, particularly exhibition birds. Piperazine affects only adult roundworms. When an embryonated egg hatches in a chicken's intestine, within 7 days the new young worm attaches itself to the bird's intestinal lining. Although this immature form does more damage than an adult roundworm, during the 10 days it remains imbedded in the lining, piperazine can't touch it. Whenever you worm your flock, repeat the worming in 7 to 10 days, giving young worms time to release their hold on the intestinal lining.

Capillary Worm

Six species of *Capillaria* or capillarids invade chickens, causing "capillariasis." Capillarids are white, hairlike or threadlike worms. Most are too small to be seen with the naked eye, but may be seen with the aid of a magnifying glass. They usually lodge in a chicken's crop, ceca, and/or intestines. In a serious infestation, worms may move into the bird's throat or mouth.

Most capillarids have an indirect cycle, with earthworms as the intermediate host. Some have a direct cycle. One species *(C. Contorta)* is both direct and indirect. Capillarid eggs are small and difficult to identify during fecal examination (described later in this chapter).

Symptoms of capillariasis are pale head, poor appetite, droopiness, weakness, emaciation, and sometimes diarrhea. Chickens may sit around with their heads drawn in. Postmortem examination (described in chapter 10) may reveal adult worms in a thickened and inflamed crop.

Capillariasis is most likely to occur in flocks kept on built-up litter. No approved treatment is readily available to small-flock owners; levamisole is often used.

Crop Worm

Easily confused with capillary worm, the threadlike crop worm *(Gonglyonema igluvicola)* invades the crop and sometimes the esophagus and proventriculus (stomach). Its indirect cycle involves beetles and cockroaches.

Unless they get out of hand, crop worms do little damage. Signs of a serious infection are droopiness, weakness, lack of activity, reduced appetite, and thickening of the crop wall. Crop worms can be controlled by controlling beetles and cockroaches.

Cecal Worm

The cecal worm *(Heterakis gallinarum)* is the most common parasitic worm in North American chickens. As its name implies, it invades a bird's ceca. Other than carrying blackhead, to which most chickens are immune, the cecal worm does not seriously affect a bird's health. Leghorns are more susceptible to this parasite than heavier breeds such as Rhode Island Red and Wyandotte.

Cecal worms are slender, white, and about ½-inch long, making them easy to see. Their cycle is direct. Eggs embryonate in 2 weeks (longer in cool weather) and survive for long periods under a wide range of environmental conditions. Phenothiazine is the approved method of treatment, although many backyard flocks are treated with levamisole.

Strongyloides avium is another parasite that invades the ceca, primarily in chickens raised in Puerto Rico. This worm is unusual for two reasons. First, rather than hatching in an animal host, it's eggs hatch in soil, where mature worms live and grow. Second, only the female worm parasitizes chickens. Infestation can be deadly to young birds, but may cause no symptoms in adult birds. No approved treatment is available for small flocks; levamisole is often used.

Stomach Worm

The stomach worm *(Tetrameres americana)* invades a chicken's proventriculus, causing anemia, emaciation, diarrhea, and in a severe infestation, death. This worm is such a bright red color that you can sometimes see it through the wall of an unopened stomach during postmortem examination (see chapter 10). On close inspection, you will find worms of two shapes: the elongated ones are male, the roundish ones are female.

T. americana has an indirect lifecycle involving cockroaches and grasshoppers. Its near relative *T. fissispina*, which is identical but considerably smaller, is carried by the same intermediate hosts and also by earthworms and sand hoppers. Control of the stomach worm involves controlling its intermediate hosts.

Eye Worm

Eye worm *(Oxyspirura mansoni)* is prevalent in the southern United States, Hawaii, the Philippines, and other tropical and subtropical areas. It is a small white worm that lodges in the corner of a chicken's eye. The eye becomes swollen, inflamed, and watery, impairing the chicken's vision. The eyelids may stick together and the eye may turn cloudy and eventually be destroyed. Meantime, the chicken scratches the eye, trying to relieve irritation.

Eye worms have an indirect cycle. Worm eggs deposited in the eye pass into the tear duct, are swallowed by the chicken and expelled in droppings, and are eaten by the Surinam cockroach *(Pycnoscelus surinamensis)*. When a chicken eats an infective cockroach, worm larvae migrate up the esophagus to the mouth, through the tear duct, and into the eye. Wild birds are also infected

CHART 5-1

Roundworms (Nematodes)

Common Name / *Scientific Name*	*Appearance*	*Intermediate Host*
capillary worm (capillarid) *Capillaria anatis*	white, threadlike, 0.3–1" (8–28mm) long	none
capillary worm (capillarid) *C. annulata*	white, threadlike, 0.04–2.4" (1–60 mm) long	earthworm
capillary worm (capillarid) *C. contorta*	white, threadlike, 0.3–2.4" (8–60 mm) long	none *or* earthworm
capillary worm (capillarid) *C. obsignata*	white, threadlike, 0.3–0.7" (7–18 mm) long	none
capillary worm, threadworm (capillarid) *C. bursata*	white, threadlike, 0.4–1.4" (11–35 mm) long	earthworm
capillary worm, threadworm (capillarid) *C. caudinflata*	white, threadlike, 0.3–1" (9–25 mm) long	earthworm
cecal worm *Heterakis gallinarum*	yellowish-white, thin, 0.3–0.6" (7–15 mm) long	none
cecal worm *Strongyloides avium*	white, free-living, tiny, 0.08" (2.2 mm) long	none
cecal worm *Subulura brumpti*	white, 0.3–0.6" (7–14 mm) long	beetle, earwig, grasshopper
cecal worm *S. strongylina*	white, 0.2–0.7" (4.5–18 mm) long	beetle, cockroach, grasshopper
crop worm *Gongylonema ingluvicola*	white, threadlike, 0.7–2.2" (17–55 mm) long	cockroach, beetle
eye worm, Manson's eye worm *Oxyspirura mansoni*	white, slender, 0.3–0.8" (8–20 mm) long	cockroach
gapeworm, forked worm, red worm *Syngamus trachea*	red, Y-shaped, 0.2–0.8" (5–20 mm) long	none *or* earthworm, slug, snail
gizzard worm *Cheilospirura hamulosa*	reddish, 0.4–1" (9–24 mm) long	beetle, grasshopper
roundworm, common *Trichostrongulus tenuis*	white, slender, 0.2–0.4" (5.5–11 mm) long	none
roundworm, large (ascarid) *Ascaridia galli*	yellowish white, thick, 2–4.5" (50–115mm) long	none
stomach worm *Tetrameres americana*	bright red, male: long, 0.2" (5 mm) female: round, 0.16" (4mm)	cockroach, grasshopper
stomach worm *T. fissiprina*	similar to *T. americana* but smaller 0.06–0.16" (1.5–4.1 mm) long	cockroach, earthworm, grasshopper, sandhopper
stomach worm, spiral *Dispharynx nasuta*	white, coiled, 0.3–0.4" (7–10 mm) long	none

*Use not approved — consult a veterinarian.

Organ Affected	*Symptoms*	*Severity*	*Treatment*
cecum, sometimes small intestine, cloaca	weakness, emaciation, possible diarrhea, death	moderate–severe	levamisole*
crop, esophagus	emaciation, death	moderate–severe	levamisole*
crop, esophagus, sometimes mouth	weakness, emaciation, reluctance to move, possible diarrhea, death	severe	levamisole*
small intestine, cecum	huddling away from flock, weakness, emaciation, possible diarrhea, death	severe	levamisole*
small intestine	pale head, inactivity, reduced appetite, slow growth, possible diarrhea, death	moderate–severe	levamisole*
small intestine	pale head, inactivity, reduced appetite, slow growth, possible diarrhea, death	moderate–severe	levamisole*
cecum	weakness, weight loss (carries blackhead)	mild	phenothiazine (Wormal) levamisole*
cecum, sometimes small intestine	none or pasty cecal discharge, turning thin and bloody (found in Puerto Rico)	mild–severe, severe in young birds	levamisole* thiabendazole*
cecum	none	mild	levamisole*
cecum	none, (found in Puerto Rico and S. America, not N. America)	mild	levamisole*
crop, sometimes esophagus, proventriculus	droopiness, weakness, inactivity, reduced appetite, slow growth, thickened crop wall	mild	control intermediate host
eye	scratching of eyes; watery, inflamed, swollen eyes; eyelids stuck together	moderate	ivermectin (3 drops in eye twice daily)
windpipe, bronchi, lungs	gasping, coughing, eyes closed, head drawn in, yawning, head shaking, death	mild–moderate in adult birds	levamisole*
gizzard	usually none	mild–moderate	control intermed. host
cecum, sometimes small intestine	primarily in young birds: weight loss, anemia, deaths peak in spring and fall	severe	thiabendazole* mebendazole*
small intestine, sometimes esophagus, crop, gizzard	pale head, inactivity, reduced appetite, slow growth, diarrhea, death	moderate	piperazine (Wormal) levamisole*
proventriculus	diarrhea, anemia, emaciation, death	moderate–severe	control intermed. host
proventriculus	diarrhea, anemia, emaciation, death	moderate–severe	control intermediate host
proventriculus, sometimes esophagus	heavily infested birds may die	moderate–severe	mebendazole*

by eye worm, and may help spread it to chicken flocks. Eye worm is controlled by controlling cockroaches around the hen house.

Veterinary treatment, usually reserved for valuable birds, involves applying a local anesthetic to the eye, carefully lifting the third eyelid, applying 1 or 2 drops of 5 percent cresol solution, and immediately flushing out the eye with clean water. If the eye is treated in the early stage of infection, it should clear up in 2 or 3 days.

An alternative (unapproved) treatment involves putting 3 drops of ivermectin into the chicken's eye, twice a day, until the eye worms are gone.

Gapeworm

The gapeworm *(Syngamus trachea)* buries its head in the lining of a bird's windpipe or other part of the respiratory system, causing "the gapes" or "gapes." Gapeworms get their name from the habit an infected bird has of continually yawning or gasping for air. These worms, which are big enough to be seen without magnification, are also called "red worms" or "forked worms" — each blood-red female has a somewhat paler male permanently attached, forming the letter Y.

Gapeworms can cause considerable losses in free-ranged flocks, particularly those associated with adult turkeys. This parasite is especially serious in young birds; older chickens become resistant.

An infected chicken coughs up worm eggs, swallows them, and expels them in droppings. The cycle is either direct or indirect, involving earthworms, slugs, and snails. Eggs take up to 2 weeks to embryonate and may survive in soil for as long as 4½ years.

Symptoms of gapes are yawning, grunting, gasping, sneezing, coughing (sometimes coughing up a detached worm), choking, loss of energy, loss of appetite, weakness, emaciation, closed eyes, head shaking, frequent throwing of head forward with mouth open to gasp for air, and convulsive shaking of the head (to dislodge worms from the windpipe). Gapeworms multiply rapidly, eventually suffocating the bird.

Infected small flocks are treated with either thiabendazole or levamisole.

Thorny-Headed Worm

The thorny-headed worm (Acanthocephalans) is more common in Asia than in North America. It invades a chicken's intestine, causing anemia and weakness. Like the nematode, it is cylindrical in shape. It can be identified by its tubular sucking appendage, or proboscis, sporting curved hooks or spines.

These worms have an indirect life cycle. Intermediate hosts include snakes, lizards, and a variety of arthropods (spiders, mites, ticks, centipedes, and insects). Mebendezole, although not approved, is used as a treatment.

Flatworms

Flatworms belong to the phylum Platyhelminthes (*platys* meaning "flat" and *helmins* meaning "worm" in Greek). Flatworms come in two versions, ribbon-shaped tapeworms (cestodes) and leaf-shaped flukes (trematodes).

Tapeworm

An estimated 50 percent of all chickens in small flocks are infested with tapeworms. Like roundworms, tapeworms come in many species. The eight species that invade chickens range in size from microscopic to 13 ½ inches (34 cm) long. Infestation is called "cestodiasis."

Most tapeworms are host specific — those infecting chickens invade only chickens and their close relatives. All tapeworms lodge in the intestinal tract, attaching their heads to the intestine wall with four pairs of suckers. Each species prefers a different portion of the intestine.

During postmortem examination (see chapter 10), most tapeworms can easily be seen without benefit of magnification. The exception is the microscopic tapeworm *Davainea proglottina.* To see it, open a portion of the duodenal loop and place it in water. The loose ends of the tapeworms will float away from the intestinal tissue.

Ironically, this smallest species is also the most deadly. As many as 3,000 have been found in one bird. Symptoms include dull feathers, slow movement, emaciation, breathing difficulty, paralysis, and death. General symptoms of cestodiasis are weight loss and decreased laying. Leghorns tend to be more resistant than Plymouth Rocks.

All tapeworms require an intermediate host; an ant, beetle, earthworm, housefly, slug, snail, or termite. Caged birds are likely to be infected by worms whose cycle involves flies. Litter-raised flocks are likely to be infected by worms whose cycle involves beetles. Free-ranged chickens are likely to be infected by worms whose cycle involves ants, earthworms, slugs, or snails.

A tapeworm's body is made up of individual segments, one or more of which break away each day. A chicken starts shedding segments within 2 to 3 weeks after eating an infective intermediate host. In a severe infestation, you may see segments in droppings or clinging to the area around the vent, looking like bits of white rice. Each segment contains hundreds of eggs — in its lifetime, each tapeworm releases millions of eggs, ensuring that some survive.

Tapeworm Control

To control tapeworm, you must control the intermediate host. Since symptoms are similar for most tapeworm species, it's important to know which species you're dealing with so you'll know which intermediate host(s) you are looking for.

Exterminating beetles is particularly troublesome, since not all beetles found in and around chicken coops are harmful. In fact some are beneficial. To complicate the matter, tapeworms are carried by numerous species including darkling, dung, and ground beetles. Ask your county Extension agent or state poultry specialist for information on problem beetles and their control in your area.

Although no drug is currently approved to combat tapeworm, a veterinarian can provide a suitable medication. Luckily, tapeworm is not a major poultry disaster.

Flukes

Trematodes or flukes belong to the same phylum (Platyhelminthes) and class (Cestoda) as tapeworms, but are in the order Galliformes. Their only similarity to tapeworms is that both are flat. The fluke is leaf-shaped rather than

CHART 5-2

Tapeworms (Cestodes)

Common Name *Scientific Name*	*Appearance*	*Intermediate Host*
large chicken tapeworm *Choanotaenia infundibulum*	very white, flat, segmented, up to 9" (23 cm) long	beetle (several species), housefly
large chicken tapeworm *Raillietina cesticillus*	white, flat, segmented, up to 6" (15 cm) long	histerid and darkling beetle
large chicken tapeworm *R. enchinobothrida*	white, flat, wide, segmented, up to 13.5" (34 cm)	ant
large chicken tapeworm *R. tetragona*	white, flat, wide, segmented, up to 10" (25 cm) long	ant
microscopic tapeworm *Davainea proglottina*	white, flat, segmented, less than .16" (4 mm) long	slug, snail
short tapeworm *Amoebotaenia cuneata*	whitish, flat, segmented, less than 0.16" (4 mm) long	earthworm
short tapeworm *Hymenolepis cantaniana*	white, flat, segmented, up to 0.8" (2 cm) long	dung beetle (S. carabeidae)
threadlike tapeworm *H. caricca*	white, flat, segmented, slender, threadlike, up to 0.5" (12 mm) long	dung and ground beetle, termite

ribbon-shaped. It is not as host specific as the tapeworm, so it may be introduced to an area by wild birds.

Flukes are rarely serious except where poor living conditions allow a massive infestation. The four species that infect chickens each prefer a different part of the body — eye, skin, oviduct, or lower excretory system — where they attach themselves with two suckers.

The oviduct fluke causes a hen's oviduct to swell and sometimes rupture, resulting in the hen's death. Early symptoms of infection include droopiness, weight loss, chalky white droppings, reduced egg production, soft-shelled eggs, and finding a fluke encased in an egg.

The skin fluke forms ⅙- to ¼-inch (4–6 mm) cysts under the skin, usually near the vent. The cysts, each containing two flukes, ooze and attract flies, leading to a possibly fatal bacterial infection. Meantime, the chicken suffers from depressed appetite and has difficulty walking. Treatment requires surgically removing the flukes.

Flukes have complicated life cycles that involve two intermediate hosts.

Part of Intestine Affected	*Symptoms*	*Severity*	*Treatment*
small intestine		moderate	
duodenal loop, small intestine		none-mild	
large intestine		severe	
large intestine	weight loss, decreased laying	moderate-severe	none approved for poultry; see your veterinarian
duodenal loop		severe	
duodenal loop		mild	
duodenal loop		none-mild	
duodenal loop		none-mild	

Breaking the cycle is therefore easier than breaking the cycles of roundworms or tapeworms. The scenario goes something like this: Fluke eggs pass out of an infected chicken, are picked up by and develop within a snail, are released by the snail in water, swim around until they're eaten by a dragonfly or mayfly, and infect a chicken that eats the dragonfly or mayfly. The easiest way to control flukes is to keep chickens away from ponds, lakes, or swamps where dragonflies and mayflies abound.

CHART 5-3

Flukes

Fluke	*Body Part Affected*
Collyriclum faba	skin
Philophthalmus gralli	eye
Prosthogonimus macrorchis (P. ovatus)	oviduct
Tanaisia bragai	lower excretory system

Fecal Test

Some internal parasites can be identified by signs that appear in the infected bird's droppings. Checking droppings may therefore help you identify the parasite so you can determine appropriate management changes and/or treatment, and so you can avoid the unnecessary use of wormers due to guesswork. You may discover that your chickens are not seriously infected with parasites, giving you reason to look for some other cause if your flock is experiencing problems.

Checking droppings, or more properly called "conducting a fecal examination," can be done by any veterinarian, usually for only a few dollars. There are, however, good reasons to learn how to do your own testing. A veterinarian's office might not be handily nearby, discouraging you from testing as often as you would like. Mailing samples doesn't solve the problem, since samples dry out and parasite eggs may hatch or disintegrate. Even when you do your own testing, if you find something that looks serious, you might then wish to have your findings confirmed by a veterinarian before making drastic management changes or initiating drug treatment.

Home Test

Conducting your own fecal examinations is not difficult. To get an idea what's involved, take a fecal sample to your veterinarian and ask to have a look when the sample is placed under a microscope. The vet will help you identify anything that is found. Once you know what you're looking for, you will have an easier time identifying signs of parasites on your own.

The parasites in a bird's digestive tract release eggs, larvae, cysts, segments, and sometimes mature adults in a bird's droppings. Parasites in the respiratory system may be coughed up and swallowed to appear in the bird's feces. Even external parasites, especially mites, are sometimes pecked by a bird and turn up in its droppings.

You can collect droppings from the ground or floor, if you're certain they're fresh. Otherwise, obtain a sample directly from a bird: place your hand inside a plastic bag, persuade the bird to do its duty, and wrap the sample by turning the bag inside out over the sample. If you're checking the whole flock rather than individual birds (for example, new birds you're just bringing in), collect about a dozen samples and mix them together.

Examine the sample for clearly visible signs of dead worms or tapeworm segments. Whether or not you find anything, the next step is to examine the sample under a microscope. The most likely thing you'll see is parasite eggs. Some eggs are unique and easy to recognize. Others are quite similar within a group, making it difficult to tell one species from another. Either way, you'll need a pictorial guide such as *Veterinary Clinical Parasitology* (listed in the appendix).

Be aware that some things a bird eats that turn up in its droppings may resemble parasites. Such "pseudo-parasites" include mold spores, pollen grains, grain mites, and corn smut spores. The latter can easily be mistaken for tapeworm eggs.

Examination Kit

To conduct a fecal examination, you'll need a microscope, preferably one that magnifies from 100 times to 400 times. A good microscope can cost hundreds of dollars, unless you find one at a flea market or garage sale. An inexpensive microscope, designed to introduce children to science, is sufficient for most home purposes. As an alternative to purchasing a microscope, you might persuade a local high school or college biology instructor to let you bring in your samples for examination.

Most of the other things you'll need are ordinary items found around the average house. If your microscope is an inexpensive one, you'll need a light for it — which can be as simple as a well-directed strong flashlight beam or a hand-held egg candler.

The most difficult to find items, though not expensive, are microscope slides and test tubes. Look for them at medical supply outlets or ask your druggist to get them for you. If you purchase a student microscope, it may come with a variety of things you need, including microslides and covers, but eventually you'll need replacement covers.

Unless you plan to test more than one sample at a time, you'll need only one test tube (it doesn't hurt to have at least one spare). To hold the test tube in an upright position, make a stand by drilling a hole in a block of wood or styrofoam so the tube fits snugly.

To speed up the separation of eggs from other fecal matter, professionals use a centrifuge (a machine that spins to separate particles of varying densities). At home, your options are to examine a simple smear or use the flotation method.

Fecal Examination Kit

Equipment	*Description*
Microscope	100X to 400X magnification
Specimen cups	3 ounce (90 ml) paper cups
Wooden sticks	tongue depressors or Popsicle sticks
Strainer	small tea strainer
15 cc test tube	½" x 4" (12 mm x 10 cm) long
Test tube holder	wooden or styrofoam block
Flotation solution	sugar and tap water
Medicine dropper	eye dropper
Microslides with cover slips	standard 3" x 1" (75 x 25 mm)
Pincers	tweezers
Identification guide	*Veterinary Clinical Parasitology*

Simple Smear Method

The simple smear method is not very accurate, but it's better than nothing, and it gives you something to do while you're waiting for eggs to separate for the flotation method.

Begin by placing your microscope on a piece of a magazine or newspaper in such a way that you can look through the microscope to read the print. Put a slide into the microscope and use an eye dropper to place a drop of water in the center of the slide.

With a toothpick, pick up a ⅛-inch (3 mm) blob of droppings and stir it into the water droplet until the water turns cloudy. You should still be able to see the printed page through the moistened sample. If necessary, use tweezers to pick out large pieces of debris. Place a cover slide over the sample and systematically examine the sample through the microscope.

Flotation Method

The aim of the flotation method is to separate out eggs or larvae so you can more readily see them. When you combine the feces sample with a flotation solution, eggs will float and heavier fecal matter will sink.

To make the flotation solution, combine 2¼ cups of sugar (454 g) with 1½ cups (355 ml) of tap water in a small saucepan. Stirring, heat the mixture until it turns clear. Pour the solution into a clean, labeled jar and keep it in the refrigerator until you need it.

When you're ready for the test, use a wooden stick to transfer a ½-inch (2-3 g) blob of fresh fecal matter into a paper cup (more is not better here — too much fecal matter will make your sample too thick to strain). Measure out one and a half test tubes of flotation solution into the cup. With the wooden stick, mix the sample and solution thoroughly, taking care not to stir up air bubbles. Pour the liquid through a strainer into a second paper cup. Stir and press out as much liquid as you can.

Important sanitation measure: *Before proceeding, seal the first cup containing solid fecal matter in a plastic bag for disposal and clean the strainer by pouring boiling water through it.*

Place the test tube in a holder and pour the liquid from the second cup into the test tube. If necessary, use an eye dropper to top off the test tube with fresh flotation solution until the liquid rises above the rim, but does not run over the edge. Using tweezers, place the slide cover slip on top, taking care not to leave an air bubble beneath the slip or jostle the tube so it overflows.

Leave the cover slip on the test tube for 3 to 6 hours, during which parasite

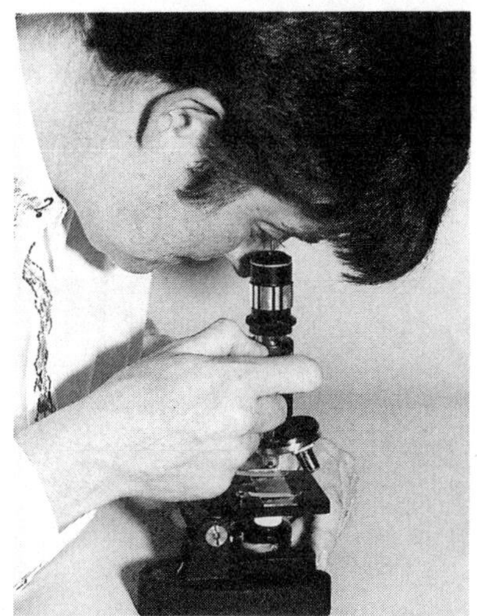

Fecal samples can be examined for nematodes and oocysts using a low-powered microscope.

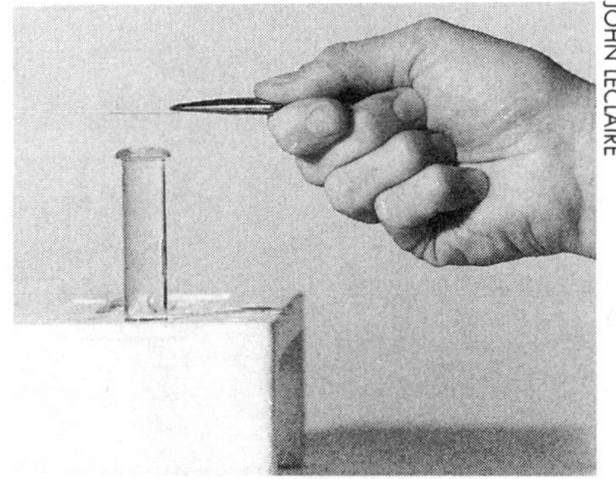

JOHN LECLAIRE

Flotation solution rising above test tube rim.

eggs will float to the top. A good thickness of material should stick to the bottom of the slip.

With tweezers, carefully lift the slip straight upward and put it in the center of a microscope slide, taking care not to create air bubbles. Avoid squeezing the slide and cover together, or you might mash the evidence.

Place the slide in the microscope and systematically examine it under 400X magnification. (For protozoan oocysts, described in chapter 6, set the microscope at 100X). Compare anything you find with photos in your identification guide.

Finding a few parasite eggs is normal and no cause for alarm. A count of more than 500 eggs per gram of feces (EPG) is considered a moderate infestation, which translates into about 1,000 eggs per ½-inch blob of droppings. A count of more than 1,000 EPG (or about 1,200 eggs per ½-inch blob) means prompt treatment is necessary. Of course, you would need a centrifuge to spin this many eggs from any sample, but you can see that there's a vast difference between finding a few eggs on your slide and even a "moderate" infestation.

When you're done with your fecal test, clean out the test tube with an old toothbrush labeled for the purpose. Rinse all your materials with boiling water and set them on a paper towel to dry before putting them away. Store your microscope away from moisture and dust.

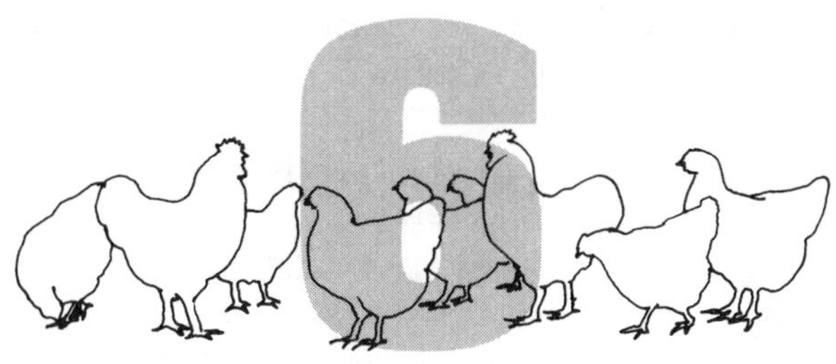

Internal Parasites: Protozoa

PROTOZOA ARE SINGLE-CELLED CREATURES that look round when viewed through a microscope. They are the simplest members of the animal kingdom and also the smallest, ranging in size from 1 to 50 microns (0.00004 inch or 1⁄1,000 mm) — too small to see with the naked eye. Many protozoa are harmless. Others are parasites, causing serious diseases.

Two phyla of protozoa affect chickens: Apicomplexa and Sarcomastigophora. Included in them are several genera that cause a variety of diseases in

CHART 6-1

Protozoan Diseases

Genera	*Disease*	*Affects*	*Prevalence*
Cryptosporidium	cryptosporidiosis	cloaca, cloacal bursa, lungs, air sacs, eye lids	common
Eimeria	coccidiosis	ceca or intestines	common
Histomonas	blackhead	ceca and liver	very rare
Leucocytozoon	leucocytozoonosis	blood, liver, lung, spleen, brain	rare
Plasmodium	malaria	blood, liver, lung, spleen, brain	rare
Toxoplasma	toxoplasmosis	central nervous system	very rare
Trichomonas	canker	mouth and throat	rare

chickens, some of them quite serious. Luckily, the worst protozoan parasites are rare or are not found in North America.

Coccidiosis

Coccidiosis is the most common and most widely known protozoal disease of poultry. It is caused by several different species of protozoa known as coccidia, most of which are in the Eimeria genera. Cocci is the most likely cause of death in growing birds, usually striking chicks 3 to 6 weeks of age. The worst cases are likely to occur at 4 to 5 weeks.

Coccidia are found wherever there are chickens. Even in the healthiest flock, coccidia are present in the intestines of most birds over 3 weeks old. Many species cause no disease or only mild disease, in which case the chickens are said to have "coccidiasis."

Gradual exposure (or surviving an infection) allows a chicken to become immune to the disease-causing coccidia in its environment, so by maturity most chickens are immune. Chickens with Marek's disease are an exception, since they don't always develop the same immunity to coccidiosis as healthy chickens do. Immune chickens won't get coccidiosis, unless their resistance is reduced by some other disease or they're exposed to a new species of coccidia.

A devastating outbreak may occur when a large number of growing or mature birds are brought together from different sources, since they may not all have been exposed to (and therefore developed immunity to) the same coccidia species. Outbreaks also occur where sanitation is poor and/or birds are stressed due to overcrowding, an abrupt change in rations, being transported, or some drastic change in the weather.

Life Cycle

Coccidia have short, complex, direct life cycles. A chicken eats an infective egg, or oocyst, containing eight coccidia in a form known as a "sporozoite." The oocyst is crushed in the bird's gizzard, releasing the eight sporozoites, which lodge in the bird's intestine wall and begin to reproduce. Within 4 to 6 days, the reproductive cycle goes through two or more generations (the length of time and number of generations vary with coccidia species), at the end of which millions of oocysts are released in the chicken's droppings.

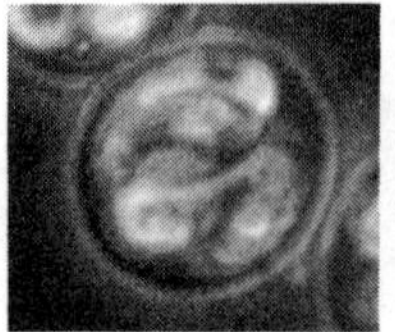
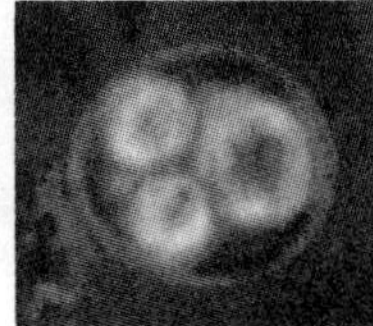
Oocysts: E. tenella (left), E. acervulina (right).

The life cycle of protozoa resulting from the first oocyst is now over, making coccidiosis a self-limiting disease with potentially inconsequential results. How seriously a bird is infected depends on the number of oocysts it eats — in a highly contaminated environment, one chicken may eat between one thousand and one million infective oocysts.

To become infective, the oocysts must develop or "sporulate" (the protozoal equivalent of embryonation in nematodes). For most species of coccidia, sporulation takes 18 hours or less. When a chicken eats a sporulated oocyst, the cycle begins again.

Infected and recovering birds shed oocysts that contaminate dust, soil, damp litter, feed, and drinking water. As birds either die or recover and the infection plays out, the number of shed oocysts decreases. Oocysts are sensitive to ammonia, molds, and bacteria, so they do not survive long in litter. Continuing litter contamination requires constant shedding by infected birds.

In soil, given the right moisture and temperature, oocysts can survive for several weeks (up to 18 months under ideal conditions). They can't survive long in dry soil, and they don't survive at temperatures below freezing or above 130°F (55°C). The danger of an outbreak is therefore greatest during warm, humid weather. Chicks hatched in late winter or early spring therefore tend to be healthier than chicks hatched during the warmer, more humid summer months.

The first outbreak of coccidiosis in a new chicken coop is usually the worst, a phenomenon known as "new-house coccidiosis syndrome." The reason is that the first birds raised on new ground have little exposure to infective oocysts. When they eventually become exposed, they have little or no immunity and the outbreak is particularly serious.

Oocysts are spread on the feet of wild birds (even though the wild birds themselves don't become infected), on the bodies of insects and other animals, on people's shoes, on the tires of feed delivery trucks, and on used equipment that hasn't been thoroughly cleaned.

Symptoms

Coccidia irritate the intestinal lining, interfering with the absorption of nutrients. Outbreaks range from so mild you don't notice your chickens are sick to so severe they die. In mature birds, the chief sign is slow or no egg production. Breeds with yellow shanks and skin may turn pale due to their reduced ability to absorb pigments from feeds. Older birds that appear healthy become a source of infection for younger birds.

In young birds, symptoms include slow growth, a change in the droppings (runny, off-color, sometimes tinged with blood), and dehydration due to diarrhea. The disease may come on slowly, or bloody diarrhea and deaths may come on fast. The weakened chickens become more susceptible to other parasites and diseases. Intestinal tissue damage causes the birds to be especially susceptible to bacterial infections such as salmonellosis or necrotic enteritis.

CHART 6-2

Coccidia Affecting Chickens

Species	Invades
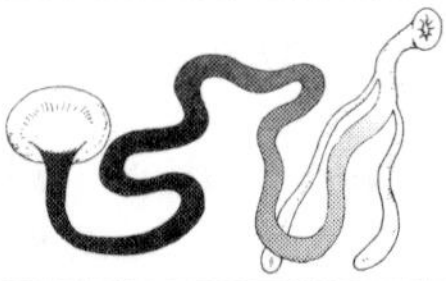 *Eimeria acervulina***	duodenal loop
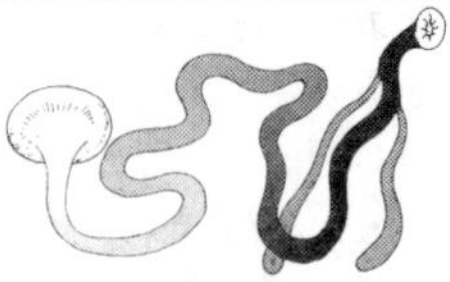 *E. brunetti***	lower small intestine and ceca
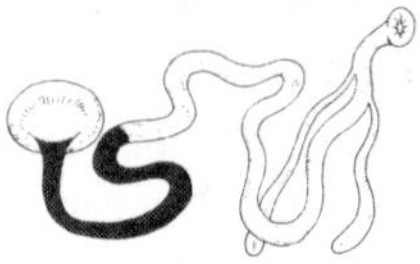 *E. hagani*	duodenal loop
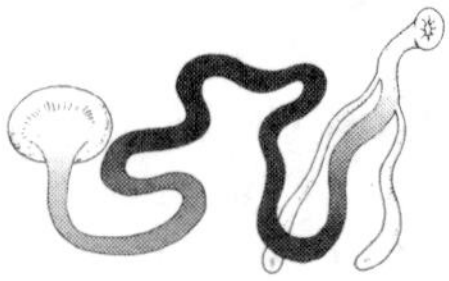 *E. maxima***	middle portion of small intestine
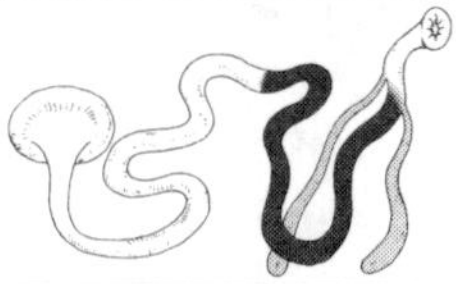 *E. mitis*	lower small intestine
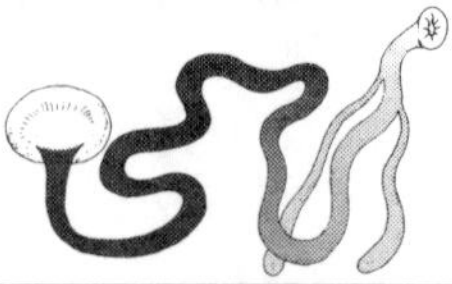 *E. mivati***	entire intestine (starts in upper portion and works its way down)
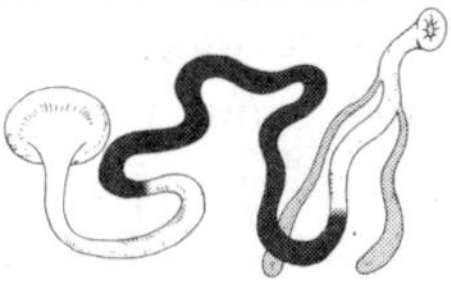 *E. necatrix***	middle portion of small intestine
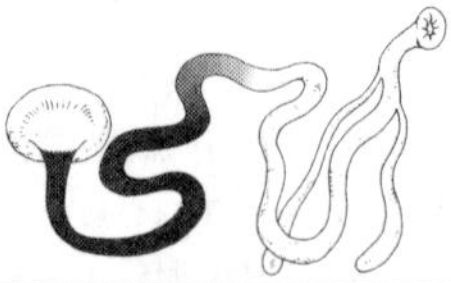 *E. praecox*	duodenal loop
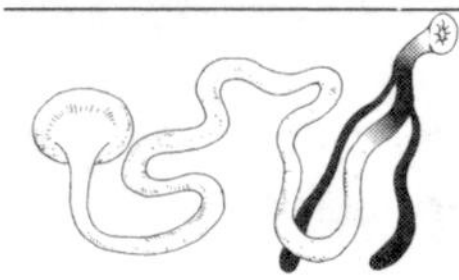 *E. tenella***	ceca

*See Chapter 10. **Main causes of clinical outbreaks.

Symptoms	*Postmortem Findings**	*Oocysts*
(usually in chicks 3 to 6 weeks old) slow growth, pale skin	roughened wall of duodenal loop with gray or white round or striped patches (under magnification), sometimes overlapping	oval
slow growth, bloody droppings, up to 30% mortality; survivors do not grow well	peeling away of intestine lining	large, oval
watery diarrhea	tiny bloody spots along duodenal loop wall	oval to round
(usually chicks 3–6 weeks old) slow growth, pale skin, rough feathers, yellow, gray, or brown diarrhea, loss of appetite, weight loss, high mortality	reddened, distended, thickened small intestine filled with grayish, pinkish, or orange brown mucus	large, yellowish, oval
slow growth, weight loss, pale skin	none significant	small, round
slow growth	thickened intestine wall with patches similar to *E. acervulina* but rounder	roundish
(usually in birds 8 to 18 weeks old) comes on fast; weight loss, watery, bloody diarrhea, up to 25% mortality	portions of intestine may be twice the normal size, filled with blackish blood clots, lining thickened, mottled with white spots or bloody (red or black) dots	roundish
slow growth, pale skin, watery diarrhea, dehydration	intestine filled with watery fluid, small red dots along lining	roundish to oval
(usually in chicks 3 to 6 weeks old) comes on fast; slow growth, weight loss, bloody diarrhea, severe anemia high mortality (bacterial infection); survivors do not grow well	ceca filled with clotted blood and dead tissue that turns blackish, hardens and is eventually expelled in droppings	large, round

Coccidiosis is worse in a flock that's combating another disease; cocci often follows an outbreak of infectious bursal disease.

In severe cases, destruction of the intestinal lining causes hemorrhaging and death. In any case, internal damage is often done before you notice the first symptoms. Seriously damaged birds never become as productive as unaffected birds. It's therefore best to manage your flock with cocci in mind, rather than to wait and treat the disease after it occurs.

If you do suspect coccidiosis, a fecal test (described in chapter 5) will tell you whether or not your birds are shedding oocysts and will help you pinpoint the species. Several tests may be required to identify the species, since an infected chicken does not shed oocysts at a steady rate. In diagnosing the cause of an outbreak, you can pretty safely eliminate any species that previously infected your flock. If you conduct a postmortem examination (see chapter 10), do so immediately after death — within an hour, changes occur that make diagnosis more difficult.

Coccidia Species

Eimeria protozoa come in many species that infect nearly every kind of livestock, but each is highly species specific — the coccidia that invade chickens do not affect other kinds of livestock, and vice versa. Even different kinds of birds are infected by different species of coccidia.

In chickens, coccidiosis is caused by nine species of Eimeria protozoa, some more serious than others. One bird may be infected with more than one species at a time. Each species is identifiable by a number of traits including the portion of a chicken's intestinal tract it prefers, the appearance of its oocysts (size, shape, and color), and the symptoms it produces.

E. acervulina is the most common cause of coccidiosis in North America. *E. tenella* and *E. necatrix* are the most serious, coming on rapidly and resulting in high death rates. *E. tenella,* a form of cecal coccidiosis, generally infects chicks 3 to 6 weeks of age. *E. necatrix,* a form of intestinal cocci, takes longer to build up and so is more likely to occur in maturing birds 8 to 18 weeks old.

Cocci Control

Measures for controlling coccidiosis involve, in order of preference:

- good management
- the use of drugs
- vaccination

Good management includes providing adequate dry litter, clean drinking water, and proper nutrition. All ground-fed chickens are exposed to infective oocysts throughout their lives. A well-managed flock quickly develops resistance. The sooner that happens, the healthier the chickens will be.

CHART 6-3

Drugs Used to Treat Coccidiosis*

Drug	*Application*	*Withdrawal Time*
Amprolium	water	none
Sulfadimethoxine	water	5 days
Sulfamethazine	water	10 days
Sulfaquinoxaline	feed	10 days

*For dosage and length of treatment, follow directions on label.

Coccidiosis is generally less of a problem in free-ranged flocks, being more serious when chickens are concentrated in a small area. Chicks raised on wire and moved to litter when they're partially grown become seriously infected, since they have not had a chance to develop resistance through gradual exposure. Resistance is not necessary for caged layers and cage-managed show stock, since they are unlikely to be exposed to coccidia (unless their drinking water becomes contaminated).

Vaccination against coccidiosis has limited success, although it is sometimes used for breeder pullets. Vaccination is seldom used for broilers — the mild infection produced by the vaccine slows growth, making the option uneconomical. Genetically engineered antigens, now on the horizon, may one day be used to immunize young chicks.

Anticoccidials

A number of drugs are available to prevent or control coccidiosis. Which one you use, if any, and how you use it depends on whether your intent is to prevent infection, permit a mild infection that allows resistance to develop, or treat an existing infection. The type of drug used and the dosage needed also vary with the species of coccidia involved — not all coccidiostats are effective against all species.

Drugs designed for treatment require high dosage levels, yet an excessive dose can poison chickens. Since the toxic level of sulfamethazine is close to the level required for treatment, poisoning can occur at normal doses if high temperature causes an increase in treated water intake. Symptoms of poisoning are depression, paleness, and slow growth. At temperatures over 80°F (27°C), avoid poisoning by using only one-third the recommended dose.

The use of some anticoccidials, particularly amprolium, causes vitamin deficiency. It's a good idea, therefore, to offer a vitamin supplement after you treat your flock. Do not use a vitamin supplement *during* treatment, because vitamin deprivation is one of the ways amprolium controls coccidia. Since coccidiosis increases a flock's susceptibility to bacterial infections, using an antibiotic along with the anticoccidial improves the rate of recovery.

Some of the same drugs used to treat cocci, plus a few additional ones, are used in low dosages to prevent a serious outbreak in young birds while (at least theoretically) allowing them to develop immunity through gradual exposure. The use of drugs for this purpose, usually from the day of hatch to 16 weeks of age, does have drawbacks:

- Although drugs used for treatment are equally effective in prevention — since they reduce the protozoa population by killing any coccidia a chicken eats — the chickens may not be exposed to adequate numbers of coccidia to become immune, so an outbreak may occur when the drug is withdrawn.
- Drugs designed specifically for control (rather than treatment) supposedly reduce the degree of infection while allowing immunity to develop, but some only arrest the development of immunity, paving the way for an outbreak when they are withdrawn. Some are toxic at high levels and/or produce side effects. Any continuous low dose of medication in water or feed can lead to the development of drug-resistant strains of coccidia, requiring rotation of drugs used.
- The medication has a withdrawal time of 30 days, so if you raise meat birds, you'll have to find a non-medicated brand of feed during that last month. That being the case, why not seek out the alternative brand and use it right from the start? Feeds containing preventive medication are designed for commercial producers who bring in as many as 30,000 broilers at a time, and raise one batch right after another. In a small flock, the use of medication is a poor substitute for good management.

Cryptosporidiosis

Cryptosporidiosis is the one form of coccidiosis that is not caused by *Eimeria,* but rather by the protozoa *Cryptosporidium baileyi.* Unlike the other forms of coccidiosis, cryptosporidiosis is not specific to chickens; it infects other birds and is possibly spread by wild species. Although *C. baileyi* does not invade mammals, it may be spread from flock to flock on the feet of animals and humans.

Like other coccidioses, cryptosporidiosis is spread by oocysts, but each contain four (rather than eight) sporozoites. The oocysts are considerably smaller than those of other coccidia, and detecting them requires special laboratory techniques.

Like other coccidia oocysts, cryptosporidia oocysts are sensitive to ammonia in litter. They are also somewhat sensitive to chlorine bleach as a disinfectant, and they cannot survive temperatures above 140° F (60°C).

Unlike *Eimeria* oocysts, those of *Cryptosporidium* are infective when they leave the host's body. Some may not leave at all, but remain and develop within the same host (called "autoinfection"). As few as 100 oocysts in one bird can quickly produce a serious infection.

Although it has not been studied as thoroughly as other forms of coccidiosis, intestinal cryptosporidiosis is apparently quite common in chickens. It is usually mild, often producing no symptoms other than pale skin in yellow-skinned breeds. Once infected, birds become immune.

Oocysts may be inhaled as well as ingested, causing respiratory infection that is less common though more severe than the intestinal form. Respiratory cryptosporidiosis is likeliest to affect birds in the 4- to 17-week age group. Survivors begin recovering in 2 to 3 weeks. *E. coli* often produces a secondary infection, and an existing infection with *E. coli* or infectious bronchitis virus makes respiratory cryptosporidiosis worse.

Cryptosporidia invade other parts of the body, including the eyelid and the cloacal bursa, from which they may travel up the urinary tract. No means of prevention or treatment is known. Chickens develop natural immunity when exposed to oocysts at low levels, leading to the possibility of a vaccine in the future.

Histomoniasis

Infection with *Histomonas meleagridis* protozoan parasites is commonly known as "blackhead" because an infected bird's face tends to darken, although this is neither a sure sign of the disease nor necessarily characteristic of it. The disease — caused by round, microscopic histomonads — is serious in turkeys, but chickens are normally immune.

Blackhead is more common in range-fed than housed or caged chickens, since the disease occurs when a chicken eats an earthworm carrying eggs of the cecal worm *(Heterakis gallinarum),* which in turn are harboring histomonads. The parasites lodge in the chicken's cecum, enter the bloodstream, and eventually migrate to the liver.

Histomonads shed by infected chickens may reinfect the same chicken or infect another chicken that picks in droppings or eats a fly, sowbug, grasshopper, or cricket carrying the parasite on its body. Once shed, histomonads cannot survive long in the environment unless they are protected by a cecal worm egg or an earthworm.

Chicks 4 to 6 weeks old are the most susceptible to histomonad infection. Mild strains produce no symptoms; virulent strains may cause deaths in the 20 to 30 percent range. Drugs approved in the United States are not particularly effective. Since survivors continue to shed histomonads, control requires controlling cecal worms (see "Cecal Worm," page 84).

Toxoplasmosis

The protozoan *Toxoplasma gondii* causes toxoplasmosis in warm-blooded animals including chickens and humans. It is mainly a disease of the central nervous system, but may also affect the reproductive system, muscles, and internal organs.

This protozoa has a complex life cycle. A chicken may become infected in many different ways: picking in infected droppings of chickens, cats, or other animals; picking at an infected chicken, live or dead; eating earthworms harboring toxoplasma oocysts. Toxoplasma may be spread from one area to another on the feet of rodents.

Control involves keeping litter dry, controlling filth flies, cockroaches, and rodents, and keeping the yard free of cats. No effective cure is known.

Trichomoniasis

The protozoan parasite *Trichomonas* occasionally infects chickens, causing a mouth and throat disease known as "canker." It is primarily a disease of pigeons that may be spread to chickens through feed or water contaminated with discharge from an infected bird's mouth. Control involves keeping pigeons away from chickens and isolating infected chickens so the parasite does not spread.

Blood Parasites

A chicken's blood may be invaded by a variety of protozoan parasites, most of which are not common in North America.

Leucocytozoon are found near swampy areas and are spread by blackflies and biting midges, causing anemia and sometimes death due to hemorrhage.

Plasmodium protozoa, transmitted by mosquitoes, cause malaria found in chickens in Africa, Asia, and South America, but so far (knock on wood) not in North America.

Avoid these blood infections by controlling biting and bloodsucking insects such as blackflies, biting midges, mosquitoes, and flies. Do not allow weeds and trash to accumulate, as they provide breeding grounds for insects.

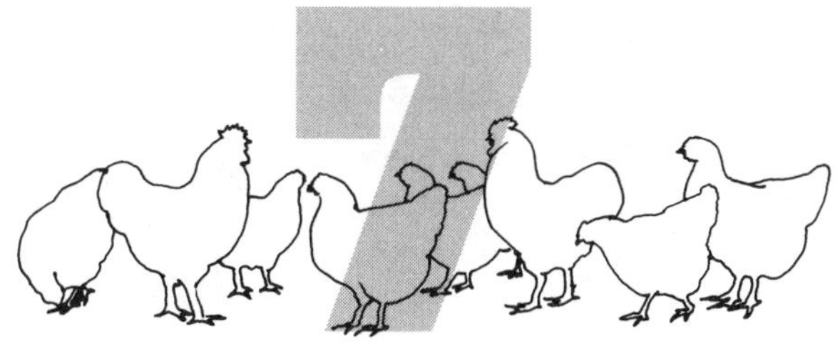

7 Infectious Diseases

THE INFECTIOUS DISEASES described in this chapter are caused by plant-like microscopic parasites — bacteria, viruses, and fungi. Some of these microflora are always present but cause disease only under certain circumstances, such as when a chicken's resistance is low due to stress. Such microbes are called "opportunists."

A few microbes produce disease wherever they occur. They are commonly known as "germs," but technically they are "pathogens," and are described as being "virulent" or "pathogenic." Variations in pathogenicity among strains cause the same disease to appear in different degrees of severity or even in different forms altogether.

The vast majority of microbes are either harmless or beneficial. Beneficial microflora may live on a chicken's skin or within its body, aiding digestion and/or enhancing the bird's immunity by fending off pathogenic microbes, a process known as "competitive exclusion."

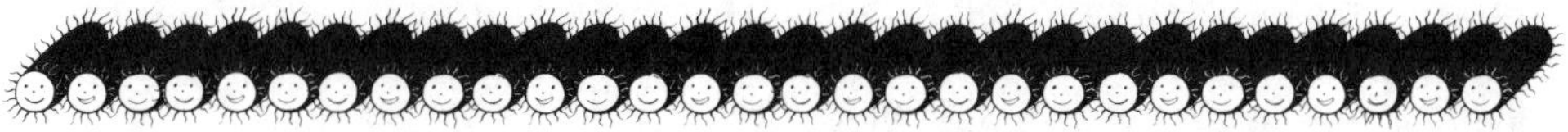

87% OF ALL MICROBES ARE BENEFICIAL OR HARMLESS

10% ARE OPPORTUNISTIC

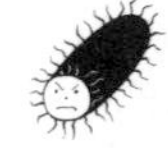

3% ARE PATHOGENIC

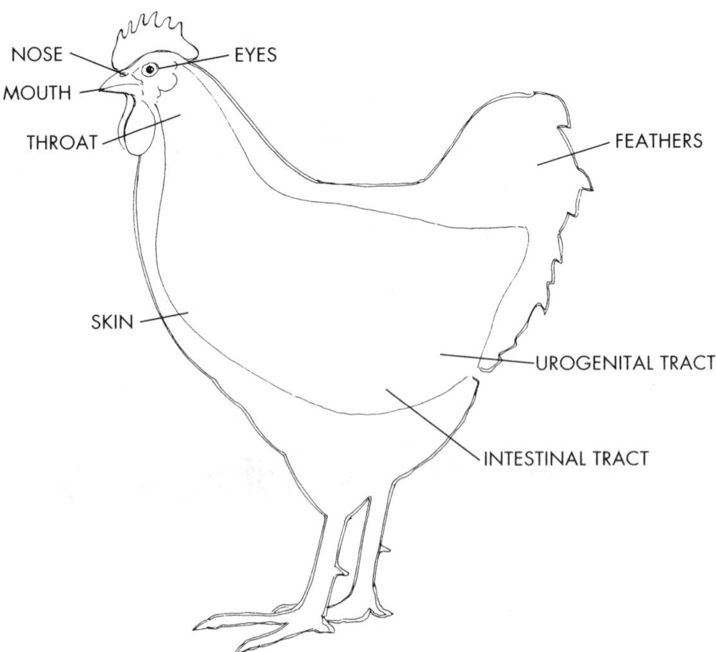

Where normal microflora reside

Bacterial Diseases

Bacteria are single-celled microbes that are abundant in the soil, water, and air. They were first discovered in the 17th century, when the microscope was invented. Some can move only on air or water currents; others (like salmonella) have tails that let them swim through liquids.

Some bacteria multiply by producing spores (individual cells encased within a tough membrane). Others multiply by dividing themselves in half; under ideal conditions, they multiply so rapidly that within hours, one bacterium becomes millions.

Pathogenic bacteria enter the body through the digestive system, respiratory system, or cuts and wounds. If they settle in an organ or tissue, the infection becomes chronic or long term. If they travel throughout the body by means of the bloodstream (a condition called "septicemia"), the infection is acute or short term, often ending in death.

Bacteria produce diseases in two ways: by causing mechanical damage to the body and by generating toxins that poison the body. Some bacterial diseases are caused by damage, some by poisoning, and some by both.

Most bacterial diseases share one or more of these four properties: they produce carriers; they are transmitted from breeders to chicks through hatch-

Bacterial Shapes

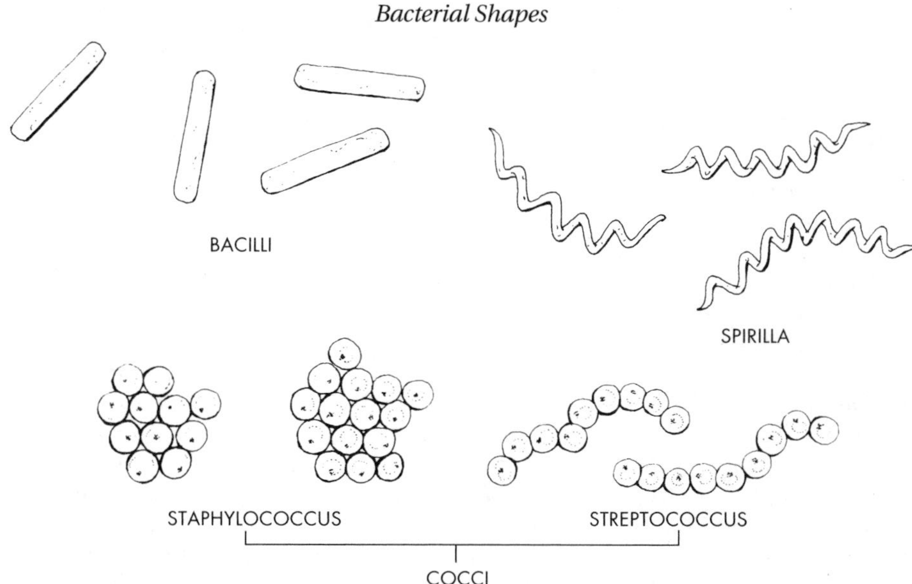

ing eggs; they are spread by rodents and wild birds; they survive for a long time in poultry housing. Owners of commercial flocks control bacteria by periodically depopulating their housing and thoroughly disinfecting before bringing in new, clean stock (all-in, all-out management).

Bacteria are divided into four related groups according to their shapes, visible by magnifying them 1,000 times under a microscope. The major ones that are harmful to chickens fall into three categories:

- rod-shaped, called "bacilli," such as the organisms that cause colibacillosis, clostridial diseases, erysipelas, infectious coryza, listeriosis, cholera, pseudomonas, salmonellosis, and tuberculosis;
- round, called "cocci," such as the organisms that cause chlamydiosis, staphylococcosis, streptococcosis, and mycoplasmosis (although mycoplasmas are unique in their ability to change shape);
- spiral, called "spirilla," such as the organisms that cause campylobacteriosis and spirochetosis.

Campylobacteriosis

Campylobacteriosis is an intestinal disease that infects a wide range of animals including dogs, humans, and especially chickens. Poultry experts estimate that 90 percent of all commercial broilers are infected.

Several species of *Campylobacter* cause the disease. The species most likely to affect chickens, as well as humans, is *C. jejuni.* Campylobacters are

CHART 7-1

Bacterial Diseases

Disease	*Cause*	*Prevalence*
Campylobacteriosis	*Campylobacter jejuni*	common
Chlamydiosis	*Chlamydia psittaci*	very rare
Clostridial diseases		
Botulism	*Clostridum botulinum*	rare
Necrotic dermatitis	*C. septicum*	rare
Necrotic enteritis	*C. perfringens*	rare
Ulcerative enteritis	*C. colinum*	common
Colibacillosis	*Escherichia coli*	common
Air-sac disease	*E. coli* and other bacteria	common
Chronic respiratory disease	*E. coli*	common
Omphalitis	*E. coli*	common
Swollen head syndrome	*E. coli*	rare
Coryza, infectious	*Haemophilus paragallinarum*	common
Erysipelas	*Erysipelothrix rhusiopathiae*	rare
Listeriosis	*Listeria monocytogenes*	very rare
Mycoplasmosis		
Air-sac disease	*Mycoplasma gallisepticum* and other bacteria	common
Chronic respiratory disease	*M. gallisepticum* and other bacteria	common
Pasteurellosis		
Cholera, (acute)	*Pasteurella multocida*	common
Cholera, (chronic)	*P. multocida*	not common
Pseudomonas		very rare
Salmonellosis		
Arizonosis	*Salmonella arizonae*	rare
Paratyphoid	*S. heidelberg* *S. enteriditis* *S. typhimurium* and other spp	very common
Pullorum	*S. pullorum*	rare
Typhoid	*S. gallinarum*	rare
Spirochetosis	*Borrelia anserina*	rare
Staphylococcosis		
Arthritis, staphylococcic	*Staphylococcus aureus*	common
Bumblefoot	*S. aureus*	common
Omphalitis	*S. aureus* and other bacteria	common
Streptococcosis	*Streptococcus zooepidemicus*	not common
Omphalitis	*Streptococcus faecalis* and other bacteria	common
Synovitis, infectious	*M. synoviae*	not common
Tuberculosis	*Mycobacterium avium*	fairly common

spread among chickens through infectious droppings in feed and water. The main symptoms are depression and watery, mucousy, or bloody diarrhea.

No effective way has been found to treat an infected flock. Campylobacters are, however, particularly sensitive to drying and can be eliminated from housing by thoroughly cleaning and disinfecting, followed by leaving the coop empty for at least a week before introducing new birds.

Clostridial Diseases

Clostridial diseases result from toxins produced by bacteria in the *Clostridium* group. Some clostridial bacteria do not cause disease unless a chicken's resistance has first been reduced by coccidiosis or by an illness (such as infectious bursal disease) that damages the immune system.

Clostridium colinum causes ulcerative enteritis, a short-term intestinal disease spread by infectious droppings in litter, feed, and water. The disease is known as "quail disease" because it was first identified in quail, the most susceptible of all avian species. The bacteria are able to survive under a variety of conditions, so once an outbreak occurs, housing is permanently contaminated. Control then involves replacing litter between flocks or keeping your birds on wire. Ulcerative enteritis may be avoided by taking care not to bring a carrier into your flock.

Clostridium septicum is commonly found in soil and in the intestines of chickens. It usually causes infection in combination with other bacteria, often after the chicken's immunity has been reduced by some other illness, especially infectious bursal disease. Alone or in combination, the bacteria cause necrotic dermatitis, characterized by patches of dead skin and/or sudden death. Necrotic dermatitis can easily be avoided through good management and proper sanitation.

Clostridium perfringens is commonly found in air, soil, water, and feces. The bacteria generate a potent toxin that causes necrotic enteritis in young and growing birds raised intensively on litter. The disease appears suddenly (often after a change in feed) and progresses rapidly, causing deaths within a few hours, sometimes without symptoms. It is easy to treat with antibiotics and easy to avoid through good management.

Clostridium botulinum, bacteria that commonly live in the intestines of chickens, are not themselves pathogenic. When they multiply in the carcasses of dead animals or in rotting solid vegetables such as cabbages, they generate some of the world's most potent toxins. Birds become poisoned after pecking at rotting organic matter or after drinking water into which it has fallen.

A poisoned bird gradually becomes paralyzed from the feet up. Initially the bird sits around or limps if you make it move. As paralysis progresses through its body, its wings droop and its neck goes limp (giving the disease its common name, "limberneck"). By the time the eyelids are paralyzed, the bird looks dead, but it continues to live until either its heart or its respiratory system becomes paralyzed.

If the bird isn't too far gone, you might bring it around with antitoxin (from a veterinarian) or by squirting cool water and an epsom salt solution into its crop (see "Flushes," page 192). Botulism is another disease that can easily be avoided through good sanitation.

Colibacillosis

Colibacillosis is a group of infectious diseases caused by one or more strains of *Escherichia coli,* the so-called "coliform" bacteria commonly found in the environment worldwide. Many strains, including some that normally live within chickens, do not cause disease. Other strains are opportunistic.

The illnesses caused by *E. coli* are varied and often complex. The bacteria may infect alone or may combine with or follow other diseases, especially chronic respiratory disease, infectious bronchitis, infectious synovitis, and Newcastle. A bird's susceptibility to coliform invasion is increased by stress and by damage to its respiratory system caused by ammonia fumes or dust.

Coliform infections range from severe and acute to mild and chronic. The susceptibility of chickens varies with the bird's strain and age — infection is more common in young birds than in older ones. The bacteria are transmitted through the shells of hatching eggs, causing dead embryos or chicks with infected navels (omphalitis). In the brooder, *E. coli* bacteria spread rapidly by means of infected droppings picked from litter, feed, or water.

The bacteria enter a chicken by way of either the digestive or the respiratory system but may eventually settle in the bird's eye, heart, liver, navel, oviduct, leg joints, or wing joints. They may get into the bloodstream, causing acute septicemia and the sudden death of an apparently healthy bird.

Coliform bacteria survive for long periods in dry litter and dust and are spread through the droppings of infected rodents and chickens. Respiratory colibacillosis can be prevented by minimizing stress, providing good ventilation, and keeping chickens free of mycoplasmal and viral infections. Intestinal colibacillosis is more difficult to avoid but can be minimized by controlling rodents and keeping feed and drinking water free of chicken droppings.

Coryza

Infectious coryza is a respiratory disease caused by *Haemophilus paragallinarum* bacteria that are prevalent in the southeastern United States and in California. The disease can be difficult to recognize because it resembles other respiratory diseases and often occurs in combination with them. Its chief symptoms are swelling of the face and, in chronic cases, the unmistakable odor of nasal discharge.

Infectious coryza is spread mainly through contact with carrier birds, which include all survivors of the disease and other birds in the same flock, even though they may never have had symptoms. The disease is easily introduced by unknowingly bringing growing or mature carriers into an established flock. A vaccine is available, but should be used only to prevent future outbreaks once Infectious coryza has been diagnosed in your flock.

The only way you can get rid of infectious coryza is by disposing of the infected flock, disinfecting the premises, and leaving housing vacant for at least 3 weeks before introducing new birds. Infectious coryza is not transmitted through hatching eggs, making it possible to start a new flock by incubating eggs from infected breeders, provided you take great care to raise the chicks in an uncontaminated environment.

Erysipelas

Erysipelas, caused by *Erysipelothrix rhusiopathiae* bacteria, is rare in chickens. It is significant as a disease chickens share with many other birds and animals, notably turkeys, pigs, sheep, and humans.

Bacteria shed in the droppings of infected birds or other animals survive for years in alkaline soil. Chickens on range that previously held infected turkeys, sheep, or pigs may become infected through open wounds that result from fighting, cannibalism, or dubbing. The disease is most likely to occur among cockerels on free range — cockerels, because they commonly wound each other in peck-order fights; free range, because it provides contact with potentially contaminated soil.

The most startling symptom is the sudden death of apparently healthy cockerels, while birds in nearby flocks (on uncontaminated soil) thrive. Since survivors continue to shed bacteria, and since this disease poses a health risk to humans, the only sensible approach is to dispose of an infected flock and start a new flock on fresh ground. Erysipelas is not transmitted through hatching eggs, making it possible to start a new flock by hatching eggs from infected breeders, provided you keep the new birds away from contaminated ground.

Mycoplasmosis

Mycoplasmosis encompasses any disease caused by mycoplasma bacteria, the smallest living organisms capable of free existence. A mycoplasma is about the same size as a virus, but (unlike a virus) can multiply outside a living cell. The two important mycoplasmas affecting chickens are *Mycoplasma synoviae,* which causes air-sac disease in young birds and infectious synovitis in all ages, and *M. gallisepticum,* which causes air-sac disease in young birds and chronic respiratory disease in growing and mature birds.

Diseases caused by mycoplasmas can be difficult to recognize without laboratory work, since they often occur in combination with other bacteria and with viruses. They are spread from infected breeders through hatching eggs and by direct contact with infected or carrier birds. Survivors become immune to future infection but remain carriers. The bacteria cannot survive long away from a bird's body.

At one time, all chickens carried mycoplasma and became infectious in response to stress. Today, mycoplasma-free strains are available among the commercial breeds. The bacteria threaten primarily commercial operations with high concentrations of large flocks in relatively confined geographic areas. The farther your flock is from an infected flock, the lower its risk of exposure.

Chlamydiosis

Chlamydia psittaci, a bacteria-like organism, affects all species of birds. It is like a virus in that it multiplies only within the cell of another life form, but otherwise it behaves like a bacteria and can be treated with antibacterial drugs. It produces an infection commonly known as "psittacosis" or "parrot fever" because it was first identified in psittacine birds (parrots). Outbreaks are cyclical and, among poultry, are more common in turkeys than in chickens, which are naturally resistant. Chlamydiosis is significant because it infects humans as well as birds.

Salmonellosis

The genus *Salmonella* contains over 2,000 different species. Although they all have the potential of causing disease in chickens, only about a dozen cause 70 percent of the salmonella outbreaks. Evidence suggests that 75 percent of all chickens are infected with one or more kinds of salmonellae at some time in their lives.

These bacteria create a serious problem for poultry keepers because chickens that appear perfectly healthy are often carriers. Symptoms may be triggered at any time by stress due to crowding, molting, feed deprivation, drug treatment, or simply being transported.

The bacteria are transmitted by carriers to their offspring through hatching eggs (a process called "transovarian" transmission) in one of two ways:

- the yolk is infected as the egg is being formed in the body of an infected hen;
- the shell is contaminated as the egg is being laid or when it lands in a

dirty nest; the bacteria then penetrate the shell (most likely because the shell gets cracked or wet) and multiply within the egg.

An infected embryo may die in the shell toward the end of incubation or may hatch into an infected chick. The disease spreads to healthy chicks or chickens that come into contact with infected chickens or other infected animals (including humans). It spreads by means of contaminated droppings in litter, drinking water, and damp soil around waterers. It is spread mechanically by flies, rodents, wild birds, used equipment, shoes, truck tires, and the like. Salmonellae may also be present in rations containing contaminated livestock by-products.

Salmonellae generally enter a bird's body by way of mouth. They cause inflammation of the intestines, or Ulcerative enteritis, and so are often referred to as "enteric" bacteria. Acute Ulcerative enteritis is indicated by watery diarrhea, sometimes smelling bad or containing blood. Symptoms of chronic Ulcerative enteritis are emaciation and persistent diarrhea, which may appear mucousy or bloody. If the disease becomes septicemic, the bird's head, comb, and wattles turn dark and purplish.

Salmonella bacteria are divided into four groups with symptoms so similar that laboratory identification is required to tell them apart.

1. *S. pullorum* causes pullorum, a disease that affects only poultry, primarily chickens. Because it is always associated with diarrhea topped with white urates, it was once called "white diarrhea." Pullorum is spread by infected breeders through hatching eggs, causing death to embryos in the shell or to chicks soon after they hatch. Since some states require exhibition birds to be blood tested, a home-testing kit is now available. Local laws may require you to pass an examination in order to test your own flock.

2. *S. gallinarum* causes typhoid that is also specific to poultry, primarily chickens. Like pullorum, typhoid is rare in North America.

3. Paratyphoid infection (*para* meaning resembles) is caused by over 150 different species of salmonellae that invade a large number of animal species. Paratyphoid is the most important bacterial disease in the hatching industry, since it causes deaths among chicks and stunts survivors. This group is also important in the meat and egg industry, since it is responsible for causing food poisoning in humans. The most common paratyphoid strains in chickens are *S. heidelberg* and *S. typhimurium;* at present, the most serious to humans is *S. enteriditis.*

4. *S. arizonae,* like the paratyphoid group, infects a large number of animal species. These salmonellae cause avian arizonosis, mainly among turkeys. Rarely do chickens get the disease, which is similar in appearance and treatment to paratyphoid.

Controlling Salmonellae

Salmonellae readily survive and multiply in the environment, making their control difficult. They survive for years in infected droppings, feathers, dust, and hatchery fluff, and for almost a year in garden soil fertilized with infected droppings. The bacteria cannot survive long at 140°F (60°C), a temperature well below that of heating compost. The bacteria thrive in fresh litter, but cannot live long in built-up litter, due to the high pH of ammonia.

Antibiotics can be used to control a salmonella outbreak, but culling is preferable to treatment for at least three reasons:

- antibiotics alter intestinal microflora, interfering with recovery;
- the use of antibiotics causes antibiotic-resistant strains of bacteria to develop;
- survivors are carriers and continue to spread the disease.

In 1935, the National Poultry Improvement Plan (NPIP) was organized to standardize pullorum blood-testing and eliminate reactors from breeding flocks. Later, tests for other salmonelloses were added to the program. Approximately two-thirds of the states are now classified as "Pullorum-Typhoid Clean." Information on NPIP, which publishes a directory of pullorum-free breeding flocks, appears in the appendix.

Avoid salmonellosis by purchasing birds from disease-free flocks and purchasing rations that do not contain slaughterhouse wastes. Keep feed and water free of droppings. Minimize stress. Clean and disinfect facilities between flocks; clean and disinfect incubators and brooders between hatches. If an outbreak occurs, cull heavily. Remember, survivors are carriers — you'll never get rid of salmonellae unless you get rid of the carriers.

Spirochetosis

Spirochetosis is rare in North America, although the tick that carries it is quite common in the Southwest. Symptoms include yellowish-green diarrhea containing large amounts of white urates, and a high rate of deaths. Control the disease by controlling fowl ticks and by keeping susceptible birds away from birds that are immune carriers due to exposure to fowl ticks.

Staphylococcosis

Staphylococcus aureus bacteria commonly live on a chicken's skin or mucous membranes. Normally they increase the bird's resistance to other infections, but will themselves cause infection if they get into the body through a break in the skin. Procedures such as dubbing, cropping, debeaking, and toe clipping open the way to a staph infection.

Staph bacteria are the most likely cause of infection in feet (bumblefoot), joints (arthritis), and breast blisters. Newly hatched chicks become infected through open navels (omphalitis). If a chicken's immune system has been permanently damaged by infectious bursal disease or Marek's disease, staph may get into the bloodstream, causing sudden death. Laying hens in hot weather are particularly susceptible. Ironically, mild stress increases a chicken's resistance to staph infections.

Streptococcosis

Streptococcus bacteria normally live within the intestines of chickens, infecting birds only if their resistance is low — usually due to infection by some other disease. *S. faecalis* is one of the causes of omphalitis, in which embryos die in the shell and chicks die soon after hatching. *S. zooepidemicus* can cause sudden death in mature birds. *S. equisimilis* causes wounds to fill with pus. Avoid strep infections by minimizing stress and practicing good sanitation.

Pasteurellosis

Pasteurellosis is a group of illnesses caused by 125 species of pasteurella bacteria. The only significant disease of chickens in this group is cholera, caused by *Pasteurella multocida,* a bacterium that both causes damage and generates toxins.

Fowl cholera can be either acute or chronic. Although the two forms are quite different, symptoms may overlap, since survivors of the acute form often become chronic. Mature chickens are more susceptible than young ones.

P. multocida bacteria survive at least 1 month in droppings, 3 months in decaying dead birds, and 2 to 3 months in moist soil. They are spread primarily through mucus discharged from the mouth, nose, and eyes of infected birds (including wild species), wild animals (rodents, raccoons, opossums), livestock (particularly pigs), pets, and humans. They may be eaten in contaminated feed or water and may be spread on contaminated equipment and shoes. They are not transmitted through hatching eggs.

Antibiotic treatment sometimes reduces the rate of death, but the disease usually returns when medication is withdrawn. At one time, cholera was very common. Today it is controlled through good management, which entails not bringing in older birds that might be carriers and not mixing birds of different ages.

Tuberculosis

Avian tuberculosis, one of the first poultry diseases ever investigated, is caused by *Mycobacterium avium,* bacteria that infect all species of birds, but more often chickens and captive exotic birds than other domestic poultry or wild species. The bacteria also infect pigs and rabbits, and to some extent people (although a different bacterium is usually responsible for human TB).

Avian tuberculosis is more likely to be found in the northcentral states than in the West or South. It spreads through contact with the droppings of infected birds. The bacteria survive in soil for up to 4 years. The concentration of bacteria in soil depends on how long infected birds have been housed there and on how crowded they are.

Since the disease requires a long period of exposure to get established, it affects primarily older birds. Symptoms are not dramatic. An infected chicken is less active than usual and gradually loses weight, even though it continues to eat well. Eventually its breast muscles shrivel, causing its keel to stick out. It may live for months or years, depending on how extensively the disease invades its body.

Prevention entails replacing each year's breeding or laying flock with young birds, keeping birds away from housing or range that formerly held an infected flock, not mixing birds of different ages, and preventing chickens from picking in their droppings.

The disease may be controlled by blood-testing or skin-testing a flock and removing positive reactors. If just one infected bird is overlooked, however, the disease will continue to spread. Since contaminated premises are difficult to decontaminate, the best approach is to dispose of an infected flock and establish a new flock in a new environment.

Uncommon Bacterial Diseases

Some bacteria commonly found in the poultry environment infect chickens only if their resistance has been reduced by some other disease or condition. Once chickens become infected, the bacteria multiply within the birds' bodies, become more numerous in the environment, and continue to cause disease. Among these opportunistic infections are two that are significant in their ability to infect humans as well as chickens.

Listeria monocytogenes bacteria are common in the soil and intestines of birds and other animals living in temperate climates. They cause listeriosis, a disease to which most chickens are resistant. The bacteria primarily infect a chicken's heart and brain (encephalitic form), but may get into the bloodstream (septicemic form) and cause death.

Pseudomonas aeruginosa bacteria live in soil, water, and other humid environments. Infection may occur in chickens treated with a vaccine or antibiotic that has been handled in an unhygienic manner. Pseudomonas spreads from breeders to chicks through hatching eggs, causing death to chicks during late incubation or early hatch.

Viral Diseases

Compared to bacteria, viruses are simpler in structure and are much smaller. They are, in fact, the smallest pathogens known — so tiny they can be seen only through a microscope that magnifies them to 100,000 times. Like bacteria, not all viruses cause disease and the diseases they do cause range from mild to fatal.

Viruses differ from bacteria in being more host specific. They are more difficult to control than bacteria because they

- break down the defenses of a healthy bird,
- do not respond readily to drugs,
- survive well in nature,
- are readily transmitted from one location to another.

Since they are so small, millions of viruses can travel on one speck of dust. Just think how many can be carried on the hair of a fly, a rat's foot, a feather, the sole of a man's shoe, or a used chicken crate.

Outside the cells of another living organism, a virus has no life — it neither breathes nor eats. Its only known activity is to take over the cell of another life form for the purpose of making copies of itself.

Pathogenic viruses usually get into a chicken's body by being inhaled or swallowed, but they may also enter through an eye or a wound (including an injection puncture). Sometimes viruses invade a cell and hide there for months or years before becoming active. Sometimes they take over cells near their point of entry, causing a skin disease such as pox. Other times they travel to another preferred site, most often the respiratory system (infectious bronchitis) or the nervous system (Marek's disease). Sometimes they travel through the bird's body, producing plague-like infections such as exotic Newcastle disease and lethal forms of avian influenza.

Viruses cause disease in five ways, by

- disrupting or destroying cells;
- invading or disrupting the immune system;
- activating the immune system, causing fatigue or fever;
- triggering development of antibodies that lead to inflammation or tissue damage;
- interacting with chromosomes to cause a tumor.

Usually when a bird is attacked by a virus, its immune system mobilizes to fight off the virus, which may take a few days to a few weeks. In the process, the bird's body becomes sensitized to the virus, and it is thereafter immune to the disease caused by that virus. The bird may, however, continue to shed the virus and infect birds that haven't yet been exposed.

CHART 7-2

Viruses Infecting Chickens

*Virus Family**	*Chicken Disease*	*Prevalence*
Adenovirus 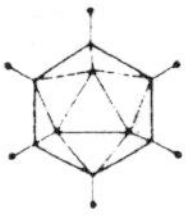	infectious anemia egg drop syndrome	rare very rare
Birnavirus 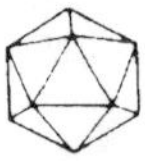	infectious bursal disease	common
Coronavirus 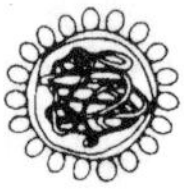	infectious bronchitis	common
Herpesvirus 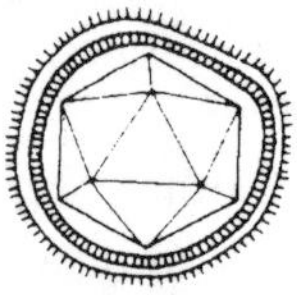	infectious laryngotracheitis Marek's disease	common very common
Orthomyxovirus 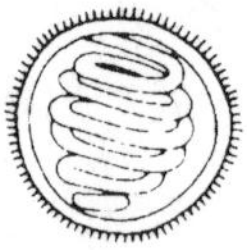	influenza	rare
Paramyxovirus 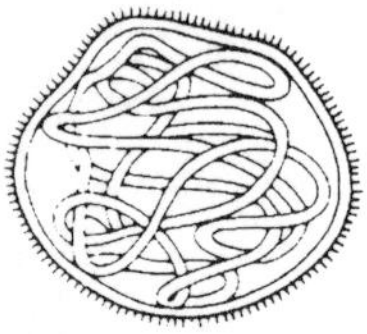	Newcastle disease (mild) Newcastle disease (exotic)	common very rare
Picornavirus	epidemic tremor	rare
Poxvirus 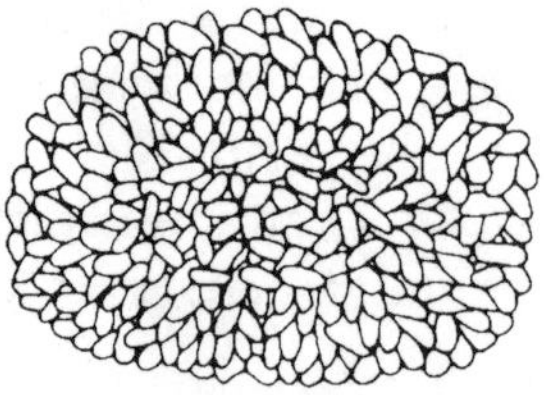	pox	common

Virus Family	Chicken Disease	Prevalence
Reovirus	arthritis	rare
	infectious stunting syndrome	rare
Retrovirus	lymphoid leukosis	common
	osteopetrosis	common
	runting syndrome	very rare
Rotavirus	rotaviral enteritis	common

* Illustrations are drawn to scale.

Some viruses, on the other hand, attack so fast the bird's body cannot respond before serious damage or death occurs. Other viruses weaken the immune system, leaving the bird open to attack by an opportunistic or secondary infection (which may cause the bird's death). If a chicken has a viral infection when it is vaccinated against some other disease, the virus may interfere with the vaccine's ability to trigger immunity.

Viruses are classified into families according to their size and shape. Each family includes numerous members, and new families are constantly being discovered.

Adenovirus Syndromes

Viruses in the adenovirus family are not yet well understood. They apparently cause a variety of infections, often in combination with other organisms. They may be the cause of infectious anemia, a fatal disease of broiler chicks intensively raised on used litter. The viruses enter a chicken's body through the digestive system and spread slowly by means of contaminated body discharges, especially droppings. Their main method of transmission is through hatching eggs laid by infected hens or placed in contaminated cartons. Iodine disinfectant slows the spread of disease. Chicks are protected by maternal antibodies for their first 2 or 3 weeks of life.

Egg drop syndrome is caused by a waterfowl adenovirus introduced to chickens either through vaccine derived from infected duck eggs or through contact with infected waterfowl or drinking water contaminated by them. The virus remains quiet and undetected until hens approach their peak of production. Eggs laid by infected hens may have thin gritty shells, soft shells, or no shells. The first sign in brown-egg layers is pale eggs. Although the virus has been found in numerous ducks and geese in North America, and has infected chickens elsewhere, so far no chickens have experienced egg drop syndrome in North America.

Arthritis

Viral arthritis, caused by the avian reovirus, is quite similar in appearance to infectious synovitis caused by mycoplasma bacteria. The main symptoms are swollen hocks and lameness, primarily in intensively raised broilers 4 to 8 weeks old. Aside from vaccination, the only known way to prevent viral arthritis is to avoid overcrowding.

Bronchitis

Infectious bronchitis, the most contagious disease of chickens, is a respiratory illness caused by a coronavirus and characterized by coughing, sneezing, and rattling sounds in the throat. It starts suddenly, spreads rapidly, and can travel through the air to a second flock more than 1,000 yards away. Deaths occur primarily in chicks. Pullets that survive may have permanent ovary damage and may not lay eggs as mature hens.

Vaccination is not foolproof, since it bestows immunity only against the strains contained in the vaccine, and new strains keep popping up. Survivors are carriers, so the only sure way to get rid of infectious bronchitis is to get rid of your flock, clean up, disinfect, and start over. Because the disease is not usually transmitted through hatching eggs, you can get clean chicks from an infected flock, but be sure to carefully clean up the environment and avoid introducing infected birds in the future.

Bursal Disease

Infectious bursal disease occurs when a birnavirus invades lymph tissue, particularly tissue of the cloacal bursa. The disease is sometimes called "Gumboro disease" because it was first studied in Gumboro, Delaware. It causes atrophy of the cloacal bursa, resulting in suppressed immunity and greater susceptibility to future infections, particularly colibacillosis and necrotic dermatitis. Another result of suppressed immunity is failure to develop an immune response to vaccines.

The disease appears suddenly, usually in large flocks of broilers, and involves most birds in the flock. The first symptoms are watery or whitish diarrhea that sticks to vent feathers, causing birds to pick at their own vents. Deaths, when they occur, peak within a week and survivors recover rapidly thereafter. A subsequent infection in the same housing may be so mild you don't notice it.

IBD virus is not egg-transmitted and survivors are not carriers, but the disease is highly contagious and difficult to get rid of in housing that once held an infected flock. Chicks exposed to the virus before they are 2 weeks old develop natural immunity. Vaccines are also available.

Viral Diarrhea

Enteritis, characterized by inflamed intestines and diarrhea, has many viral causes, some of which have yet to be discovered. Viral enteritis in chickens is becoming more common than ever, and can be divided into three main groups:

Bluecomb— cause unknown. The disease affects pullets just coming into production. It is similar to bluecomb in turkeys, caused by a coronavirus to which chickens are resistant.

Infectious stunting syndrome— cause unknown, but likely involves one or more reoviruses. This disease primarily infects intensively raised broilers.

Rotaviral enteritis— rotaviruses are common in the poultry environment and do not always cause disease. When infection does occur, massive amounts of new viruses are released in the droppings of infected birds, causing the disease to spread.

Avoid viral diarrhea through good sanitation and not crowding birds. Thoroughly clean up and disinfect between flocks, and don't reuse old litter.

Epidemic Tremor

Avian encephalomyelitis is a relatively rare infectious disease of chicks caused by a picornavirus. Its chief symptoms are loss of coordination and rapid trembling of the head and neck, giving the disease its common name, epidemic tremor. The disease is transmitted from breeders to chicks through hatching eggs. An adult outbreak is so mild it is likely to go unnoticed, lasts less than a month, and leaves birds immune without making them carriers. Survivors of a chick outbreak should be culled, since they rarely develop into good layers or breeders.

Influenza

Avian influenza was among the first diseases known to be caused by a virus. It is caused by several different orthomyxoviruses and comes in many forms, ranging from mild to rapidly fatal. Symptoms vary widely and may relate to respiration (coughing, sneezing), digestion (appetite loss, diarrhea), reproduction (reduced fertility, soft-shelled eggs), or nerves (twisted neck, wing paralysis). Sometimes the first symptom is numerous sudden deaths of apparently healthy birds.

In North America, outbreaks among chickens are rare and widely spread in both time and place: the disease appeared in Alabama in 1975, Minnesota in 1979, and (the worst case) in Pennsylvania in 1983-84. If avian influenza occurs in your area, stay away from infected flocks and their handlers until the infection is under control.

Laryngotracheitis

Infectious laryngotracheitis, or "laryngo," is a highly contagious respiratory disease caused by a virus in the herpes family. Its chief symptoms are moist respiratory sounds (gurgling, choking, rattling, whistling, or "cawing") and coughing up bloody mucus. In a serious case, a large percentage of birds die.

Vaccination keeps the disease from spreading, but causes birds to become carriers. Vaccinating therefore doesn't make sense unless laryngo is prevalent in your area. Vaccination is usually recommended for those who show or who regularly bring in adult birds, but since vaccinated birds are carriers, if you vaccinate, you run the risk of having your birds infect any unvaccinated birds they come into contact with. (In the old days, flocks were immunized by bringing in an infected bird — survivors of the ensuing infection became immune.)

The virus does not live long off birds and is not spread through hatching eggs. You can safely start a new flock from infected breeders if, and only if, you dispose of the old flock and carefully clean and disinfect housing before moving the young birds in.

Newcastle Disease

Newcastle disease gets its name from the British town of Newcastle-upon-Tyne, one of the first places where it was studied. The disease comes in many different forms, ranging from mild to devastating. Mild forms are quite common, not particularly serious, and can be controlled by vaccination where the virus is prevalent. Virulent or so-called "exotic" forms will infect even a properly vaccinated flock, but fortunately are relatively rare.

Vaccination in the face of an exotic outbreak slows the spread of disease and reduces the number of deaths, but won't keep birds from getting the disease. Furthermore, vaccinated survivors are likely to be carriers.

Exotic Newcastle is usually introduced by illegally imported cage birds that have not gone through official quarantine. It is spread by contaminated droppings on used equipment and the shoes of humans, and causes a rapid, high number of deaths. The disease can easily be confused with other serious respiratory infections.

Symptoms include a sharp drop in laying accompanied by breathing difficulties, soon followed by muscular tremors, twisted neck, and wing or leg paralysis, and sometimes watery, greenish diarrhea. If an exotic infection occurs in your area, stay away from infected birds and keep their handlers away from your flock until the outbreak has been controlled.

CHART 7-3

Forms of Newcastle Disease

Form	*Characteristic*	*Symptoms*	*Formal Name*
MILD:			
Beaudettes	affects all ages, mild respiratory infection	drop in laying, slight wheezing, few deaths	mesogenic Newcastle disease
Hitchner's	affects young birds, mild to serious respiratory infection	wheezing, some deaths	lentogenic Newcastle disease
enteric	mild intestinal infection	none	asymptomatic - enteric lentogenic Newcastle disease
EXOTIC:			
Beach's	affects all ages, acute, lethal, nervous & respiratory infection	appears suddenly, gasping & coughing, drop in laying, wing or leg paralysis, 100% affected, up to 50% adults die, up to 90% young die	neurotropic velogenic Newcastle disease
Doyle's	affects all ages, acute, lethal nervous, respiratory & intestinal infection	sudden death or listlessness, rapid breathing, drop in laying, watery greenish diarrhea, 100% affected, nearly 100% die, bloody digestive tract	viscerotropic velogenic Newcastle disease

Pox

Pox in chickens (not at all the same as chicken pox in humans) occurs when the pox virus gets into wounds caused by insect bites, dubbing, fighting, cannibalism, or injury on poorly designed equipment. Fowl pox appears in two forms: dry pox affecting the skin (cutaneous form) and wet pox affecting the upper respiratory tract (diphtheric form).

Dry pox causes clear or whitish bumps on the comb, wattles, and other unfeathered portions of the body. The bumps eventually come together to form scabs, fall off, and leave scars. Wet pox causes yellowish bumps in the mouth, throat, and windpipe, sometimes affecting the bird's ability to breathe so that it dies from suffocation. In either case, survivors recover in 4 to 5 weeks.

In pox-prone areas, disease may be controlled through vaccination and by controlling mites and mosquitoes.

Viral Tumors

Some viruses are nearly identical to the growth-promoting chromosomes in a chicken's cells, and have the ability to invade cells and modify those chromosomes. The resulting mutation induces the cells to multiply out of control, causing a tumor.

Tumors can occur in any part of a chicken's body. They may be benign (starting and developing in one place) or malignant (spreading to other parts of the body). External benign tumors may be removed surgically (assuming the bird is worth the cost); malignant tumors usually come back after surgery. Interior tumors, whether benign or malignant, are rarely discovered until after the bird dies.

In veterinary jargon, a tumor is called a neoplasm (from *neo* meaning new and *plasm* meaning shape). Miscellaneous viruses occasionally cause neoplasms in a hen's ovary or oviduct (most often in hens over one year old) or along the backs and thighs of broilers (appearing as crater-like ulcers that may clump together).

By far the most important tumors in chickens are in the avian leukosis complex, an interrelated group of viral diseases that affect few other birds (or animals) besides chickens and that fall into two categories based on their causes:

- Marek's disease, caused by six different herpesviruses that primarily affect the nerves of growing birds;
- the leukosis/sarcoma group (leukosis means "whitening," sarcoma being a malignant tumor), caused by retroviruses that primarily affect older birds.

Marek's Disease

The Marek's virus kills more chickens than any other disease. It's so common, you can safely assume your flock is infected, even if your chickens don't show any symptoms. Stress due to crowding, moving, or even the natural process of maturing can weaken a flock's immunity, causing an outbreak of the dormant virus. The virus attacks various parts of a chicken's body, resulting in an array of symptoms — droopy wing, paralyzed leg, head held low, twisted neck, blindness, sudden death.

CHART 7-4

Forms of Marek's Disease

Form	*Characteristics*
Cutaneous (skin form)	enlarged feather follicles
Neural (nerve form)	progressive paralysis weight loss anemia labored breathing diarrhea few or insignificant postmortem findings
Ocular (eye form)	graying, shrunken iris irregular-shaped pupil emaciation diarrhea blindness death
Visceral(internal organs)	tumors in ovary, heart, lung, and other organs

The virus is not transmitted by means of hatching eggs. In fact, a newly hatched chick is briefly protected if its dam transmits a high antibody level through her eggs. Chicks should be brooded away from adult birds, however, since the first few weeks of life are the most critical time for infection. Chicks that are isolated until the age of 5 months develop a natural immunity that helps them overcome exposure to Marek's virus as adults. Some chicken strains are genetically more resistant than others.

Turkeys carry a non-tumor-forming virus that prevents the Marek's virus from developing tumors. Chickens that are run with turkeys therefore develop some measure of immunity (although keeping the two together creates other problems, such as the possibility of the turkeys getting blackhead from the chickens).

Marek's vaccine for chicks is derived from the turkey virus, making it one vaccine that does not cause a mild case of disease in order for birds to build up antibodies. To become immune, chicks must be exposed to the turkey virus before they are exposed to Marek's virus. Vaccination should therefore occur as soon after hatch as possible and chicks should be isolated until immunity develops in about a week. A single vaccination confers lifelong immunity, but is not 100 percent foolproof — about 5 percent of all vaccinated chickens get the disease anyway.

Marek's disease in chickens has been used as a model for studying cancer in humans, and Marek's vaccine has become a model for developing a human cancer vaccine. There is no evidence, however, that the Marek's virus causes cancer in humans.

Leukosis

Like Marek's disease, the neoplasms in the leukosis/sarcoma group infect all chickens by the time they reach maturity. Rarely, however, do they cause disease.

The viruses in this group are most likely to cause lymphoid leukosis, occasionally osteopetrosis (thickening of the leg bones that affects primarily cockerels and cocks), only rarely erythroid leukosis (causing enlarged, bright red liver and spleen) or myeloid leukosis (causing chalky white internal tumors along the spinal column and beneath the keel). The latter two are so infrequent that they warrant only brief mention.

Lymphoid leukosis usually strikes chickens just reaching maturity. The symptoms are not particularly dramatic and are so similar to those of Marek's disease that the two are easily confused. Unlike Marek's disease, lymphoid leukosis cannot be prevented by vaccination.

CHART 7-5

Differences Between Lymphoid Leukosis and Marek's Disease

Characteristic	*Lymphoid Leukosis*	*Marek's Disease*
Incubation period	14 weeks	2 weeks
Earliest age	14 weeks	4 weeks
Usual age	over 6 months	under 6 months
Peak age	4 to 10 months	2 to 7 months
Peak age for deaths	24 to 40 weeks	10 to 20 weeks
Paralysis	no	yes
Eye tumors	no	possible
Skin tumors	rare	possible
Nerve tumors	no	yes
Liver tumors	yes	yes
Heart tumors	yes	yes
Intestinal tumors	yes	yes
Bursal tumors	yes	no
Muscle tumors	rare	possible

Runting Syndrome

Runting syndrome, like lymphoid leukosis, is caused by a retrovirus and can be easily mistaken for Marek's disease. The virus that causes runting syndrome seems to be more prevalent than the disease, but since it doesn't always produce symptoms, it's considered relatively rare and not much is known about it. In North America, it is most likely to occur in southeastern states, especially Florida, Mississippi, and North Carolina.

Fungal Diseases

Fungi are parasitic plants that lack chlorophyll and live on decaying organic matter. They include molds, mildews, yeasts, mushrooms, and toadstools. Of more than 100,000 different species, most are either beneficial or harmless. Two kinds of fungi cause disease — yeast-like and mold-like. They cause disease of four types:

- allergic reaction to inhaled spores in moldy litter;
- poisoning due to toxins released by fruiting bodies (i.e. poisonous mushrooms and toadstools);
- poisoning due to toxins generated through invasion of stored feed (e.g. aflatoxicosis or ergotism) — this type of poisoning is called "mycotoxicosis" (discussed on page 140);
- infection due to invasion of skin, lungs, or other body tissue (e.g. favus or thrush) — this type of infection is called a "mycotic disease" or a "mycosis."

Mycoses

Mycoses are grouped according to whether they are:

- superficial — affecting the skin or mucous membranes (e.g. favus);
- deep — affecting internal organs, usually the lungs (e.g. aspergillosis, dactylariosis, histoplasmosis, thrush). Deep infections are opportunistic, taking advantage of a chicken's low resistance due to stress or the presence of some other disease.

Fungal infections have gotten more common since the use of antibiotics became widespread, because antibiotics destroy normal body flora, making it easier for pathogenic fungi to take over. Still, mycoses are rare enough in chickens that methods for their control and treatment remain less advanced than those for bacterial and viral diseases.

Chart 7-6

Fungal Diseases

Disease	*Cause*	*Prevalence*
Aspergillosis	*Aspergillus* spp	rare
Dactylariosis	*Dactylaria gallopava*	very rare
Favus	*Microsporum gallinae*	rare
Histoplasmosis	*Histoplasma capsulatum*	very rare
Thrush	*Candida albicans*	common

Aspergillosis

Aspergillosis refers to any disease caused by the spores of *Aspergillus* spp fungus commonly found in the environment, especially in soil, grains, and decaying vegetative matter including litter. These molds are capable of infecting all birds, more commonly turkeys than chickens. They produce a form of pneumonia that is acute in chicks and chronic in mature birds.

Infection is rare in North America and may easily be prevented through good sanitation (especially in the incubator and brooder), avoiding moldy grain and litter, periodically moving feeders and waterers or placing them on droppings boards, providing good ventilation to minimize dust, and keeping stress to a minimum.

Thrush

Candida albicans causes thrush or candidiasis in many species of birds and animals, including humans. Thrush probably occurs among chickens more often than we know, since its symptoms are not particularly distinctive. Thrush is primarily a disease of chicks and growing birds. It can be prevented by controlling coccidiosis and by avoiding the overuse of antibiotics.

Rare Mycoses

Uncommon fungi that occasionally invade chickens include:

Microsporum gallinae that causes a superficial infection called "favus," in which the comb of a mature cock looks like it's been sprinkled with flour;

Dactylaria gallopava in moldy sawdust used as litter, causing a brain disease called "dactylariosis" that makes chicks tremble and walk in circles;

Histoplasma capsulatum, a fungus that causes histoplasmosis, a rare but potentially fatal disease chickens share with other birds and with humans living along the Mississippi, Missouri, and Ohio rivers.

Syndromes

A syndrome is a group of symptoms that occur in combination and appear as a particular disease. In most cases, the disease is poorly defined — its symptoms are not always the same and/or its cause is not yet known. These diseases are so poorly defined that one disease may have several names (malabsorption syndrome, pale bird syndrome, infectious stunting syndrome) or the same name may be applied to more than one disease (e.g. runting syndrome). The diseases in this group are described more fully in chapter 15:

- air-sac syndrome (air-sac disease)
- egg drop syndrome
- fatty liver syndrome
- infectious anemia
- infectious stunting syndrome
- runting syndrome
- star-gazing syndrome (epidemic tremor)
- sudden death syndrome
- swollen head syndrome

Diseases of Unknown Cause

Syndromes are not alone among diseases for which we've not yet found a cause, despite all our modern technology. The following conditions (described in chapter 15) have unknown causes:

- bluecomb
- broiler ascites
- crop impaction
- gout (visceral)
- round heart disease
- twisted leg

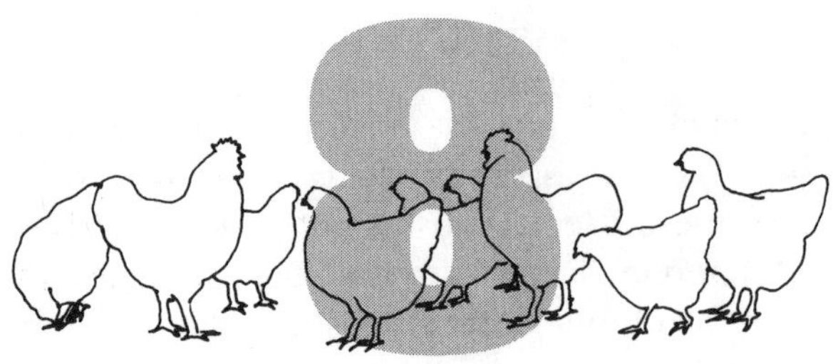

8 Environment-Related Problems

THE ENVIRONMENT CANNOT BE OVERLOOKED as a source of health problems for chickens. Extremely cold weather can lead to frostbite. Steamy weather can cause heat stress. Crowded conditions often lead to cannibalism. Unsafe chemicals or vegetation cause poisoning. Rodents spread diseases and, on occasion, attack chickens. Happily, each of these problems can be avoided through awareness and good management.

Frostbite

All chickens can tolerate quite a bit of cold weather, provided you see that their drinking water doesn't freeze and their housing is neither drafty nor damp. Draftiness removes warm air trapped by ruffled feathers. Moisture in the air makes chickens cold by absorbing body heat. Combs and wattles are therefore more likely to freeze in damp housing than in dry housing.

Since cocks don't sleep with their heads tucked under a wing, as hens do, cocks are more likely than hens to have their combs and wattles frozen when temperatures dip during the night. Cocks with large combs are more likely than others to be frostbitten.

Frozen combs and wattles look pale. If you discover the condition while

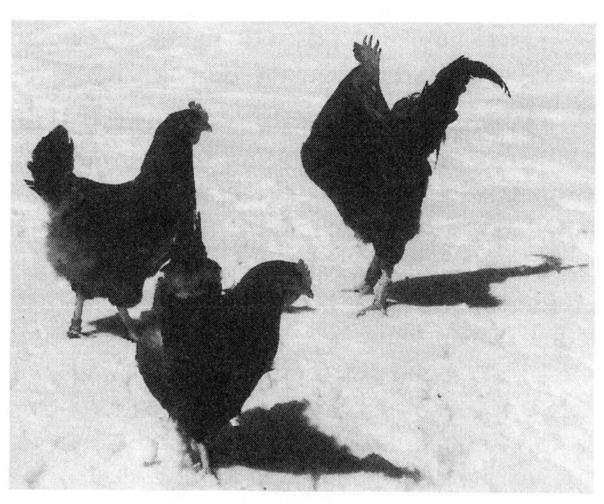

Heavily feathered birds like these New Hampshires adapt better to winter weather than lightly feathered birds.

the part is still frozen, apply a damp, warm cloth (105°F, 40.5°C) to the frozen part for 15 minutes or until it thaws. Do not rub. After the part has thawed, gently apply an antiseptic ointment such as Neosporin. Isolate the bird and keep an eye on it to see that the comb heals properly.

Frozen combs and wattles are more likely to be discovered after they have thawed and become red, hot, swollen, and painful. The bird doesn't feel like moving, is listless, and loses interest in eating. If the part has already thawed, warming it is no longer necessary. Gently coat the part with Neosporin and isolate the bird.

After the swelling goes down, the skin may peel, the part may itch, and it may be sensitive to cold for a while. It may turn scabby, develop pus, and eventually fall off. The suffering cock will continue to lose weight and may become infertile.

If the comb or wattles were seriously frozen, instead of swelling they may remain cold, begin to shrivel, and eventually die back. Other chickens may peck at the affected part, making matters worse.

If a comb or wattle turns black, the affected tissue has died and gangrene has set in — the comb or wattle is no longer receiving a blood supply and must be surgically removed.

Dubbing and Cropping

Surgical removal of the comb (dubbing) and wattles (cropping) is done for one of several reasons:

- to remove injured or infected tissue
- to keep combs and wattles from freezing
- to increase egg production and reduce feed costs

- to minimize blood loss in fighting cocks
- because show regulations require it

Modern and Old English game cocks must be dubbed and cropped in order to avoid disqualification from some shows (other breeds may be disqualified if they *are* dubbed or cropped). Fighting cocks are dubbed to minimize blood loss due to injuries. In cold climates, large-combed hens may be dubbed to minimize heat loss, thereby reducing feed costs and improving egg production; cocks are dubbed to avoid frostbitten combs and wattles that interfere with fertility.

Dubbing and cropping are stressful and should be avoided immediately before or after birds are vaccinated. Neither should breeders be dubbed before or during hatching season, or low fertility may result. Birds can be dubbed at any age after their combs and wattles develop, but those in the 8- to 12-week-old bracket bleed less than older birds.

Regardless of a bird's age, it can bleed to death as a result of improper dubbing. Feeding each bird a vitamin K tablet daily for 5 days preceding the operation aids clotting. The surgery is painful and should be done under veterinary supervision so an anesthetic can be used.

Use small tin snips or 6-inch (12 cm) curved surgical scissors, available from a medical supplier, and heat the instrument to destroy any bacteria that might be present. Snip off the comb ½ inch (1 cm) above the head. Cauterize the surface by searing it with a hot iron to minimize bleeding. If the wattles are to be cropped at the same time, snip them off and coat them with an astringent such as iron subsulfate.

To prevent infection, either inject ½ cc penicillin into the bird's breast muscle daily for 10 days or add 1 teaspoon (5 ml) tetracycline or bacitracin per gallon to the drinking water for 10 days. The comb and wattles should heal within 30 days.

Heat Stress

Lightly feathered breeds like Leghorns, Hamburgs, and Minorcas suffer less in warm weather than heavily feathered breeds like Brahmas, Cochins, Rocks, and Reds. Laying hens are more susceptible to heat stress than birds not in production. Closed nests make matters worse. Avoid using trapnests during hot weather. If hens must be trapnested, check nests frequently and release hens before they suffocate in the close confines of a too-hot nest. Outdoors, white birds are less subject to heat stroke than dark birds because they reflect sunlight better.

Any chicken's body operates most efficiently when the outside temperature is 70-75°F (21-24°C). Chickens cannot sweat to keep cool. Instead, they hold their wings away from their bodies and pant. Holding the wings away from the body exposes more skin surface under the wings, thereby increasing evaporation and radiational cooling. Panting releases heat through evaporation from the lungs.

A mature chicken starts panting when the temperature reaches 85°F (29.5°C). A chick pants when the temperature is 100°F (38°C) or more. Panting causes a chicken to exhale large quantities of carbon dioxide, which raises its blood pH. The resulting changes in physiology cause stress. The chicken stops eating and lays fewer and smaller eggs with thinner shells. A young bird stops growing.

When the temperature reaches 104°F (40°C), even panting is not enough and deaths may occur. Cool things down by increasing air circulation — open doors and windows or install a fan. Among the least expensive fans is a variable-speed paddle or Casablanca fan. Be sure the coop is properly vented so hot air doesn't get trapped against the ceiling.

Hosing down the outside walls and roof improves cooling through evaporation, as does occasionally misting or fogging chickens. Take care not to mist so much that water puddles on the floor. Mist only adult chickens and only when the temperature is above 95°F (35°C) and the humidity is below 75 percent. Cooling won't occur if the air is already so humid that no more water can evaporate. Mist only when the fan is running or air circulation is otherwise sufficient to dry the birds.

Chickens eat less when they're hot. To ensure adequate nutrition, feed only fresh rations. Chickens also drink more in hot weather so they can expel extra moisture in their droppings as an additional cooling mechanism (causing droppings to be looser in hot weather). Encourage drinking by supplying cool water and extra watering stations. If the water supply remains the same when a flock's water requirements go up, water deprivation may result (see "Dehydration," page 40).

Walking among your birds will encourage them to move, stimulating drinking, but don't disturb them at peak heat periods, which only increases stress. Symptoms of serious heat stress include drinking excessive amounts of water, labored breathing, and weakness. If a heat-stressed bird becomes prostrate, but is still alive, move it into the shade. Dunk it in cool water and use a plastic tube attached to a funnel to fill its crop with cool water. If the bird survives, it may remain weak for several days.

Cannibalism

Light, high-strung laying breeds, especially Leghorns and other Mediterraneans, are more likely to engage in cannibalism than the heavier American and Asiatic breeds. Within a breed, some strains are more cannibalistic than others. Birds of the same strain may be cannibalistic when raised in one place but not another, proving that you can discourage cannibalism by providing a proper environment.

The problem has many causes, often working in combination. Conditions that can trigger cannibalism include:

- heat without adequate ventilation
- nests not dark enough
- bright lights in the brooder house (lights on all night or sunlight coming through windows)
- crowding (especially in fast-growing chicks that quickly fill the available space and can't get away from each other)
- boredom or lack of exercise (more likely in caged or housed birds than in free-ranged flocks)
- feed and water troughs too few or too close together (failure to increase the number of feed and water stations as chicks grow)
- feed too high in calories and too low in fiber (chickens quickly satisfy their nutritional needs and get bored)
- external parasites (a chicken pulls out its own feathers, drawing blood that attracts other birds to pick)
- injury or bleeding (e.g. from an injured comb or a broken feather quill)

Toe Picking

Cannibalism often starts with toe picking, a common problem among chicks, especially those reared on paper to prevent litter eating. Toe picking can also occur in chicks brooded on wire — sharp wire edges cut their toes and the bleeding attracts toe pickers. Toe picking may start when chicks can't find anything else to eat because the feeder is poorly designed, is too high, is too far away, or is too small for the number of chicks involved.

To get chicks picking at feed instead of feet, sprinkle a little starter ration on paper, or place shallow containers of starter close to the heat source where the chicks can easily find it. If toes are injured from picking, light the brooder with a red light so chicks can't easily detect blood while the toes heal.

Head Picking

Head picking generally occurs in older birds, especially when combs or wattles bleed due to fighting or frostbite. Cocks or hens housed in adjoining cages may pick each other's heads, even if the birds have been debeaked. When possible, space cages far enough apart to prevent picking. Cardboard or paper feed sacks wedged between cages are not the answer, since a solid barrier reduces air circulation, causing caged birds to suffer in warm weather. Isolate any bleeding bird until the wound heals.

Feather Picking

Evidence of feather picking is dull, broken feathers and bare patches on a bird's neck, breast, back, and below the vent. Tail-feather picking is especially common in growing birds, when new feathers filled with blood attract pickers before enough plumage grows to cover the area. But it can start at any time, triggered by crowding, lack of exercise, irritation due to parasites, or low-protein diet and other nutritional deficiencies. Picked birds must continually grow new feathers, causing the same stress reactions associated with molting, including a drop in laying.

Feather loss doesn't necessarily indicate feather picking. Layers often have broken or missing feathers, especially on their necks and tails, rubbed off on feeders and nests. Mating cocks frequently wear the feathers off a hen's back. The annual molt also causes feather loss. Some birds drop and replace their feathers gradually, others lose many feathers at a time. During the molt, encourage feather growth and discourage feather picking by increasing dietary protein.

Vent Picking

Vent picking is the worst form of cannibalism because it escalates quickly and often ends in death. It can start if nests are too light, so that a hen's vent gets picked while she's laying. But it is most likely to occur among pullets just coming into lay, usually after one tears tissue or prolapses while passing an unusually large egg (see "Prolapsed Oviduct," page 53).

Egg Eating

Egg eating occurs when not enough nests are provided, nests are too light, housing is too light in general, or hens are crowded and bored. Egg eating is also encouraged by anything that causes egg breakage — eggs aren't collected often enough, have soft or thin shells, or become cracked due to insufficient nesting material. Once chickens find out how good eggs taste, they will break eggs on purpose to eat them.

A nutritional deficiency, especially vitamin D or calcium, can cause soft shells that lead to egg eating. A laying hen's calcium needs are increased by warm weather and by age. Appropriate nutritional supplements include free-choice feeding of limestone or ground oyster shell, or adding vitamin AD&E powder to drinking water three times a week.

Controlling Cannibalism

The first step in controlling cannibalism is to remove the injured bird. The next step is to try to identify and remove the picker. Cannibalism usually starts with just one bird, who teaches the bad habit to others. If you can't catch the instigator(s) in the act, look for blood or egg yolk on beaks and face feathers.

In the brooder, start heat at 95°F (35°C) and reduce it 5°F (3°C) per week. After the first week, turn off lights at night. Increase ventilation as birds grow and become more active, and when the weather turns warm.

At the first sign of cannibalism, smear red anti-pick solution on wounded birds and a few others, install red lights, and paint windows red or cover them with red plastic (imitation stained glass). Red lighting gives everything a rosy hue, making it more difficult for birds to identify bloody sores that encourage more picking.

Add oats, barley, or alfalfa to the ration so birds will have something to pick at. Salt and manganese are other nutritional additives that may help.

Alleviate boredom by feeding less at a time but feeding more often. Hang a bunch of greens or a shiny pie tin from the ceiling. Install swinging perches for bantams and light breeds to play on (but never for heavy breeds prone to foot injuries). Darken nests by tacking or stapling curtains in front, pinning up one edge for a few days until the hens learn to go behind the curtains.

High-strung birds may be fitted with "specs" or clip-on eyeshields that reduce their ability to accurately aim their beaks. The disadvantages to using specs are that they don't fit young birds and they are expensive for a large flock.

If all else fails, debeak.

Debeaking

Debeaking involves removing the tip of the upper portion of the beak. It is routine in commercial operations as a means of controlling cannibalism and reducing fighting among cocks. Debeaking does not inhibit a bird's ability to eat or drink, but it does disfigure the bird. For that reason, show birds should never be debeaked.

Some hatcheries offer debeaked chicks as an option. Electric debeakers are used by those who handle large numbers of chicks. On a small scale, birds can be debeaked at any age, but care must be taken to avoid damage to chicks. Regardless of a bird's age, improper debeaking can cause permanent injury.

Removing one-fifth of the upper beak of day-old chicks with nail clippers keeps cannibalism from getting started but is not permanent, as the beak will grow back within 6 weeks. Any beak will grow back if you trim too little the first time. If you remove too much from the upper beak, the lower beak may grow long and require occasional trimming.

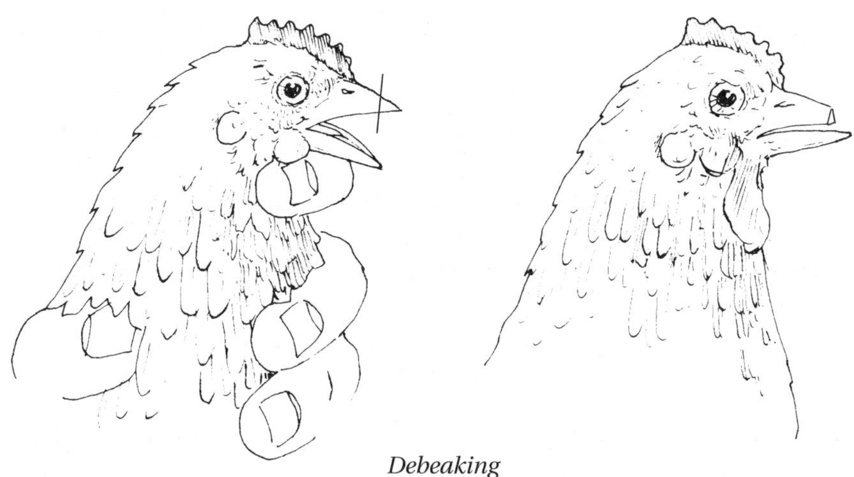

Debeaking

Small-scale debeaking may be done in one of three ways:

1. Use toenail clippers to remove one-third of the upper beak. Hold the bird's tongue away from the clippers by pressing it against the lower beak with a finger. Stop bleeding by cauterizing the cut with a styptic pencil or with heat. Take care: if you burn too little, bleeding will continue; if you burn too much, the beak will be sensitive or interfere with the bird's ability to eat and drink.

2. Use a hot instrument (livestock disbudding iron, hot-gun for gluing, vehicle cigarette lighter, etc.) to burn back one-third of the upper beak of a chick or ¼ inch from the upper beak of an adult bird. This method debeaks and cauterizes at the same time.

3. Use a knife to nick the upper beak of an adult bird ¼ inch from the end. With your thumb, hold the cut portion against the blade and roll the knife against the tip to tear the horny portion and expose the quick. This method causes little or no bleeding, but is only temporary as the beak will eventually grow back.

Poisoning

Poisoning is not often a problem in chickens, especially where common sense is used in keeping the flock away from pesticides, herbicides, rodenticides, fungicide-treated seed (intended for planting), wood preservatives, rock salt, and antifreeze.

Poisoning can result from misguided management, especially in an effort to repel lice and mites. Some people put mothballs in nests, for example, without knowing that naphthalene is toxic to chickens. Others use nicotine sulfate (Black Leaf-40) to paint roosts or treat individual birds, causing birds to become depressed and go into a coma, or to die suddenly of respiratory failure.

Toxic seeds are sometimes accidentally harvested along with feed grains. Such seeds include:

- coffee weed (*Cassia obtusefolia)* in corn and soybeans, causing a drop in egg production, diarrhea, paralysis, and death;
- gossypol in cottonseed meal, causing bluish combs and wattles, emaciation, low egg production, and low egg quality;
- crotalaria seeds and stems, causing bright yellowish-green droppings and inactivity;
- sorghum seed, causing depressed growth and leg deformity;
- rye seed, causing poor growth, pasting, soft bones, and lameness.

Other naturally occurring toxins in the environment cause selenium poisoning (see page 32), blue-green algae poisoning (see "Algae Poisoning," page 246), botulism (see "Clostridial Diseases," page 111), and mycotoxicosis.

Mycotoxicosis

Unlike infectious fungal diseases, which occur when fungi or their spores invade body tissue, fungal poisoning occurs when chickens consume toxic byproducts generated by mold growing in feed. A number of poisons or mycotoxins are produced by molds that grow naturally in grains, and some molds generate more than one kind of poison.

Aspergillus flavus, the same fungus that causes aspergillosis, also causes aflatoxicosis, a disease that increases a bird's susceptibility to heat stress and infection. In the United States, aflatoxins are the only feed-borne mycotoxins regulated by law.

Fusarium sporotrichioides, along with other species of *Fusarium,* causes fusariotoxicosis, a digestive disorder that interferes with egg production, growth, and feathering.

Claviceps purpurea produces a highly toxic alkaloid that causes ergotism, the oldest known mycotoxicosis. It is characterized by shriveled combs, sores on legs, convulsions, and death.

Aspergillus spp and other fungi generate ochratoxin, one of the most poisonous of all mycotoxins. The fungi that cause ochratoxicosis prefer high temperatures and so, in contrast to ergot and fusarium molds, they thrive in pelleted feed (which is manufactured under intense heat) unless it contains mold inhibitors.

All mycotoxicoses increase a chicken's need for vitamins, trace elements (especially selenium), and protein. Poisoning is difficult to identify and diagnose, in part because one feed source may contain more than one kind of mycotoxin. A positive diagnosis usually requires analysis of the feed to identify any fungi present. Since small-flock owners generally buy feed in small quantities, it's likely that a given batch will be used up before anyone thinks of analyzing it. Once the contaminated feed is removed, chickens usually recover.

Fungal poisoning can be avoided by using commercially prepared feeds containing mold inhibitors and by storing feeds away from humid conditions. Use plastic storage cans rather than metal ones, which generate moisture by sweating. Never give chickens feed that has gone moldy. If you buy moldy feed, take it back and insist on a refund.

CHART 8-1

Fungal Poisoning

Disease	*Caused By*	*Grain Source*
Aflatoxicosis	*Aspergillus flavus* and other fungi	all grains
Ergotism	*Claviceps purpurea*	wheat, rye, cereal grains
Fusariotoxicosis	*Fusarium sporotrichioides* and others	corn, wheat, barley, millet, safflower seed
Ochratoxicosis	*Aspergillus ochraceous* and other fungi	barley, corn, sorghum, wheat

Antifreeze Poisoning

Nearly all animals are attracted to ethylene-glycol because it tastes sweet and it doesn't freeze, thereby becoming the only "water" available to drink in cold weather. Poisoning is most likely to occur due to antifreeze spillage in fall, winter, and early spring. The lethal dose is 0.1 ounce per pound (8 ml/kg) of body weight, or about 3 tablespoons of antifreeze per mature chicken.

Antifreeze destroys a bird's liver and kidneys. The bird appears drowsy and uncoordinated, twists its head back, has trouble breathing, and has watery droppings. It ruffles its feathers, lies down, and dies. Few people would recognize antifreeze poisoning unless they actually saw the bird drinking antifreeze.

Chick Poisoning

Chicks are especially susceptible to certain toxins, including:

- carbon monoxide, from being transported in the poorly ventilated trunk of a car (chicks die);

Chart 8-2

Toxic Plants*

Common Name	*Botanical Name*	*Toxic Parts*	*Symptoms*
Castor bean	*Ricinus communis*	bean	diarrhea and progressive paralysis
Corn cockle	*Argrostemma githago*	seed	rough feathers, diarrhea, and slow growth
Daubentonia	*Daubentonia longifolia*	seed	diarrhea, staggering, droopy wing, and death
Death camas	*Zygadenus* spp	leaf, stem, and root	diarrhea, salivation, and muscular weakness
Glottidium	*Glottidium vesicarium*	seed	bluish comb and wattles, diarrhea, and prostration
Milkweed	*Asclepias* spp	leaves	incoordination, convulsions, and death
Nightshade	*Solanum nigrum*	immature berries	irregular movements, paralysis, and death
Oleander	*Nerium oleander*	all parts	weakness and diarrhea
Pokeberry	*Phytolacca americana*	berries	incoordination
Potato	*Solanum tuberosum*	green tubers	incoordination
		raw peels, and sprouts	prostration
Vetch	*Vicia* spp	pea	convulsions
Yew	*Taxus* spp	all parts	bluish combs and wattles, labored breathing, incoordination, and collapse

*Most toxic plants don't taste good and chickens won't normally eat them unless the birds are starving.

- disinfectant overuse, especially in a poorly ventilated brooder (chicks huddle with ruffled feathers);
- fungicide, eaten on coated seeds intended for planting (chicks rest on hocks or walk stiff-legged);
- pesticides, used to rid housing of insects (chicks die);
- rose chafers, occurring in late spring and early summer in eastern and central North America (chicks become drowsy, weak, and prostrate, go into convulsions, and die or recover within 24 hours);
- nitrofurazone, used to treat some bacterial diseases (chicks squawk loudly, move rapidly, fall forward);
- coccidiostats (nicarbazin, monensin, sulfaquinoxaline), added to water in warm weather, when chicks drink more and thereby obtain a toxic dosage.

Rodents

Rodents are attracted to chicken houses by feed in troughs, spilled grain, availability of water, and protection from the elements. They spread diseases on their feet and fur and through droppings left in troughs or grain bins. They are especially a problem where the floor is raised above dirt, providing a darkened airspace, and where wall cavities and trash piles offer nesting sites.

The most common rodents in chicken houses are:

- Norway rat (*Rattus norvegicus*)
- roof rat (*Rattus rattus alexandrinus*)
- house mouse (*Mus musculus*)

Don't assume that just because you rarely see rodents you don't have them. Rodent experts say that for every 1 you do see, 300 to 1,000 are hiding somewhere. Despite your best management efforts, always assume you have rodents. Wage a constant battle and increase your efforts if you spot any of these signs: holes through walls, tunnels (in soil, litter, or under floors), droppings around feed storage.

CHART 8-3

Rodent Droppings

Rodent	*Droppings*
Mouse	small, dark brown or black, rod-shaped
Rat	large, various colors, capsule-shaped

Rats

Rats start fires by gnawing through the tough insulation of electrical wires to keep their teeth filed down. They also attack chickens. If you find dead, chewed-up chicks, suspect rats.

Rats are active at night. If you see a rat in the daytime, you have a *bad* rat problem — the rats have overpopulated and the dominant ones are keeping the weaker ones away from feed, forcing them to eat during the day.

Feed loss is one of the worse consequences of an infestation. Eight rats eat 1 pound (2.2 kg) of feed each day. One pair of rats produces four to seven litters each year. Even though not all of the offspring reach breeding age, within a year one pair can easily become 1,500 rats.

Mice

Chickens are the natural enemies of mice, but the agile little rodents are good at scurrying away. Mice reproduce even faster than rats — each pair has five to eight litters per year. Mice are most active at dusk and dawn, but they feed all day long. It takes 305 mice to chow down on 1 pound (2.2 kg) of feed per day.

Rodent Control

Despite all our modern technology, we still haven't found a better mousetrap. The best way to discourage rodents is to make the chicken house unattractive to them. Since rats and mice shun open areas, keep the land around your coop clear of weeds and trash. If the floor is raised, make sure it's at least 1 foot (30 cm) above ground so rodents don't feel protected. Use hang-

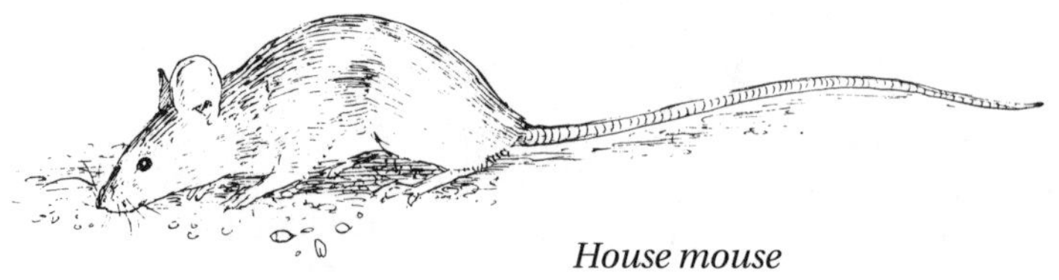

House mouse

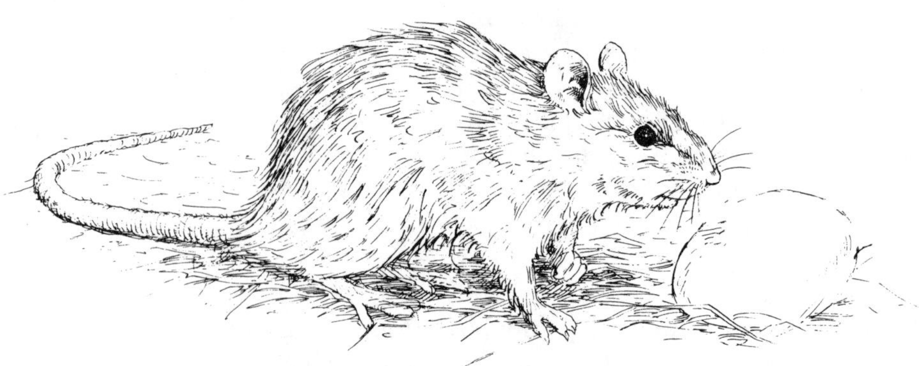

Norway rat

ing feeders that are difficult for rodents to reach, store feed in containers with tight-fitting lids, and avoid spillage.

Keep a cat. A cat's advantage for rodent patrol far outweighs any disadvantages it may have as a potential disease carrier.

If you have a serious rodent problem, set traps. Use spring traps, placed at right angles to the wall with the trigger and bait close to wall. Since mice run along sills, rafters, and other high places, set traps high as well as on the ground. As clichéd as it may sound, Swiss cheese is still the best trap bait.

Identify tunnels and fill them in. Place poisoned bait near tunnels that are reopened within a day or so (the unopened tunnels have become inactive). After a course of baiting (which varies with the type of bait you use), reclose the active tunnels. Rebait any that are opened again. Continue until tunnels are no longer reopened.

Rodent Bait

The most common rodent poison contains an anticoagulant that competes with vitamin K and thereby interferes with blood clotting. A multiple-dose anticoagulant must be eaten several times to be effective. A

Rodent bait station

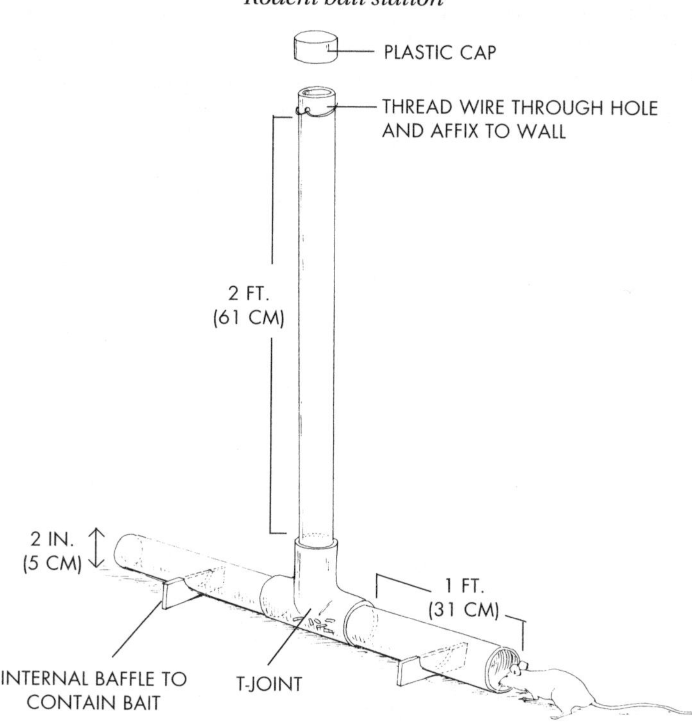

CHART 8-4

Rodenticides

Multiple-Dose	*Single-Dose*
Chlorophacinone	Brodifacoum
Diphacinone	Bromadiolon
Pival	Bromethalin*
Warfarin	Cholecalciferol

*Unlike other baits (which are relatively safe), Bromethalin affects the central nervous system and is fairly toxic to all animals.

single-dose anticoagulant kills after only one feeding.

Since a multiple-dose bait requires several days to take effect, be sure to put out enough bait to accomplish your purpose. Keep the bait out until no more is eaten. Multiple-dose bait is relatively safe for pets and other animals, since a single dose is ineffective.

Single-dose anticoagulants are also relatively safe for other animals, since a large dose is needed to be lethal to animals larger than a rodent. Even though single-dose anticoagulants require only one feeding, leave the bait out for at least 2 days to make sure all rodents consume some.

Not all baits are anticoagulants. Some contain vitamin D3, which causes death through an imbalance of blood-calcium levels. This type of bait is fairly safe to animals other than rodents, since they must eat a large amount to be affected. Single-dose bait that attacks the nervous system is toxic to all animals.

Regardless of a bait's level of safety, take care when putting it out so that chickens, pets, and children can't get into it. Never just scatter bait around or drop it into tunnels — rodents may kick it out where chickens or other animals will find it and eat it. No bait is effective if an abundance of other feed is available, so carefully clean up spilled grain before putting out bait.

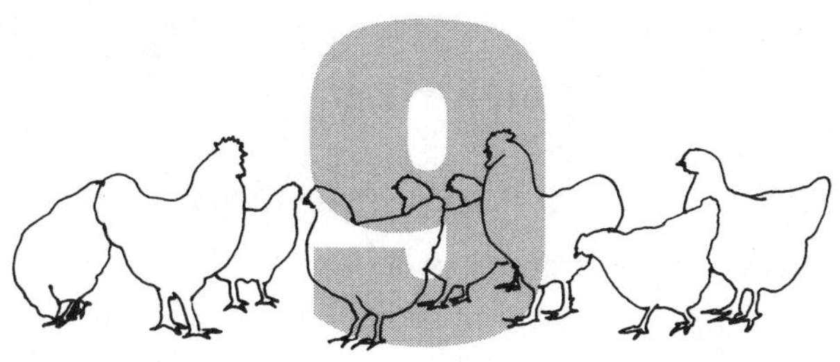

Diagnostic Guides

TRYING TO FIGURE OUT WHAT DISEASE your chickens have, or diagnosing the disease, involves four basic steps:

- examining flock history
- considering the symptoms
- conducting a postmortem examination
- performing laboratory procedures

Home laboratory procedures are pretty much limited to investigating internal parasites, as described in chapter 5. Postmortem examination is discussed in detail in the next chapter, as is the process of submitting specimens to a pathology laboratory. Consider enlisting the help of your state lab if, after going through the first three steps, you're still not sure what disease you're dealing with.

Flock History

When you experience a problem, suddenly all those little details you thought you'd never forget, but now can't quite remember, become immensely important. You'll be happy you took a few moments to write down events as they occurred. If you neglected to keep accurate records as you went along, try to reconstruct your flock's history based on the accompanying chart.

CHART 9-1

Flock History

This:	*Can Help You Determine This:*
Other diseased flocks	Diseases prevalent in your area
Previous diseases	Disease-causing agents already present on your property
Contacts	Diseases possibly transmitted by carrier chickens, visitors, dirty equipment, etc.
Flock age	Diagnosis based on age group involved (approximation only)
Time of year	Relationship to weather or to carriers such as mosquitoes
Feed changes	Diseases due to improper nutrition or toxins in feed
Duration of disease	Diagnosis based on how long symptoms last
Rate of spread	Diagnosis based on how fast symptoms spread
Past vaccinations	Diseases not likely to be involved
Medications used	Diagnosis based on flock response to drugs
Percentage involved	Diagnosis based on percentage of sick birds
Mortality rate	Diagnosis based on percentage of dead birds

Symptoms

CHART 9-2

Signs of Health

Body Part	*Appearance*
Comb & wattles	bright, full, waxy
Eyes	bright, shiny, alert
Nostrils	clean, no rasping
Head & tail	held high
Breast	full & plump
Abdomen	firm but not hard
Posture	erect, active, alert
Feathers	smooth & clean
Vent	clean, slightly moist
Droppings	firm, gray-brown with white caps

Symptoms are visible signs of disease. In order to readily recognize symptoms, you need to be thoroughly familiar with how a healthy flock looks, acts, and smells. Be observant when you tend your flock. Each time you enter your coop, stand quietly for a moment and watch.

Any change you detect, including a change in the amount of feed your birds eat, the amount of water they drink, their posture, their droppings, and the condition of their plumage may all be first signs of disease.

Signs of Disease

If you notice anything unusual in your flock, follow these steps in checking for signs of disease.

1. Watch from a distance to see what each bird is doing, how it moves, and

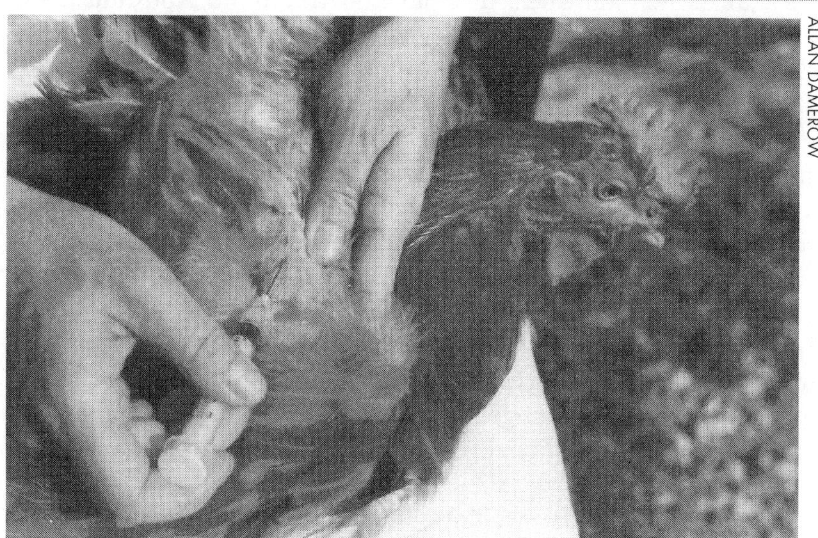

ALLAN DAMEROW

Taking Blood Samples

Your veterinarian or pathologist may ask you to bring in blood samples from live birds. Blood samples are usually taken from a main wing vein or brachial. Begin by pulling a few feathers from the depression in the upper part of the underside of the wing to expose the main vein. Disinfect the skin with 70 percent alcohol.

In one hand, hold both wings over the chicken's back so it can't flap. Insert a sharp 20-gauge needle (¾-inch for chicks, 2-inch for mature birds) into the vein with the needle pointing away from the chicken's body and toward the wing tip. Starting with the plunger pulled back slightly to allow an initial air space in the syringe, slowly but steadily pull back on the plunger until the syringe contains at least 2 ml of blood.

Take care to neither go through the vein nor nick the vein at the top, both of which will prevent you from drawing a sample. The first time you need a blood sample, try to get a veterinarian or other experienced person to show you how.

When you withdraw the needle, if the bird bleeds internally, press the spot with your thumb for a few moments. Unless the chicken has a clotting problem, drawing blood should pose no threat to its health.

Without jostling or rotating the syringe, place it in a clean container where it will remain horizontal. Do not refrigerate or freeze it, but take the sample to the lab for analysis the same day it was drawn. If the lab needs a whole blood sample (rather than one in which water-like serum separates from the blood) your veterinarian or pathologist will give you an anticoagulant to keep the blood from separating.

how it stands when still. Check droppings on the ground. Note unusual smells. Listen for unusual sounds: if you whistle, the birds will stop their activities to listen, and you can more easily hear respiratory sounds.

2. Count the number of affected birds. Come back a few hours later and count again. How fast the illness sweeps or creeps through a flock can provide an important clue as to what the disease might be. Since different diseases progress at different rates, if more than one disease is involved, how fast individual symptoms move through a flock can be especially important.

3. Keep track of the number of birds that die. Note how and where they die, and how soon they die after they first show symptoms.

4. For a closer look, catch birds with a minimum of fuss. Symptoms can change when you pick up a bird, especially if the bird had to be chased to be caught. Check body openings for unusual excretions: discharge from the mouth, clogged nostrils, sticky eyes, diarrhea. Note any unusual smell coming from these discharges.

5. Check for wounds, swellings, blindness, and external parasites. (See chapter 4 for instructions on checking for parasites.) To check for blindness, move a finger toward the bird's eye. If the bird blinks, it is not blind. Don't wave your hand, or air movement may make the bird blink.

6. If symptoms lead you to suspect a disease that involves a change in body temperature, take the bird's temperature: shake down the thermometer, insert it into the bird's vent, and hold it there for 3 minutes or until the thermometer beeps if its electronic. The normal temperature for an adult bird is 103°F (40°C); normal body temperature for a chick is 106.7°F (42°C).

7. Use the diagnostic charts in this chapter to help you identify the disease. Then look up each possibility in the alphabetic list in chapter 15 (or, in the case of parasites, chapters 4-6) and find the condition whose combination of symptoms most closely matches those of your flock.

Matching Symptoms to Diseases

General symptoms appear in nearly any illness, whether it results from an infection, parasitic invasion, nutritional deficiency, or poisoning. General symptoms include droopiness, ruffled feathers, weight loss, and reduced egg production.

Each disease group has its own set of general symptoms as well. Coughing, sneezing, and labored breathing are general symptoms of respiratory diseases. Diarrhea, increased thirst, and dehydration are general symptoms of intestinal diseases. Inability to stand or walk are general symptoms of muscular or skeletal disorders. Twitching, trembling, and convulsions are general symptoms of diseases that attack the nervous system.

Specific symptoms are produced by specific diseases. Facial swelling with reddish, bad smelling nasal discharge is specific to infectious coryza. An inflamed foot with a hard, swollen abscess is specific to bumblefoot. Distended abdomen and an unhealed or mushy navel in a newly hatched chick is specific to omphalitis.

Your chickens may not have all the symptoms listed in chapter 15 under the disease you suspect, or your flock may have symptoms in addition to those listed. Some diseases are caused by different strains of the same pathogen, affecting different birds in different ways. Some pathogens affect different birds in different parts of their bodies. Diseases may occur in combinations of two or more, causing a confusing array of symptoms.

Veterinarians arrive at a probable diagnosis (otherwise known as an educated guess) in part by considering the accumulation of symptoms. The rest of us are more likely to work by the process of elimination — decide what the problem is not, and you may eventually determine what it probably is.

Start with the obvious. Consider management errors causing your birds to run out of feed or water, get too hot or too cold, become injured, or be attacked by a predator. If your chickens seem a little droopy or they aren't growing well, they most likely have worms, external parasites, or coccidiosis. Before you start considering rare diseases, eliminate common diseases as the probable cause.

Scatology

To some extent, diseases can be diagnosed by the appearance of a bird's droppings. But remember, variations in droppings are quite normal. Light brown (or sometimes copper green), pasty droppings, usually bad smelling, are normal cecal droppings deposited by each chicken two or three times a day.

Chickens don't usually produce liquid urine, as humans do. Instead, they expel solid urine in the form of salts or urates that look like chalky white caps on top of their droppings. An excessive amount of urates can be a sign that the kidneys are not functioning properly, perhaps because the chicken isn't getting enough to drink or has a kidney disease.

Watery droppings are a sign of increased urine output. They often appear as a pool of liquid surrounding solid matter that's slightly greenish in color, and can occur when chickens eat lots of succulent spring grass or drink extra water during warm weather. Watery droppings can also be a sign of disease caused by such things as kidney failure and fever.

Intestinal diseases often cause diarrhea. Based on the specific disease involved, the diarrhea may be foamy, bloody, sticky, pasty, mucousy, off-colored, smelly, or any combination thereof.

CHART 9-3

Diseases Causing a Change in Droppings

Age	*Characteristics*	*Disease*	*Prevalence*
0–10 days	vent pasting	pasted vent	common
0–3 weeks	vent pasting	arizonosis	rare
	diarrhea	omphalitis	common
0–4 weeks	watery diarrhea	campylobacteriosis	common
	white or greenish brown diarrhea	pullorum	rare
1–6 weeks	diarrhea with undigested feed	infectious stunting syndrome	common
2–6 weeks	diarrhea	necrotic enteritis	rare
3–14 weeks	diarrhea	infectious anemia	not common
3–18 weeks	whitish or water diarrhea, may be bloody	infectious bursal disease	common
4–6 weeks	bloody diarrhea	blackhead	rare
4–12 weeks	diarrhea (may be bloody)	ulcerative enteritis	common
	white-capped greenish droppings	infectious synovitis	not common
12 weeks +	diarrhea	typhoid	rare
up to 5 weeks	watery diarrhea with pasting	paratyphoid	common
chicks and growing	bloody diarrhea	coccidiosis (cecal)	common
	diarrhea	listeriosis	rare
	profuse, watery diarrhea	rotaviral enteritis	common
	white droppings, sometimes diarrhea	toxoplasmosis	rare
Growing cockerels	greenish yellow diarrhea	erysipelas	rare
Growing	watery, mucousy, pasty, tan or bloody diarrhea	coccidiosis (intestinal)	common
	green diarrhea	leucocytozoonosis	rare
	diarrhea, sour crop	thrush	common
Growing & mature	mucousy, bloody diarrhea	campylobacteriosis	common
	yellowish droppings	chronic respiratory disease	common
6 months +	loose white or green droppings	lymphoid leukosis	common

Age	*Characteristics*	*Disease*	*Prevalence*
Maturing pullets	greenish, watery, pasty diarrhea	bluecomb	rare
Maturing & mature	diarrhea, first watery and white then greenish yellow	cholera (acute)	not common
Mature hens	diarrhea	fatty liver syndrome	not common
Mature	watery, greenish, blood-stained diarrhea	Newcastle (exotic)	very rare
	yellow, watery, foamy diarrhea	colibacillosis	common
	yellowish or greenish-yellow diarrhea	ochratoxicosis	sporadic
	yellow diarrhea	streptococcosis	not common
	green diarrhea	pullorum	rare
2 years +	persistent diarrhea	tuberculosis	common
Any	greenish-yellow diarrhea	chlamydiosis	rare
	greenish-yellow diarrhea capped with white	spirochetosis	rare
	chalky white	oviduct flukes	rare
	greenish diarrhea	influenza	rare
	foamy diarrhea	worms	very common
	blue or green fluorescent droppings	moldy grain	not common
	bright yellow green droppings	crotalaria seed poisoning	rare
	pasting	rye seed poisoning	rare
	diarrhea	coffee-weed seed poisoning	rare
	diarrhea	ergotism	rare
	diarrhea	histoplasmosis	rare
	diarrhea	pseudomonas	rare
	watery diarrhea	antifreeze poisoning	not common
	brown, pasty, smelly droppings	none — normal cecal discharge	common
	loose, watery droppings	none — cooling mechanism in hot weather	common

CHART 9-4

Diseases Interfering with Movement

Age	*Characteristics*	*Disease*	*Prevalence*
At hatch	backward somersaulting	congenital tremor	rare
Chicks	uncoordinated, circling	dactylariosis	rare
	inability to stand	fatty liver syndrome	rare
	droopy wings, draggy legs	Newcastle (exotic)	very rare
0–3 weeks	leg paralysis, twisted neck	arizonosis	rare
1–3 weeks	jerky movements, falling over	epidemic tremor	rare
1–8 weeks	lost balance, outstretched legs	encephalomalacia	rare
1–12 weeks	flapping wings, flipping onto back, death	sudden death syndrome	common
3–6 weeks	squatting, feet up, weight on hocks	kinky back	not common
3–20 weeks	lameness, incoordination	necrotic dermatitis	rare
3–18 weeks	incoordination	infectious bursal disease	common
4 weeks	degenerated leg muscles	white muscle disease	not common
4–8 weeks	lameness	viral arthritis	rare
4–10 weeks	paralysis	runting syndrome	rare
4–12 weeks	lameness, swollen hocks and feet	infectious synovitis	not common
4–17 weeks	weight on keel, reluctant to move	cryptosporidiosis	not common
6 weeks +	lameness, swollen joints	cholera (chronic)	not common
Chicks & growing	lameness, weakness	leucocytozoonosis	rare
	circling, twisted neck	listeriosis	rare
	unable to stand, twisted legs and wings	rickets	rare
	circling, head twisted back	toxoplasmosis	rare
	one or both legs bent outward	twisted leg	common
Growing cockerels	lameness, swollen joints	erysipelas	rare

Age	*Characteristics*	*Disease*	*Prevalence*
Growing	droopy wing, draggy leg, twisted neck	Newcastle	common
	twisted legs with swollen joints	slipped tendon	common
Maturing cockerels	abscess on foot pad	bumblefoot	common
Maturing pullets	inability to stand	cage fatigue	not common
	inability to stand	rickets	not common
Maturing	wing or leg paralysis	Marek's disease	common
Young or mature	lameness, stilted gait, thick leg bones	osteopetrosis	common
	lameness, swollen hocks and feet	pseudomonas	rare
	stilted gait, thickened legs	scaly leg mite	very common
	weakness, paralysis	tapeworm	not common
	paralysis	fowl tick	rare
Mature	tremors, twisted neck, paralyzed wing or leg	Newcastle (exotic)	very rare
	lameness, head tremors	streptococcosis	not common
Any	convulsions, paralysis	algae poisoning	rare
	progressive flaccid paralysis	botulism	rare
	swollen joints	staphylococcic arthritis	common
	swollen, white foot joints	gout (articular)	not common
	weak legs, lost coordination	spirochetosis	rare
	leg deformity	sorghum seed poisoning	rare
	lameness	rye seed poisoning	rare
	incoordination, twisted neck	antifreeze poisoning	not common

CHART 9-5

Diseases and Conditions Affecting Egg Production

Change in Eggs	*Disease*	*Other characteristics*	*Prevalence*
Fewer	aflatoxicosis	small eggs, low hatchability	rare
	campylobacteriosis	35% drop	common
	cholera (chronic)	increase in blood spots	not common
	chronic respiratory disease	coughing, weight loss	common
	coccidiosis (intestinal)	thin breast, weak legs	rare
	egg drop syndrome	in brown-egg layers	rare
	encephalomalacia	15–30% drop for 2 weeks	rare
	epidemic tremor	temporary drop	rare
	erysipelas	70% drop	rare
	fatty liver syndrome	sudden drop	not common
	fusariotoxicosis	sudden drastic drop	rare
	infectious coryza	watery eyes, swollen face	common
	infectious laryngotracheitis	temporary drop	common
	influenza	sudden drop, broodiness	rare
	lymphoid leukosis	tumors in ovary	common
	Newcastle	temporary drop	common
	paratyphoid	often no other symptoms	common
	pox (dry)	bumps on combs & wattles	not common
	swollen head syndrome	swollen head & wattles	rare
	tuberculosis	prominent, deformed keel	common
	water deprivation	dehydration	
Watery whites	infectious bronchitis	very low production	common
	Newcastle (exotic)	very low production	very common
Blood-stained yolks	Newcastle (exotic)	very low production	very rare
	cholera (chronic)	wrinkled, off-color yolks	not common
Blood spots	cholera (chronic)	low production	not common
	heredity	no other symptoms	common
	vitamin A deficiency	clutches farther apart	not common
Smaller	aflatoxicosis	drop in production	rare
	salt deficiency	drop in production	not common

Change in Eggs	*Disease*	*Other characteristics*	*Prevalence*
Misshapen shells	Newcastle (exotic)	very low production	very rare
	infectious bronchitis	very low production	common
Pale shells	egg drop syndrome	low production	rare
Pimpled shells	vitamin D excess	leave holes if scraped off	not common
Ridged shells	infectious bronchitis	very low production	common
Soft shells	egg drop syndrome	low production	rare
	infectious bronchitis	very low production	common
	infectious laryngotracheitis	low production	common
	influenza	low production	rare
	vitamin D deficiency	cycles of low production	not common
Thin shells	cage fatigue	soon stop laying	not common
	egg drop syndrome	shells are gritty	rare
	fusariotoxicosis	high death rate	rare
	infectious bronchitis	very low production	common
	ochratoxicosis	yellow diarrhea	sporadic
No shells	egg drop syndrome	egg eating	rare
	influenza	low production	rare
No eggs	cage fatigue	followed by paralysis, death	not common
	colibacillosis	no other symptoms or death	common
	Newcastle (exotic)	drop within 3 days	very rare
	gout (visceral)	soon followed by death	common
	infectious bronchitis	gasping, coughing	common

CHART 9-6

Diseases Causing Breathing Difficulties

Age	*Characteristics*	*Disease*	*Prevalence*
chicks	gasping, sneezing, "chirping"	Newcastle (exotic)	very rare
	labored breathing, droopy head	typhoid	rare
0–1 week	gasping, swollen eyes	aspergillosis	rare
0–4 weeks	gasping	pullorum	rare
1–7 weeks	swollen eyes and sinuses	roup (nutritional)	rare
4 weeks +	nasal discharge, swollen face	infectious coryza	common
4–12 weeks	slight rattling	infectious synovitis	not common
4–17 weeks	coughing, extending neck	cryptosporidiosis	not common
5–12 weeks	rattling	air-sac disease	common
6 weeks +	sneezing, rattling, nasal discharge	cholera (chronic)	not common
Young	rapid labored breathing	leucocytozoonosis	rare
Growing cockerels	breathing difficulty, nasal discharge	erysipelas	rare
Growing & mature	rapid breathing, mucus discharge mouth and nose	cholera (acute)	not common
	gasping, rattling, coughing, bloody mucus, nasal discharge	infectious laryngotracheitis	common
Mature	gasping, coughing	aspergillosis	rare
	difficult breathing, nervous signs	Newcastle (exotic)	very rare
Any	nasal discharge	chlamydiosis	rare
	gasping, rattling, wet eyes	infectious bronchitis	common
	coughing, sneezing, rattling	influenza	rare
	sneezing, progressive swelling of head and wattles	swollen head syndrome	rare

CHART 9-7

Diseases Causing Discoloration

Age	*Characteristics*	*Disease*	*Prevalence*
1–4 weeks	greenish blue breast and legs	exudative diathesis	rare
1–6 weeks	pale skin	infectious stunting syndrome	common
3–12 weeks	reddish black skin patches	necrotic dermatitis	rare
3–14 weeks	pale comb, wattles, skin, legs	infectious anemia	not common
4–6 weeks	dark face	blackhead	rare
4–12 weeks	bluish comb	infectious synovitis	not common
4–17 weeks	pale skin	cryptosporidiosis	not common
6 weeks +	bluish, hot comb	cholera (chronic)	not common
Chicks & growing	darkened head	canker	rare
	pale, shriveled comb	toxoplasmosis	rare
	black feathers in red or buff breed	rickets	rare
Over 6 months	pale, shriveled, sometimes bluish comb	lymphoid leukosis	common
Growing & mature cocks	grayish white patches on comb	favus	rare
Growing & mature	darkened head	chronic respiratory disease	common
	pale head	cholera	rare
Maturing pullets	bluish comb	bluecomb	rare
Maturing	pale skin	Marek's disease	common
Maturing & Mature	pale head	cholera (acute)	not common
Mature	blackish, swollen eyes draining straw-colored fluid	Newcastle (exotic)	very rare
	purplish head, comb, wattles	paratyphoid	common
	pale, shriveled comb	pullorum	rare
	bluish comb	aspergillosis (chronic)	rare
Mature Hens	pale, swollen comb and wattles	fatty liver syndrome	not common
	darkened head and shanks	gout (visceral)	common
2 years +	pale or bluish comb and wattles	tuberculosis	common

(chart continues over)

Diseases Causing Discoloration (cont.)

Age	*Characteristics*	*Disease*	*Prevalence*
Any	bluish, wilted, cold comb	ergotism	rare
	bluish comb and wattles	gossypol seed poisoning	rare
	pale comb, skin, shanks	coccidiosis (intestinal)	common
	pale head	worms/lice/mites	very common
	darkened head, comb, and wattles	influenza	rare
	white bumps on comb and wattles	pox (dry)	not common
	pale or purplish comb	spirochetosis	rare

Chart 9-8

Diseases Causing Off Odors

Age	*Characteristics*	*Disease*	*Prevalence*
Hatched chicks	smelly unabsorbed yolk sac	omphalitis	common
Chicks & growing	smelly mouth discharge	canker	rare
Growing	distended, sour crop	thrush	rare
Maturing pullets	sour crop	bluecomb	rare
Growing & mature cocks	moldy smelling, scabby comb	favus	rare
Growing & mature	smelly nasal discharge	infectious coryza	common
Mature	smelly droppings on vent	pasted vent	not common
	sour-smelling, distended crop	crop impaction	rare

Chart 9-9

Diseases Affecting the Eyes

Age	*Characteristics*	*Disease*	*Prevalence*
0–1 week	swollen with yellow cheesy matter	aspergillosis (acute)	rare
1–3 weeks	dull eyes	epidemic tremor	rare
1–8 weeks	one or both eyes blind	encephalomalacia	rare
4 weeks +	one or both eyes swollen shut	infectious coryza	common
Up to 5 weeks	one or both eyes swollen or blind	paratyphoid	common
6 weeks +	swollen, sticky eyes	cholera (chronic)	not common
Growing	watery eyes	canker	rare
	swollen eyelids with sticky or cheesy discharge	roup (nutritional)	rare
	blindness	toxoplasmosis	rare
Growing & mature	frothy eyes	chronic respiratory disease	common
Maturing pullets	sunken eyes	bluecomb	rare
Maturing & mature	mucousy eyes	cholera (acute)	not common
	watery, swollen eyes	infectious laryngotracheitis	common
Mature	clear eye becomes blind	colibacillosis	common
Any	cloudy eye	Newcastle	common
	cloudy eye, sunlight avoidance	conjunctivitis	common
	watery eyes	infectious bronchitis	common
	watery and/or swollen eyes	influenza	rare
	cloudy grayish, dilated, irregular pupil; distorted or blinded eye	Marek's disease	common
	blackish eyes draining straw-colored fluid	Newcastle (exotic)	common
	red swollen eyes	swollen head syndrome	very rare
	swollen, inflamed, watery	eye worm	not common

CHART 9-10

Diseases Causing Sores in the Mouth

Age	*Characteristics*	*Disease*	*Prevalence*
Chicks & growing	white or yellow sores	canker	rare
Growing	whitish yellow sores	roup (nutritional)	rare
	grayish white circular sores	thrush	common
Any	yellow patches on roof	Newcastle (exotic)	very rare
	sores at corners of mouth	fusariotoxicosis	very rare
	white, yellow, or brown patches	pox	rare
	sores in roof of mouth	red mites	rare

CHART 9-11

Diseases Causing Temperature Changes*

Age	*Characteristics*	*Disease*	*Prevalence*
3–18 weeks	fever, then drop to below normal	infectious bursal disease	common
4–12 weeks	hot, swollen legs and feet	infectious synovitis	not common
6 weeks +	hot, bluish comb	cholera (chronic)	not common
12 weeks +	1–5 °F (1–3°C) above normal	cholera	rare
Young or mature	warm, puffy legs	osteopetrosis	common
Growing	fever, weakness	leucocytozoonosis	rare
Maturing cockerels	hot, inflamed foot	bumblefoot	common
Maturing pullets	body feels cold	bluecomb	rare
Maturing & mature	fever	cholera (acute)	not common
Mature	fever, depression, weight loss	streptococcosis	not common
	fever, purplish head	paratyphoid	common
Any	hot swollen joints	staphylococcic arthritis	common
	fever, weight loss	aspergillosis	rare
	fever, sneezing, rattling	influenza	rare
	fever, dropping to below normal just before death	spirochetosis	rare
	fever, pale head, diarrhea	typhoid	rare

*The normal body temperature for adult chickens is 103°F. (39.5°C); for chicks, it's 106.7°F (41.5°C).

Chart 9-12

Diseases Causing a High Rate of Death

Age	*Symptoms*	*Disease*	*Prevalence*
0–3 weeks	rapid deaths	carbon monoxide poisoning	not common
	diarrhea, leg paralysis	arizonosis	rare
	diarrhea, gasping	pullorum	rare
1–3 weeks	jerky movements, falling over	epidemic tremor	rare
3–18 weeks	diarrhea, vent picking	infectious bursal disease	common
Over 3 weeks	growing thin while eating well	Marek's disease	common
2–6 weeks	reluctant to move, diarrhea	necrotic enteritis	rare
3–6 weeks	can't walk, dehydration	kinky back	not common
3–20 weeks	huddling, ruffled feathers	infectious anemia	not common
	lameness, loose feathers & skin	necrotic dermatitis	rare
4–6 weeks	no symptoms or droopiness	blackhead	rare
4–17 weeks	reluctant to move	cryptosporidiosis	not common
Up to 5 weeks	droopy, thirsty, huddling	paratyphoid	common
Young & growing	bloody diarrhea	coccidiosus (cecal)	common
	gasping, watery nose and eyes	infectious bronchitis	common
	weakness, rapid deaths	leucocytozoonosis	rare
	diarrhea, inflamed vent	rotaviral enteritis	common
	emaciation, incoordination	toxoplasmosis	rare
Growing cockerels	diarrhea, nasal discharge, lameness	erysipelas	rare
Growing	slow growth, diarrhea	coccidiosus (intestinal)	common
	diarrhea, sour crop	thrush	rare
Broiler Cockerels	ruffled feathers, slow growth	broiler ascites	common
Maturing pullets	sour crop, diarrhea	bluecomb	rare
Maturing & mature	rapid death	cholera (acute)	not common
	coughing, gasping	infectious laryngotracheitis	common
Mature	thin-shelled eggs	fusariotoxicosis	very rare
	depression, weight loss	streptococcosis	not common
Any	convulsions, paralysis	algae poisoning	rare
	progressive flaccid paralysis	botulism	rare
	ruffled feathers, no appetite	typhoid	rare

(chart continues over)

Diseases Causing a High Rate of Death (cont.)

Age	*Symptoms*	*Disease*	*Prevalence*
Any (cont.)	sudden death	gout (visceral)	not common
	coughing, huddling	influenza	rare
	respiratory problems &/or paralysis &/or sudden deaths	Newcastle (exotic)	very rare
	bumps or scabs on face, mouth	pox (wet)	rare
	lameness, diarrhea, rapid deaths	pseudomonas	rare
	diarrhea, weakness, convulsions	spirochetosis	rare

CHART 9-13

Diseases Causing Sudden Death

Age	*Disease*	*Prevalence*
At hatch	typhoid	rare
1–12 weeks	sudden death syndrome	common
0–4 weeks	pullorum	rare
3–14 weeks	infectious anemia	not common
3–20 weeks	necrotic dermatitis	rare
2–6 weeks	necrotic enteritis	rare
4–12 weeks	ulcerative enteritis	common
4–8 months	round heart disease	very rare
Over 6 months	lymphoid leukosis	common
Growing	aflatoxicosis	rare
Broiler cockerels	broiler ascites	common
Maturing pullets	bluecomb	rare
Growing & mature	campylobacteriosis	common
	colibacillosis	common
Mature hens	fatty liver syndrome	not common
Mature	streptococcosis	not common
Any	malaria	rare
	botulism	not common
	cholera	not common
	erysipelas	rare
	gout (visceral)	common
	influenza	very rare
	listeriosis	rare
	Marek's disease	common
	Newcastle (exotic)	very rare
	choking (too rapid eating)	not common
	pesticide poisoning	not common
	anaphylactic shock	rare

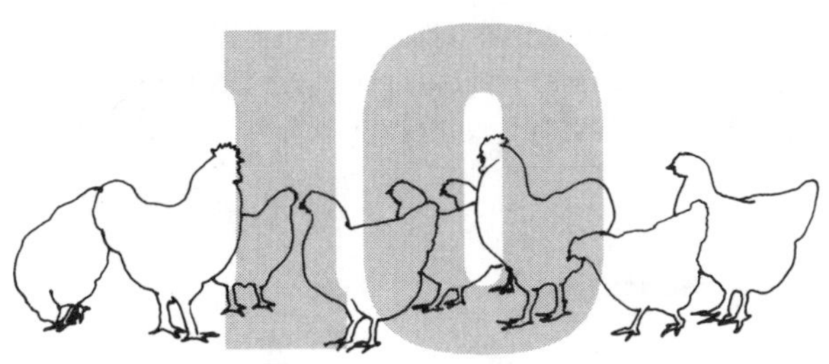

10 Postmortem Examination

MANY DISEASES, in addition to causing easily observable symptoms, cause less obvious changes inside the body. Studying the insides of a bird for signs of disease is called postmortem examination ("post" meaning after and "mortem" meaning death).

Conducting a postmortem is sometimes called "posting," or more scientifically, "necropsy" (the animal equivalent of an autopsy). Posting gives you clues to help you determine the cause of a disease outbreak.

Laboratory Analysis

If you have a sudden, severe disease outbreak, or you find several dead birds in a short time, the best way to get a rapid, positive diagnosis is to have a few birds posted at your state poultry pathology laboratory (you'll find a list of state labs in the appendix). Since the pathologist will want to know the disease's progression, submit either three live birds in various stages of illness or one bird that has recently died, one that is very sick, and one just beginning to show symptoms.

When you bring live birds to the lab, be prepared to leave them behind. The pathologist will not help you try to save any birds you bring in for examination. Taking chickens to the lab is a one-way street for two reasons:

- A pathologist's job is to examine a bird's innards, which means the bird must be dead before the examination can proceed.

- You wouldn't want to return a bird to your flock after it has been exposed to all the disease-causing organisms floating around the average lab, some of which may be worse than what your chickens already have.

Submitting Specimens

When you plan to submit a dead bird for examination, as soon as you find one dead, wet its feathers with cold water and a little detergent, taking care not to get any into the mouth or nose. Bag the bird in plastic and refrigerate it until you're ready to leave for the lab. Whether you're submitting dead or live birds, identify each with a numbered leg band (or wrap a piece of tape several times around its leg and write a number on it with an indelible marker).

Write a detailed history of the disease, how it affected each bird you are submitting, and anything else about your chickens you think might be important. The lab will provide a form for you to fill out. Attach your history to the form.

If the lab is far from your home, you may wish to ship your birds. Call first for shipping instructions. It's a good idea to call ahead, anyway, instead of just

Disease History

When you submit a sample to a diagnostic laboratory, provide this information:

- **your name, address, and phone number**
- **housing type (cage, floor, range)**
- **feed used (sources and types)**
- **breed of your birds**
- **number in your flock**
- **birds' age(s)**
- **where you got them**
- **symptoms you have observed**
- **date symptoms started**
- **approximate number sick**
- **number that have died**
- **when, where, and how they died**
- **approximate days from first symptoms to death**
- **any medications you have tried**
- **recent changes (new rations, new chickens brought in, toxic spraying in your area, etc.)**
- **additional history (vaccinations, nearby flocks, previous disease problems, etc.)**

showing up with sick or dead chickens. You may be asked to consult your veterinarian and get a referral to the lab. If there are no veterinarians nearby, or your vet is not willing to examine chickens, say so.

Unfortunately, most veterinarians know little about chickens. Even if you're lucky enough to find one with poultry experience, the fee you will be charged may be more than the cost of buying new, healthy birds. State poultry pathology laboratories, on the other hand, charge little or nothing for an initial examination.

What to Expect

Within a few days, the pathologist should call you with a preliminary report, then follow up with a written report. Don't be bashful about asking questions if you don't understand something — pathologists tend to use words only a veterinarian or other trained person can understand. If you submit your birds under a veterinarian's referral, your vet will explain the report to you.

Not all path labs are equipped to diagnose all poultry diseases. If the initial report is inconclusive, the pathologist may take an educated guess as to what the problem might be and ask if you want the diagnosis confirmed by further laboratory tests such as tissue examination, bacterial cultures, virus isolation, or sensitivity tests (to determine which drug, if any, will kill the particular pathogen in question). These tests can be time-consuming and expensive.

Even if the diagnosis is certain, the pathologist is unlikely to suggest a specific treatment. The job of a pathologist is to identify diseases, not recommend treatments. You should, however, be given enough information to obtain details on treatment options from your veterinarian, your state Extension poultry veterinarian, or your state Extension poultry specialist. Armed with this information, you can decide whether to treat the remainder of your chickens or get rid of them and start over.

Do-It-Yourself Posting

Running to the path lab with every dead bird you find is neither feasible nor even necessary. A 5 percent death rate is considered normal in any flock. Still, it's a good idea to examine dead birds and record the results in your flock history. You may see an emerging pattern that can help you discover and treat a disease in its early stages of development.

Every flock includes weak birds that have lower resistance than others to disease as a result of stress, genetic factors, or insufficient nourishment due to being far down in the peck order. These weaker birds become indicators of impending problems. If you do find signs of a disease in progress, you can take

Caution

If you suspect a chicken of having chlamydiosis or any other disease that is contagious to humans (see chapter 14) *do not* post it yourself. Take it to the state pathology laboratory.

future samples to a qualified pathologist for a confirmed diagnosis.

Another reason to do your own posting is that, if the lab is particularly busy, the pathologist may not get back to you for several days or even weeks. Meanwhile, if your chickens are getting sicker or are dying fast, you might tentatively identify the problem yourself and take appropriate action. The lab report, when it comes, will then serve as a confirming diagnosis.

Posting a chicken makes sense only if you know what the insides of a healthy bird look like — something you can easily learn by paying attention when you butcher chickens for eating. The more often you post chickens, the more observant you will become. To help sharpen your skills, get a good reference book of color photos, such as *Color Atlas of Diseases and Disorders of the Domestic Fowl and Turkey* or the less expensive *Solvay Manual of Poultry Diseases* (both books are listed in Recommended Reading, page 333).

Preparing the Specimen

Your goal is to find abnormalities such as abscesses, tumors, inflammation, fluid accumulation, foreign materials, changes in muscle or bone condition, and irregularity in the size, shape, or color of internal organs. Examine not just dead birds but at least one bird that recently began showing symptoms and one in which the disease is quite far along.

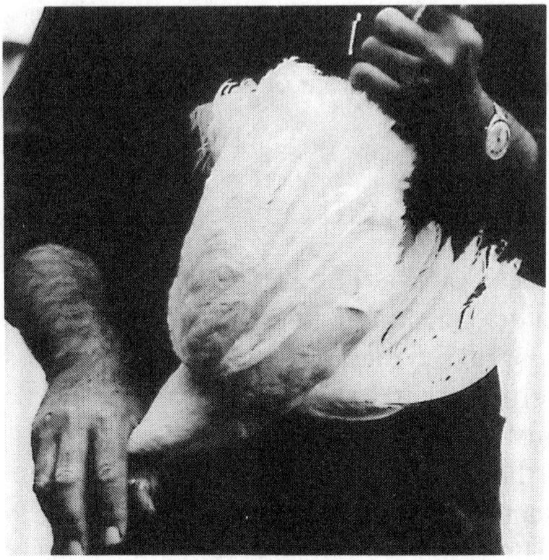

THE OHIO STATE UNIVERSITY EXTENSION

Kill a bird for posting by stretching its neck.

Examining birds in various stages of illness shows how this particular disease progresses, which may help you determine what the disease might be. Checking more than one bird also helps you determine which signs are specific to individuals (therefore possibly insignificant) and which are flock-wide occurrences (likely signs of disease).

When a bird is not already

dead, you will have to kill it. If that sounds like a drastic measure, remember you're doing it out of concern for the rest of your chickens. If a serious illness is gripping your flock, this and other birds may die anyway. Your goal is to determine the cause so you can prevent additional deaths.

The best way to kill a chicken for posting is to stretch its neck, which painlessly breaks the neck and spinal cord. With one hand, hold the bird's feet. Grasp the bird's head with the other hand, your thumb behind its comb and your little finger beneath its beak. Tilt the head back and pull steadily until the head is separated from the neck.

Continue to hold the head up until the bird stops struggling. Otherwise, it may spit up and inhale crop contents, leaving the false impression that the disease caused the respiratory system to fill with foreign matter.

Wait a few minutes while blood collects and clots beneath the neck skin, and the body tissues firm up. Meantime, examine external openings and run your hands over feathered areas to find lumps or other irregularities.

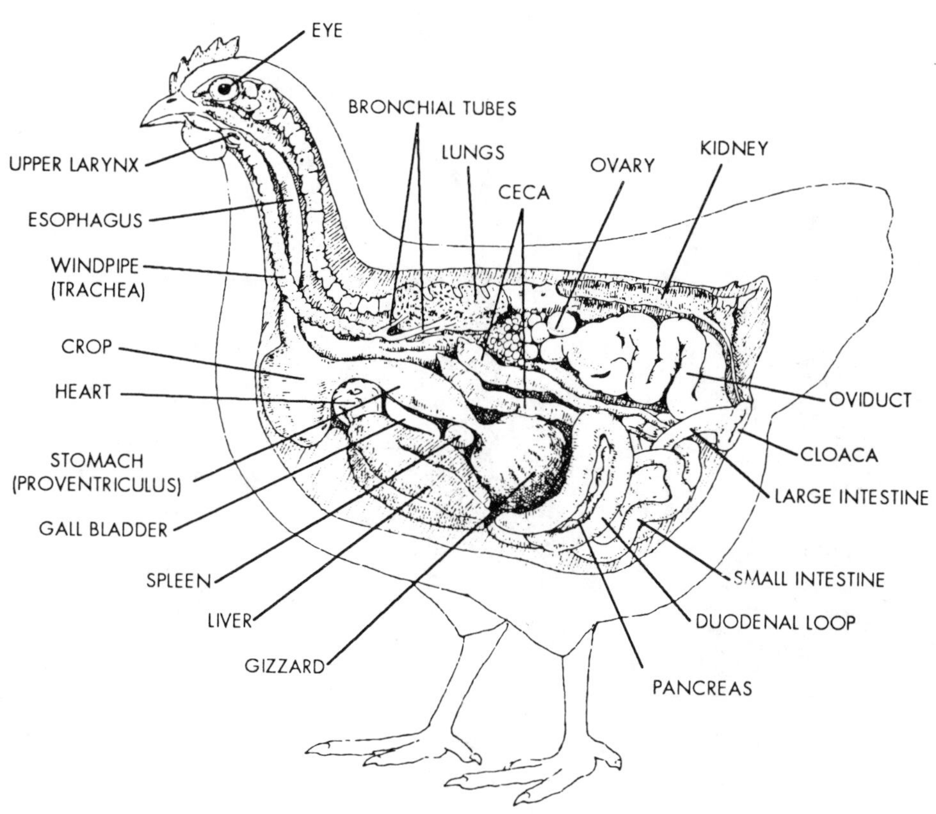

Position of internal organs - Horizontal

Opening the Bird

Conduct your postmortem outdoors or in a garage or carport, using a table or the tailgate of a pickup truck as your work surface. (Posting a diseased bird in a kitchen where food is prepared is not a sensible idea.) Cover your work surface with clean paper. Wear rubber gloves and an apron.

Use water and detergent in a spray bottle, or a wet cloth, to dampen the bird's feathers so they won't blow around. Lay the bird on its back. Holding one leg away from the body, cut the skin between the leg and the abdomen. Do the same on the other leg.

Stabilize the bird by bending the legs back, one at a time, until the joints snap to let the legs lay flat against the table. Cut the skin from the vent to the throat. Note any bloody spots or streaks in the breast or thigh muscles.

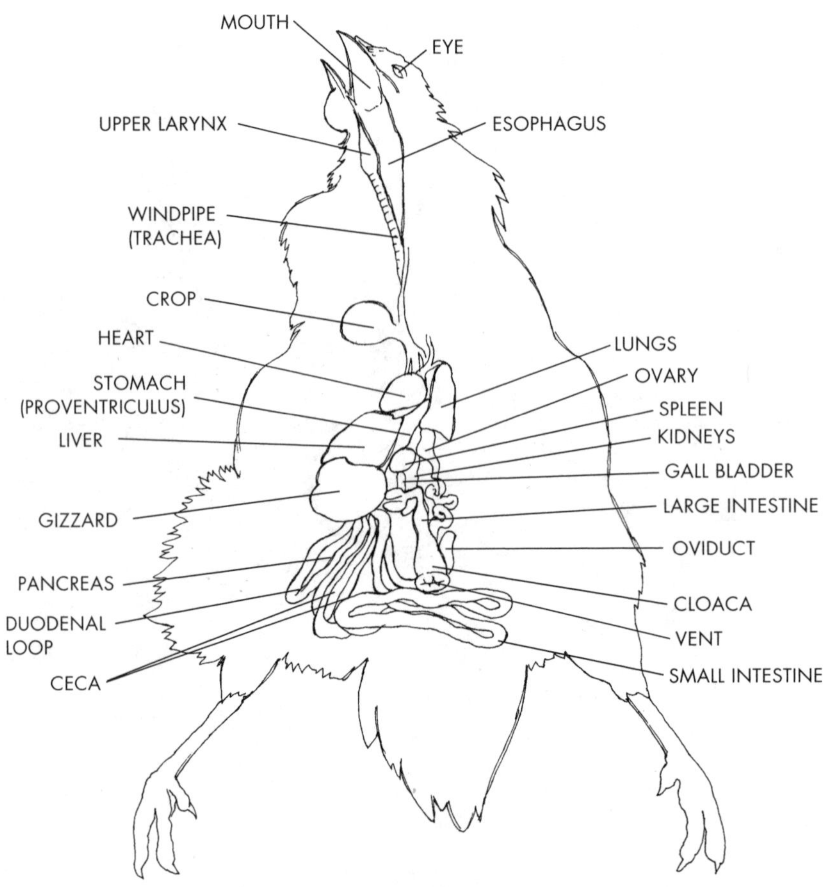

Position of internal organs - Vertical

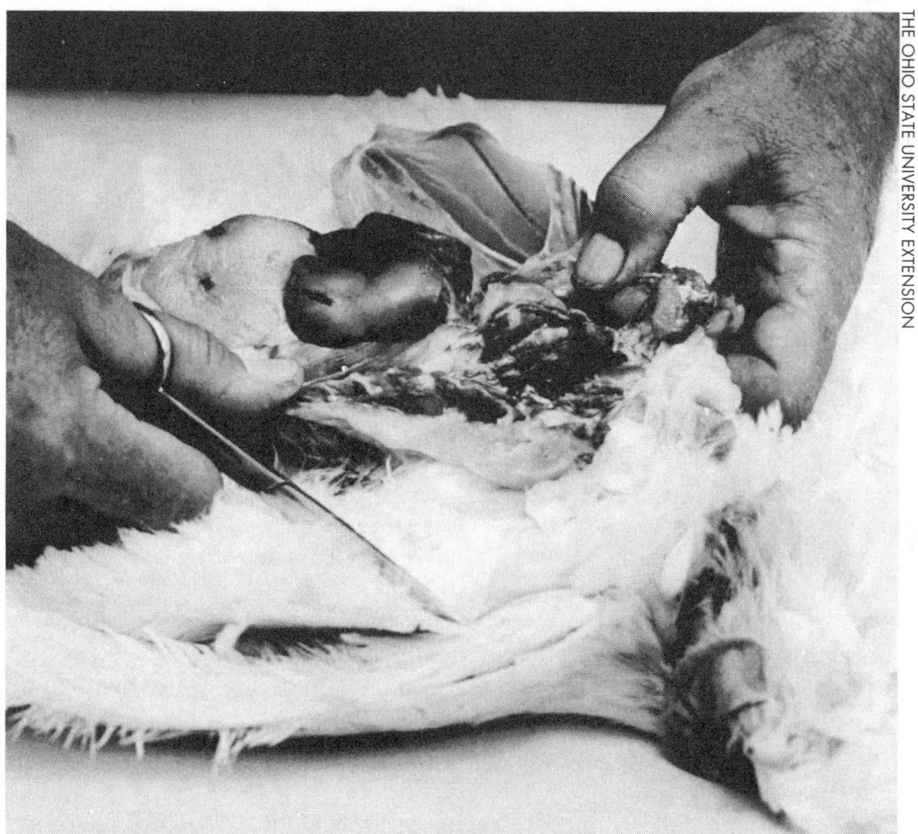
THE OHIO STATE UNIVERSITY EXTENSION

Use scissors to cut through the abdominal wall just behind the point of the keel.

About halfway from the vent to the keel, cut through the abdomen wall crosswise from one leg joint to the other. Use a pair of heavy scissors, kitchen shears, or tin snips to cut upward on one side, through the rib cage and other bones, taking care not to cut into or disturb the internal organs. Stop cutting just short of the wing joint. Make a similar cut on the other side, only this time cut all the way through the wing joint. Note how easy or difficult it is to cut the bones — an indication of their condition.

Lift the breast and rotate it on the uncut joint as if it were a hinged cover. Now you can see the internal organs in their natural position.

Examining the Organs

Take hold of the gizzard in the palm of one hand, your thumb and forefinger grasping the stomach (proventriculus), and make a cut between the stomach and the crop. With one hand, lift the stomach away. With the other hand, loosen and remove the gizzard, liver, spleen, and intestine. Set them

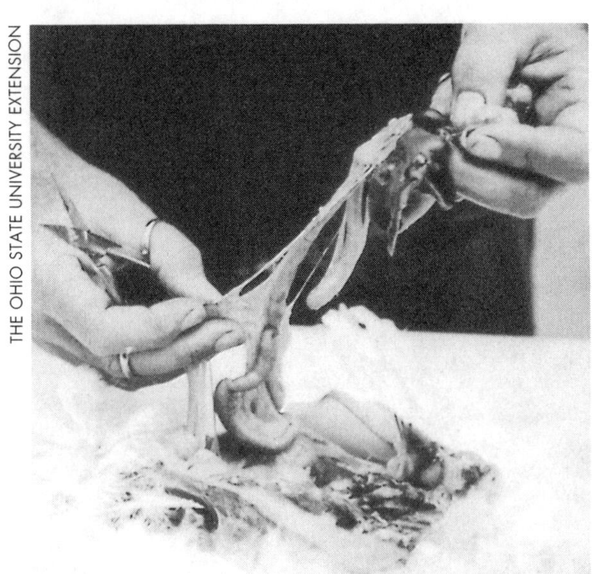

THE OHIO STATE UNIVERSITY EXTENSION

Carefully separate the gizzard from the stomach (proventriculus).

aside, leaving the intestine attached to the vent. Examine the heart, lungs, reproductive organs, kidneys, and nerves still in place.

To examine the contents of the digestive system, use your shears to cut longways through the stomach, gizzard, intestine, and ceca. Note any parasites present. Also note any unusual odor, especially related to the crop or intestines.

To examine the respiratory system, cut through the corner of the mouth

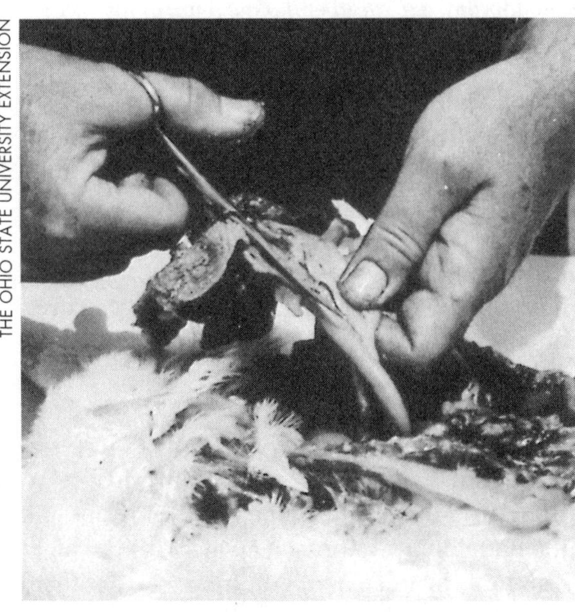

THE OHIO STATE UNIVERSITY EXTENSION

Examine the digestive system by cutting longways through the stomach, gizzard, intestine, and ceca.

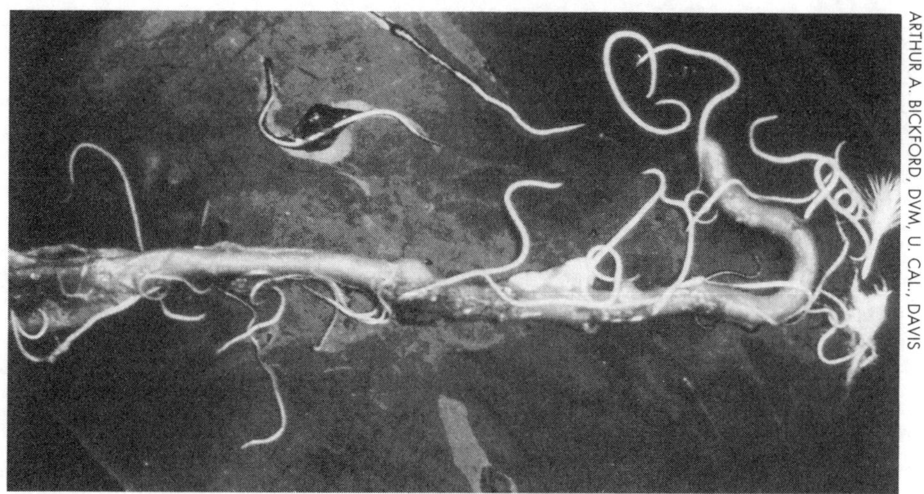
ARTHUR A. BICKFORD, DVM, U. CAL., DAVIS

Digestive tract infected with large roundworms (Ascaridia galli)

and expose the throat and crop. Then cut down the windpipe from the back of the mouth to the lungs.

To examine the head, cut across the face, half-way between the nostrils and the eye. Note any unusual odor coming from the nose area.

If the bird was lame or paralyzed, cut through the ligaments of one hock joint and twist the leg until the joint pops open. Break the leg bone, both to examine the marrow cavity and to test the bone's strength. A healthy bone makes a snapping sound when it breaks.

Interpretation

Without using a microscope and staining techniques to examine tissue, you will not be able to observe minute changes caused by illness. There are, however, plenty of obvious changes to look for.

In technical terminology, easily observable changes are called "gross lesions" ("gross" meaning large and "lesion" being medical jargon for alteration). A gross lesion is any visible change in the color, size, shape, or structure of an organ. Examples of lesions are: tumors, inflammations, accumulations of fluid, dead tissue, and enlarged organs.

Pay attention to:

- the location of the lesion (note specific organs)
- the nature of the lesion (its size, shape, color, and consistency)
- the possibility that the lesion killed the bird (by blocking airways or intestines, through extensive bleeding, by destroying a vital organ, by causing paralysis)

Try to determine the possible cause of the lesion — infection, nutritional deficiency, poisoning, injury, or whatever. Determining the cause often requires microscopic analysis, but some causes are fairly obvious, such as worms or injury due to cannibalism.

Lesions, like symptoms, may be general or specific. A general lesion can be caused by any of several diseases. A specific lesion is characteristic of a particu-

Chart 10-1

Postmortem Findings

Body Part	*Finding*	*Age/Sex*	*Possible Cause*
Bones	fragile, thin, soft	hen	cage fatigue
	soft, rubbery	young	rickets
	thickened	all	osteopetrosis
Bone marrow	tumors in marrow	2 years	tuberculosis
		all	lymphoid leukosis
	fatty marrow	broiler	infectious anemia
Body cavity	broken yolk	pullets	bluecomb, cholera, colibacillosis, infectious bronchitis, pullorum
Breast	dried out	chicks	infectious bursal disease
		young	ulcerative enteritis
		hens	gout (visceral)
		2 years	tuberculosis
	blood spotted	all	erysipelas
	white streaks	chicks	white muscle disease
		pullets	bluecomb
Ceca	cheesy core	chicks	arizonosis, blackhead, coccidiosis, salmonellosis
	bloody	chicks	coccidiosis
	yellow nodules	young	ulcerative enteritis
		all	erysipelas
	yellowish, watery	young	rotaviral enteritis
Cloacal bursa	swollen, cheesy	chicks	infectious bursal disease
	shriveled	young	infectious anemia
		young	runting syndrome
	tumors	any	lymphoid leukosis
Crop	empty or foul fluid	young	canker
	sour	growing	thrush
		pullets	bluecomb
		mature	crop impaction
	maggots	all	botulism
	sticky mucus	mature	cholera
	Turkish-towel look	growing	thrush

Body Part	*Finding*	*Age/Sex*	*Possible Cause*
Heart	film covered	young	air-sac disease
		all	chronic respiratory disease
	discolored	chicks	arizonosis
	pale, yellowish	all	fatty liver syndrome
	pale, enlarged	young	listeriosis
		mature	streptococcosis
		all	spirochetosis
	yellow, enlarged	growing	round heart disease
	spotted, enlarged	chicks	pullorum
	enlarged right side	growing	broiler ascites
	surrounded with fluid	all	cholera
	tumors	all	lymphoid leukosis
Intestine	mucus filled	young	infectious bursal disease
		pullets	bluecomb
		all	ochratoxicosis
	greenish mucus	all	spirochetosis
	watery mucus	all	campylobacteriosis
	sticky mucus	mature	cholera
	bloody mucus	all	colibacillosis
	bloody	chicks	coccidiosis
		all	leucocytozoonosis
	foul brown fluid	young	necrotic enteritis
	yellowish buttons	young	ulcerative enteritis
	yellowish, watery	young	rotaviral enteritis
	inflamed, slimy	all	typhoid
	inflamed	all	ergotism
		all	paratyphoid
	spotted	chicks	coccidiosis
		all	pullorum
	pale, distended	young	infectious stunting syndrome
	feed-filled	young	sudden death syndrome
	yellow or gray knobs	2 years	tuberculosis
Kidneys	grayish dots	all	colibacillosis
	spotted, pale	growing	infectious synovitis
	swollen	chicks	salmonellosis
		mature	lymphoid leukosis
		all	paratyphoid, typhoid, erysipelas
	swollen, spotted	growing	Marek's disease
		all	pseudomonas
	swollen, dark	pullets	bluecomb
	swollen, pale	chicks	infectious bursal disease
		all	gout (visceral), infectious bronchitis, ochractoxicosis, spirochetosis

(chart continues, over)

Chart 10-1

Postmortem Findings (cont.)

Body Part	*Finding*	*Age/Sex*	*Possible Cause*
Kidneys (cont.)	blood-filled	growing	infectious anemia
	tumors	mature	lymphoid leukosis
	shriveled or enlarged	mature	gout (visceral)
Liver	film-covered	all	air-sac disease, chronic respiratory disease
	swollen	young	necrotic dermatitis
		mature	lymphoid leukosis
		all	algae poisoning, erysipelas
	swollen, mottled, yellow	chicks	arizonosis
	swollen, discolored	growing	broiler ascites
		all	chlamydiosis
	swollen, gray spots	all	cholera
	swollen, gray areas	all	Marek's disease
	swollen, bronze or green	mature	typhoid
	swollen, greenish	growing	infectious synovitis
	swollen, red	chicks	typhoid
	swollen, red streaks/white dots	chicks	paratyphoid
	swollen, white or gray nodules	chicks	pullorum
	swollen, spotted	young	toxoplasmosis
		all	ochratoxicosis, pseudomonas, spirochetosis
	patchy	young	infectious anemia, blackhead, listeriosis
	patchy red or pale	mature	streptococcosis
	mottled with yellow	young	ulcerative enteritis
	mushy	all	histoplasmosis
	mushy, yellow	all	fatty liver syndrome
	dark	pullets	bluecomb
	greenish	all	colibacillosis
	greenish with red spots	growing	infectious anemia
	yellow "stars"	pullet	campylobacteriosis
	needle-like crystals	chicks	gout (visceral)
	tumors	growing	Marek's disease
		mature	lymphoid leukosis
	gray or yellow nodules	2 years	tuberculosis
Lungs	green, furry balls	all	aspergillosis
	grayish	chicks	salmonellosis
	grayish yellow	chicks	aspergillosis
	yellow "pearls"	all	aspergillosis
	brownish	all	typhoid
	red, bloated	all	sudden death syndrome
	bloody	young	toxoplasmosis
		growing	broiler ascites
		mature	cholera

Body Part	Finding	Age/Sex	Possible Cause
Lungs (cont.)	white or gray nodules	chicks	pullorum
	tumors	mature	lymphoid leukosis
	solidified	mature	Marek's disease
Spleen	gray or white nodules	2 years	tuberculosis
	gray white tumors	growing	Marek's disease
	swollen	chicks	pullorum
		all	erysipelas, leucocytozoonosis
	swollen, red	young	typhoid
	swollen, dark, soft	all	chlamydiosis
	swollen, spotted	young	ulcerative enteritis, infectious bursal disease
		all	colibacillosis
		all	pseudomonas
	swollen, patchy	all	Marek's disease, spirochetosis
	mushy	all	histoplasmosis
	shriveled	growing	infectious anemia
	tumors	mature	lymphoid leukosis
	gray or yellow nodules	2 years	tuberculosis
Stomach	gray white tumors	growing	Marek's disease
	swollen, bloody	young	infectious stunting syndrome
Ureter	crystals	mature	infectious bronchitis, gout (visceral)

lar disease. Few lesions are specific; most are general, testing your power of observation.

Sometimes you can identify a disease by the organ on which a lesion occurs. Other times you might identify a disease by the combination of lesions you find. When more than one disease is involved, as is often the case, the combination of lesions they produce can be confusing.

As a starting place, look up any lesion you find in the charts in this chapter. Then look up the indicated disease in the alphabetic list in chapter 15 to see if the overall description of that disease matches the condition of your birds.

Documentation

Each time you post a chicken, write down your findings in your flock history, even if you aren't sure what disease the bird might have. The information may become helpful later on, especially if a serious disease is progressing through your flock.

Veterinarian Arthur A. Bickford, a poultry pathologist in California, suggests that you not worry about trying to use proper technical jargon. Just write down what you see. If you're not sure what you're looking at, but you know something isn't right, jot down the location and describe it as "abnormal." If you don't know whether you're looking at a tumor or an abscess, write "lump." Getting too specific when you're not sure may cause confusion if you later submit your notes to a diagnostic lab.

Tissue Samples

If you find similar lesions in several birds, you might send tissue samples to the path lab for examination. Sending samples is particularly handy if the lab is not close enough for you to conveniently drop off whole birds. As with submitting whole birds, call the lab in advance to make sure you include everything the pathologist will need.

To make a tissue sample of the organ involved, take a slice at least ¼ inch (1 cm) thick. Include healthy-looking tissue as well as abnormal tissue. Place the sample in a clean, unbreakable container and cover the sample with 10 percent formaldehyde solution. (If you can't get formaldehyde from your druggist or veterinarian, you might get a little from a local high school or college biology lab or from a funeral home. Call first, and bring your own container — these sources are not in the business of distributing formaldehyde.)

Be sure the container holding the sample is sealed well so it won't leak. Pack it in a carton surrounded by plastic peanuts or an ample amount of other packing material. Include the same detailed history of the disease you would prepare if you were submitting whole birds.

Inflammation

An inflammation or swelling is only one kind of lesion, but the most common one. Inflamed conditions are identified by the suffix "itis" following the technical name for the body part that's inflamed. If it all sounds like Greek to you, that's because it is — the medical terms for various body parts are derived from the Greek language.

Words ending in "itis" are not necessarily diseases, but are often caused by several different diseases. It's helpful to know the names of the various "itises" when you're trying to understand a pathology report or a disease description in a technical poultry manual. (See next page for a list of inflamed conditions.)

Diagnosing Nutritional Deficiencies

Like infectious diseases, nutritional deficiencies may cause gross lesions that, together with other symptoms, can be used to identify the cause. Since nutritional deficiencies are no longer common, their characteristic lesions are listed separately here, along with additional symptoms as a diagnostic aid. For a fuller description of nutritional problems, see the section on nutritional diseases in chapter 2.

CHART 10-2

Inflamed Conditions

Condition	*Body Part*	*Common Cause*
Airsacculitis	air sacs	chlamydiosis colibacillosis mycoplasmosis
Arthritis	joints ("arthron")	colibacillosis mycoplasmosis salmonellosis staphylococcosis viruses
Conjunctivitis	eye lining ("conjunctiva")	ammonia fumes eye worm
Encephalitis	brain ("enkephalos")	encephalomalacia listeriosis
Enteritis	intestine ("enteron")	colibacillosis salmonellosis
Hepatitis	liver ("hepatos")	blackhead campylobacteriosis infectious anemia
Nephritis	kidney ("nephros")	colibacillosis gout (visceral) viruses
Pericarditis	membrane surrounding abdominal organs ("peritoneum")	colibacillosis cholera
Rhinitis	nasal passage lining ("rhinos")	streptococcosis
Salpingitis	oviduct ("salpinx")	*Escherichia coli*
Septicemia	blood ("septikos" = putrefaction; "hamia" = blood)	*Escherichia coli* pasteurellosis salmonellosis streptococcosis
Sinusitis	sinus cavities	*Mycoplasma gallisepticum*
Synovitus	membranes lining joints ("synovium")	*Escherichia coli* mycoplasmosis salmonellosis *Streptobacillus moniliformis* viruses

Chart 10-3

Nutritionally Related Findings

Age/Sex	*Finding*	*Additional Symptoms*	*Deficiency*
chicks	swollen hip nerve, toes curved inward	walking on hocks	riboflavin
	blue green gelatinous fluid under skin	bluish breast and legs	selenium
	soft, swollen, greenish yellow brain; *or* bluish green fluid under skin and blood spots in leg and breast muscles; *or* light streaks in breast muscles	retracted head, prostration, death	vitamin E
growing	blood spots in muscles, slow blood clotting, pale marrow	pale comb, bleeding wattles, bleeding eye	vitamin K
hen	broken yolks in body cavity	shrunken, bluish combs, wattles, prominent leg tendons on back of legs	water
all	swollen kidney, crystals in ureter	off-color droppings, shrunken muscles	water
	white sores in mouth and throat	watery diarrhea, sticky eyes and nose	vitamin A
	soft keel, collapsed ribs	weak legs, soft beak	vitamin D

Disposing of Dead Birds

Before you dispose of a dead bird, check local laws. Legal methods for disposing of animal bodies vary from place to place. For public health reasons, depositing them in a dumpster or local landfill is illegal nearly everywhere.

When the bodies are those of diseased birds, find a disposal method that prevents the spread of infectious agents or toxins. Do not bury them in a compost pile — the warm, moist environment may provide perfect conditions for pathogens to keep multiplying, and flies and rodents may spread the disease.

The two best disposal methods are burial and burning. Bury bodies deeply so they can't be dug up by dogs or wild animals. Find a spot far from wells, streams, and other water sources. While you're at it, bury all contaminated litter, feed, and droppings associated with the diseased birds.

Burning may be necessary where the water table is high, the soil is rocky or frozen, or burying is prohibited by law but burning is not. You'll need a heap of combustible materials — scrap wood or tree prunings, along with dry straw for a hot blaze. Make sure the carcasses are fully burned, then bury the ashes.

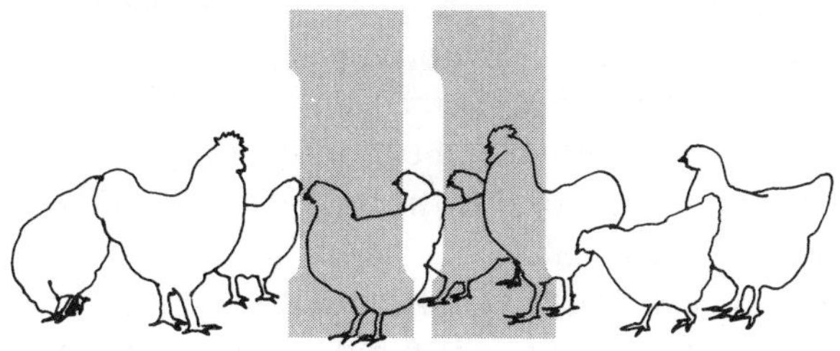

Therapy

SOME CHICKEN DISEASES CAN BE CURED if treatment starts early. Others are irreversible or fatal. By the time chickens show obvious signs of illness, the disease is usually pretty far along. Recognizing a disease as soon as it starts is the first step toward curing the ones that are temporary and dealing effectively with those that are permanent or irreversible. The longer you wait before you take action, the more difficult treatment or control becomes, and the more losses you may incur.

Treating Sick Birds

Attempting to treat a flock without knowing what's wrong can be costly, may result in continuing losses, and could make the disease worse. For example, if you treat chickens with a drug that's appropriate for coccidiosis when in fact they have infectious anemia (a disease with similar symptoms), you will make matters significantly worse.

Once you identify the problem, you have three choices:

- cull the affected birds
- wait until the disease goes away
- embark on a course of therapy

In this context, cull means kill. When a condition is serious, sometimes the only humane approach is to put the birds out of their misery. Some serious diseases should not be cured because recovered birds will be carriers, continuing to spread disease intermittently or continuously, for the rest of their lives. Other diseases are so contagious that the only way to keep them from spreading is to destroy the diseased flock.

If you are raising chickens to get healthful meat, you may prefer to cull diseased birds and start over, rather than run the risk of eating meat containing drug residue or disease-causing microbes — some of which can harm humans. By contrast, a commercial producer tries to bring as many birds as possible to market with a minimum of downgraded or condemned carcasses.

If you're raising an endangered or exhibition breed, you'll likely wish to preserve the gene pool by keeping breeders going until you can hatch enough eggs to perpetuate the flock — an approach that works only if the disease does not spread through hatching eggs. You must, of course, raise the new chicks away from diseased adults, cull the diseased breeder flock as soon as possible, and meticulously clean up their housing with an appropriate disinfectant.

Waiting until the problem goes away works only if the disease is self-limiting, meaning it naturally runs its course in a short time and birds recover on their own. Few diseases fall into that category. A good number of diseases lie somewhere between serious and self-limiting, and can be effectively treated with drugs.

Drug Use

Many non-prescription drugs are available from farm and feed stores and through mail-order catalogs. Such over-the-counter drugs are considered safe when they are used according to directions on the label. Whether you obtain a drug over the counter or by a veterinarian's prescription, it will be effective only if you have selected the right drug for the disease and know when to use it, how to use it, how often to use it, and how much to use. In addition:

- Avoid out-of-date drugs.
- Store drugs at 35 to 55°F (1.5-12.5°C), away from sunlight.
- Administer a drug only as directed — If it's supposed to be given by mouth, for example, it may be toxic as an injection.
- Observe the safe dosage level — The drug won't be effective in an amount less than the label specifies, and may be toxic in greater amounts.
- Observe the withdrawal time when treating meat birds or laying hens.
- Do not combine drugs or use more than one at a time, unless such a combination is approved by a veterinarian.

Administering Drugs

For a drug to be effective, it must reach the infectious microbes in sufficient quantity and remain in contact long enough to do the job. Most drugs should be administered for at least 3 days, or for 2 days after the symptoms disappear, whichever is longest. As a general rule, if you do not see some improvement within 2 days, you are using the wrong drug.

How you administer a drug depends on the drug you use, the disease you're treating, the number of birds involved, their condition, and the length of time the drug must be administered. Drugs can be applied:

- topically
- orally
- by inhalation
- by injection

Topical or local medications are applied directly to the skin, eyes, nose, or other external organs. Examples of topical drugs are antibiotic powders or ointments used to prevent infection of wounds, and liquids applied to an infected eye.

Oral medications are given by mouth. They work either by controlling microbes in the intestine or by being absorbed through the intestine to be distributed to other parts of the body. Oral drugs take effect slowly, usually in 4 to 12 hours, depending on the drug used, the bird's metabolic rate, and the amount of feed in its crop. Oral drugs are convenient and safe, but can be unpredictable in their absorption rates, especially when a bird has diarrhea. Examples of oral medications are tablets, capsules, feed or water additives, and drenches.

Drenching

A liquid medication, or "drench," is inserted into a chicken's mouth by means of a syringe fitted with a short piece of plastic tubing that lets you squirt the liquid into the bird's throat—taking care not to get any into the windpipe.

Inhaled medications work against microbes in the respiratory system or are absorbed through the respiratory system to be carried to other parts of the body. Such a drug may be a liquid solution applied by means of a fine mist or a dust puffed into the air. Specialized equipment is needed to put particles of just the right size and density into the air, making the use of inhaled drugs impractical for small flocks.

Injected medications, which take effect rapidly, are inserted with a needle and syringe into one of three places: beneath the skin, into the muscle, or into the bloodstream.

Shots, tablets, and drenches are suitable for treating individual chickens.

They ensure that each bird gets an adequate dose, but administering them is time-consuming and handling each bird can increase stress and aggravate the disease.

Drugs administered by feed, water, or through the air are suitable where a large number of birds are involved or the drug must be administered over a long period of time. Although flock administration saves time, you can never be sure each bird gets an adequate dose.

Feed and Water Additives

When medications are added to feed or water, low birds in the peck order may not spend enough time at the trough to obtain a sufficient dose. Furthermore, there's always the danger that birds won't eat or drink at all, or will eat or drink to excess and overdose.

If a medication must be administered by means of feed or water, adding it to water is preferable for two reasons:

- many diseases cause appetite loss and increased thirst;
- on a small scale, diluting a drug in water is easier than trying to stir it evenly into feed.

Some small-scale flock owners medicate feed or drinking water either routinely or during times of stress as a precaution against disease. The practice is not only expensive but counterproductive, since it has little or no effect in preventing disease, and can cause resistant strains of microbes to develop so that drugs won't work if a disease does strike.

Commercial growers add low levels of drugs to rations to improve egg pro-

Diluting Medications

When a drug label calls for medicating feed at a level of 200 parts per million (ppm), an equivalent amount in drinking water would be 400 milligrams per gallon (assuming chickens consume twice as much water as feed).

When instructions call for diluting a drug 1:2000 in water, combine:

drug	*with water*
2 tablespoons (1 ounce)	**16 gallons**
1 tablespoon (½ ounce)	**8 gallons**
½ tablespoon* (¼ ounce)	**4 gallons**
1 teaspoon	**2½ gallons**
½ teaspoon	**5 quarts**

*You can find a ½ tablespoon measure with the canning and freezing supplies at most discount department stores. An equivilent measure is 1½ teaspoons.

duction and to stimulate the growth rate and feed-conversion efficiency of broilers. For unknown reasons, antibiotics cause a bird's intestinal wall to thin, improving nutrient absorption. But the routine non-medicinal use of antibiotics in food-producing flocks leads to antibiotic resistance in humans as well as in the chickens (see "Antibiotic Residues," page 191).

Injections

Whenever you administer a drug by injection, use a fresh or sterile needle and syringe. To sterilize a used needle and syringe, separate them, boil them in clean water for 15 minutes, dry them on a clean paper towel, and store them in a clean, dust-free place.

If you use the same needle to inject more than one bird, before refilling the syringe between birds, dip the needle in alcohol (unless you are applying a live-virus vaccine), or pass the needle through a match flame. Keep extra needles on hand in case the one you're using gets too dull to pierce easily.

Use a 20-gauge needle, ¾ inch (.75 cm) long for chicks, 2-inches (5 cm) long for mature birds. Syringes are marked off in cubic centimeters (cc) and portions thereof. Drug dosages are specified either in ccs or in ccs per pound of weight. To determine how many ccs you need, multiply the bird's weight by the number of ccs per pound. Sometimes dosages are given in milliliters (ml). Since 1 ml equals 1.000027 cc, for practical purposes they are the same. Use a syringe large enough to hold the entire dose in one shot.

Subcutaneous injections (SC or SQ) are given directly under the skin, usually at the breast or the nape of the neck where the skin is loose. Pick up a pinch of skin and insert the needle at an angle. If you're injecting chicks, take care not to push the needle all the way through the skin and squirt the drug out the other side (or into your thumb). A subcutaneous injection is easy and safe to administer and lasts a long time — up to 2 days. On the other hand, the drug takes effect slowly because it requires a long time to migrate to the bloodstream for distribution throughout the body.

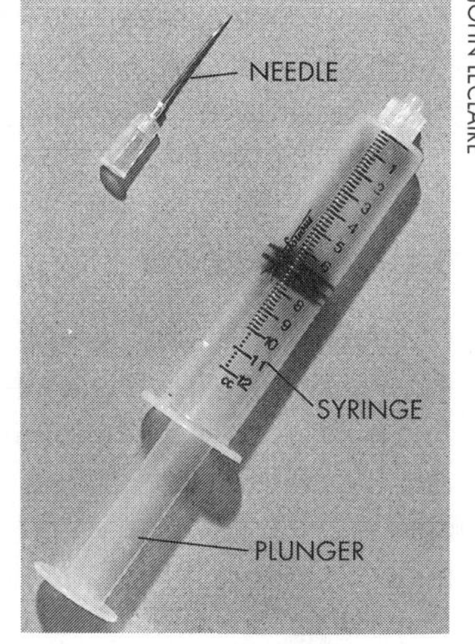

JOHN LECLAIRE

Intramuscular injections (IM) go into the meaty portion of the breast. They take effect fast — in about an hour — and last about 8 hours, but you must take care not to touch a bone or nerve, or deposit the drug into fat or the bloodstream. Insert the needle straight into the breast muscle, at a right angle. Before injecting the drug, pull back on the plunger. If blood appears in the syringe, move the needle to another spot. Otherwise, you may kill the bird by inserting the drug directly into its bloodstream.

Intravenous injections (IV) insert medication directly into the bloodstream, where it takes effect almost immediately. They are the trickiest shots to give and should be used only for drugs designed for IV administration, and only on a bird that's comatose, paralyzed, or otherwise in imminent danger of dying— IV administration of *C. botulinum* antitoxin, for example, might be used on a valuable breeder that's been paralyzed by botulism.

An IV injection goes into the main wing vein or brachial (see the box on page 149). First, pull a few feathers from the depression in the upper part of the underside of one wing, so you can better see the main vein. Insert the needle into the vein, pointed toward the wing tip (away from the chicken's body) and depress the plunger to release the drug *very* slowly.

Antibiotics

All drugs derived from fungi or bacteria and used against other living organisms are called antibiotics (*anti* meaning against and *biotic* referring to living organisms), or sometimes antimicrobials. The use of antibiotics and other chemicals is controlled by the FDA (Food and Drug Administration), USDA (United States Department of Agriculture), and EPA (Environmental Protection Agency). With all these agencies involved, it's not surprising that regulations change constantly. If you want to know the current status of any drug to be used on chickens, consult the *Code of Federal Regulations, The Federal Register,* and the *Feed Additives Compendium* (all listed in the appendix).

Antibiotics fall into six basic categories:

- anthelmintic — against worms (discussed in chapter 5)
- anti-protozoal — against protozoa (see chapter 6)
- antiviral — against viruses
- anti-fungal — against mold and fungi
- antibacterial — against bacteria

Antiviral Agents

Viruses are difficult to treat with drugs, and to date no safe, broad-spectrum antiviral drug has been discovered. A virus in the environment neither eats nor breathes, and is therefore impervious. Once a virus attaches itself to a cell in a chicken's body, any drug that harms the virus tends also to harm the infected cell. Treatment of viral diseases largely involves alleviating symptoms (in a respiratory infection, for example, using a product such as Vicks or VetRx to open up blocked airways) and keeping the bird as comfortable as possible while its immune system fights the virus.

Antiviral drugs may soon become available that either keep viruses from invading cells or interfere with their replication within a cell. The most promising of these is interferon. When a virus attacks a cell, the cell produces the natural protein, interferon, that keeps the virus from multiplying and infecting additional cells. The problem is that insufficient amounts of interferon are within the body produced to stop an especially virulent virus.

Interferon can be artificially produced and has successfully been used in massive doses to treat a variety of viral diseases, including influenza and Newcastle. It may also be combined with vaccines to provide temporary protection while immunity is developing. Interferon may soon become less expensive and more readily available.

Anti-fungal Agents

Fungal diseases, like viral diseases, do not respond well to drug treatment. Not only are fungi somewhat impervious to drugs, but drugs interfere with a chicken's natural microflora, making room for fungi to run rampant — the reason fungal infections commonly follow the use of antibiotics in treating other diseases.

Copper sulfate ($CuSO_4$), also known as "powdered bluestone," is toxic to fungi and can be used to prevent or control many fungal diseases. Clean feeders, waterers, and other equipment with an 0.5 percent solution. Treat birds with a 1:2000 concentration in drinking water (½ teaspoon per gallon) every other day for a week. *Take care* — a concentration of 1:500 or greater is toxic to chickens. Due to the possibility of a chemical reaction between copper sulfate and galvanized metal, **do not use a metal waterer.**

Superficial mycotic infections are treated with topical medications such as amphotericin B (trade name Fungizone), gentian violet, iodine, and nystatin (trade name Mycostatin, among others). Any drug used to treat a fungal infection (ringworm, athlete's foot, etc.) of pets or humans can be tried on a chicken. You can't tell in advance what will work, since fungi are resistant to many drugs. Furthermore successful treatment requires persistence, since a chicken with a superficial fungal disease infects other birds and reinfects itself.

Antibacterials

Most antibiotics are antibacterials, and some antibacterials work against fungi and protozoa as well as bacteria, so the two words are often considered synonymous. A narrow-spectrum antibacterial is effective against a specific bacteria or group of bacteria. A broad-spectrum antibacterial is effective against numerous kinds.

Whether an antibacterial is narrow-spectrum or broad-spectrum, its effectiveness will be reduced in a bird that has been infected for a long time or whose immunity has been weakened due to poor sanitation, malnutrition, or the presence of a viral infection. Although antibacterials have no effect against viruses, they are often used in treating viral diseases to keep weakened birds from getting a secondary bacterial infection.

Antibacterials that destroy bacteria are called "bactericidal." Antibacterials that retard the growth of bacteria, thereby giving the immune system time to produce antibodies and otherwise rally its own defenses, are called "bacteriostatic."

Sulfonamides or sulfa drugs were introduced in the 1930s as the first medications used to treat infection. Originally they were effective against a wide range of bacteria. Many bacteria have since become resistant, particularly staphylococci, clostridia, and pseudomonas. Nevertheless, sulfa drugs are still used today because of their low cost relative to their effectiveness. They should not, however, be used to treat laying hens.

The sulfonamide group includes several related drugs, easily identified because their names almost always start with "sulfa." They fall into two categories:

- rapidly absorbed and rapidly excreted, requiring treatment one to four times a day;
- rapidly absorbed and slowly excreted, allowing treatment only once every second or third day.

Most sulfonamides are bacteriostatic, but some can be bactericidal, depending on the drug, the dose, and the bacteria involved. Sometimes three different sulfonamides are combined to create a more effective tablet or liquid medication called "triple sulfa."

Sulfa drugs are added to drinking water for the treatment of bumblefoot, toxoplasmosis, a variety of respiratory infections, systemic colibacillosis (often in combination with penicillin G), and coccidiosis (see "Drugs Used to Treat Coccidiosis," page 103). The sulfas work best when treatment starts in the early stages of infection. A chicken usually shows improvement within 3 days, but should be treated for an additional 2 days after symptoms disappear.

In any case, sulfa treatment should not go on longer than 7 days or the result may be kidney damage and/or vitamin K deficiency (interfering with blood clotting). In addition, if a chicken does not drink enough water during treatment, its pH balance becomes too acidic. If prolonged treatment is necessary, add 1 tablespoon of sodium bicarbonate (baking soda) per gallon to the drinking water.

The *penicillins* are a large group of antibiotics derived from mold and identified by names ending in "cillin." The first penicillin was discovered in

1928 by a bacteriologist named Fleming who wanted to know why bacteria do not grow in the presence of mold. When penicillin was first used in 1941, it was considered a miracle drug and was administered so indiscriminately that many strains of bacteria have become resistant.

The penicillins may be bactericidal or bacteriostatic — depending on the sensitivity or resistance of the bacteria involved — and are used to treat a variety of acute infections. They fall into two types:

- Natural penicillin (such as penicillin G) works against a narrow spectrum of bacteria, including some strains of staphylococci, streptococci, and *E. coli.* It is sensitive to light and heat, so is usually mixed just before it is used. Natural penicillin is poorly absorbed by the intestine, and so must be administered by intramuscular injection.
- Semi-synthetic derivatives (such as ampicillin and amoxicillin) absorb better than natural penicillins and can be given orally. They work against a broader spectrum of bacteria that have become resistant to natural penicillins, including most strains of *E. coli* and *Salmonella.*

Tetracyclines, the first broad-spectrum antibiotics, all have names ending in "cycline." There are three naturally occurring tetracyclines and a number of their derivatives, all bacteriostatic against the same kinds of microbe — some chlamydia, staphylococci, streptococci, mycoplasmas, and a few other groups (but not most strains of *E. coli).*

The tetracycline most often used for chickens is oxytetracycline (trade name Terramycin), which comes both in injectable form and in a powder to be added to drinking water. Since it works best in an acidic environment, its absorption rate can be improved by adding 1 cup of cranberry juice, ½ cup of vinegar, or 2 teaspoons of citric acid (from the canning department of a grocery store) to each gallon of drinking water. To further increase the drug's effectiveness, discontinue calcium supplements during treatment. Despite the broad spectrum of tetracyclines, they work rather poorly and are used in industry primarily as growth promoters.

Aminoglycosides get their name from the fact that each contains at least one sugar (glycoside) attached to one or more amino groups. They kill bacteria that multiply rapidly — such as those causing enteric and septicemic diseases — after only brief contact, but the drugs have no lasting effect. The group includes:

- Gentamicin (trade name Garasol), a very broad spectrum antibacterial administered as an intramuscular or subcutaneous injection to treat systemic infections, particularly those caused by *E. coli.*
- Neomycin, used for staphylococcal skin infections such as bumblefoot and infected breast blister. As a topical antibiotic, neomycin comes in powder form (trade name Neo-Predef) or as an ointment (trade name

Neosporin, among others). Neomycin sulfate is used orally to treat diarrhea caused by susceptible *E. coli* and *Salmonella.*

- Streptomycin, given as an intramuscular or subcutaneous injection, works against a fairly narrow range of susceptible *E. coli, Pasteurella, Salmonella,* and staphylococci.

Aminoglycosides are often combined with penicillin to create synergism — a phenomenon whereby two drugs applied together have a greater total effect than the sum of their individual effects. An example of a synergistic combination is penicillin and streptomycin (trade name Combiotic, among others).

Erythromycin (trade name Gallimycin) belongs to a group of broad-spectrum drugs called "macrolides". It is so similar to penicillin that it is often considered an alternative. It is basically a bacteriostat, but in large doses can be bacteriocidal. Erythromycin is used to treat superficial staphylococcal and streptococcal infections, as well as chlamydiosis, mycoplasmosis, and salmonellosis. It is usually given orally, but absorption is poor unless the stomach is empty. An intramuscular injection absorbs more rapidly, but causes swelling and pain.

Bacitracin (trade name Solu-tracin 50) is similar in range to penicillin G, but does not absorb well in the intestine and is relatively toxic when given as an injection. It is mainly used topically to treat staphylococcal and streptococcal infections of the skin and mucous membranes. (It is also used in industry as a growth promoter.) Besides being bacteriocidal, bacitracin is also both fungistatic and fungicidal. Combined with neomycin, it's sold as the antibacterial ointment, Neosporin.

Antibiotic Reactions

Antibiotics can cause reactions that are as bad as, or worse than, the disease they're used to treat. For starters, they upset the balance of normal microflora in a chicken's body, particularly in its digestive tract, paving the way for entry by additional disease-causing bacteria and fungi. A classic symptom is diarrhea, which can be fatal if the drug is not discontinued.

Long-term use of sulfa drugs can cause vitamin K deficiency due to inhibition of the microflora that normally synthesize this important vitamin responsible for normal blood clotting. Infectious anemia may result unless the drug is either discontinued or supplemented with vitamin K.

Anaphylactic shock, a violent allergic reaction, may result from repeated antibiotic injections. Symptoms are paleness and rapid loss of consciousness. Swelling within the respiratory system may cause death through asphyxiation.

Antibiotic Resistance

The routine use by commercial growers of low levels of antibiotics, particularly penicillin and tetracycline, has caused more and more bacteria to become resistant to these drugs. The drug-resistant strains are spread through the use of slaughterhouse wastes as protein in rations. Since slaughterhouse wastes also contain antibiotic residues, feeding a flock rations that contain them encourages the further mutation of drug-resistant strains.

When a diseased flock is treated with a drug, strains that are sensitive to that drug are destroyed, while resistant strains survive. As a result, bacterial diseases, particularly cholera, colibacillosis, pseudomonas, salmonellosis, and staphylococcosis, are becoming more difficult to treat. Successful treatment requires a sensitivity test to determine which drug will work against the strain causing the disease.

Antibiotic Residues

When you medicate birds raised for meat or eggs, take special care to observe any precautions highlighted with the double Arrow Universal Warning Symbol. One important piece of information you'll find in the "warning" section of the label is the drug's withdrawal time.

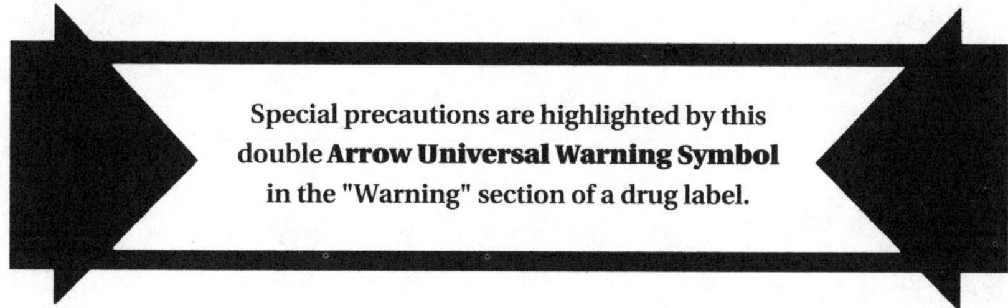

When a drug is absorbed, it is first distributed throughout the chicken's body tissue and fluid, and then is gradually eliminated through the filtering processes of the kidneys and liver. Different drugs are eliminated at different rates.

The withdrawal time on a drug label tells you the drug's elimination rate, or the number of days that must pass between the time you discontinue the drug and the time you butcher the birds for food. Remember, the withdrawal time is the minimum required by law — it doesn't hurt to err on the side of caution and add a few extra days. Before you start collecting eggs to eat, add 10 days to any withdrawal time specified for meat birds, since substances can be deposited in an egg as long as 10 days before it is laid.

Antibiotic residues in meat and eggs are harmful to humans in at least three ways:

1. They disturb the natural balance of microflora in the intestines and elsewhere.

2. They may cause microbes to become resistant to drugs prescribed by a physician.

3. They can cause a severe reaction in people who are allergic to penicillin or sulfa drugs.

Flushes

When a chicken suffers from an intestinal disease or from food poisoning, you can hasten its recovery by flushing its system with a laxative that absorbs toxins and removes them from the body. Although Epsom salts make the best flush, chickens must be handled individually, since they don't like the taste of an Epsom-salt solution and won't readily drink it. When a number of birds are involved, or handling the birds would cause undue stress, use molasses in a flock flush. Flush only adult birds, never chicks.

Epsom-salt flush: 1 teaspoon Epsom salts (magnesium sulfate) in ½ cup water, poured or squirted down the bird's throat twice daily for 2 or 3 days, or until the bird recovers.

Molasses flush: 1 pint molasses per 5 gallons water, given for no longer than 8 hours.

Supportive Therapy

Any time you treat diseased birds, isolate them away from the rest of the flock. After they have been moved, avoid moving them again to minimize stress. When you tend your flock, take care of healthy birds first, so you won't spread disease from the sick ones to the healthy ones.

Be sure the sick birds get plenty of clean water and fresh feed. Since many diseases cause a chicken to eat less, feed often to stimulate appetites. If necessary, move feed and water troughs so they'll be easier for the birds to reach. Increase the number of waterers so the birds won't run out of water during the day, and so those crowded around a waterer won't discourage others from drinking. Encourage drinking by providing cool water in summer and warm water in winter.

Provide good ventilation so the chickens won't keep breathing the same stale air, but avoid cold drafts that cause chilling. In cool weather, supply additional heat, especially if the birds are young. Pay special attention to sanitation so the population of pathogens can't build up and reduce the birds' resistance even further — drain puddles from the yard, keep droppings out of feed and water, and make sure litter is deep and clean.

Vitamin Therapy

Boost a flock's ability to fight disease, and minimize the chance of a secondary infection, by adding a vitamin supplement to the drinking water. A vitamin supplement can also be used to guard against disease in times of stress, such as during a move, before and after a show, during breeding season, or when the weather is particularly unpleasant. Chicks will get a healthy start if you treat them to a vitamin supplement throughout their first 3 weeks of life.

Electrolytes

Dehydration caused by diarrhea, worms, and other conditions depletes body fluids of certain minerals known as "electrolytes." They are called electrolytes because, when dissolved in water, they split into electrically charged particles (ions) that transmit electrical impulses. The electrolytes — calcium, chloride, magnesium, phosphorus, potassium, and sodium — play a vital role in regulating body processes and in maintaining both hydration and the body's acid/base balance.

Any time a chicken has diarrhea, or otherwise suffers from dehydration, help its body replace and retain fluids by adding an electrolyte supplement (brand name Vita-Tone, among others) to its drinking water at the rate of 1 teaspoon per gallon for at least a week.

Homemade Electrolyte Solution

If you do not have an electrolyte supplement on hand, this homemade version will get you through in a pinch.

Ingredient	*Source*
⅓ teaspoon potassium chloride	**salt substitute**
½ teaspoon sodium bicarbonate	**baking soda**
1 teaspoon sodium chloride	**table salt**
1 quart water	

Use this solution in place of drinking water for at least 1 week.

Competitive Exclusion

Antibiotics disrupt the microflora that normally live in a chicken's intestines and work in cooperation with the bird's immune system. To restore the balance of microflora following drug treatment, feed each chicken a heaping tablespoon of plain active-culture yogurt every day for a week. The process of controlling beneficial microflora to help fend off disease is called "competitive exclusion" — the beneficial microflora provide stiff *competition* that *excludes* pathogens.

A relatively new idea in the poultry world is the use of competitive exclusion to minimize bacterial diseases by feeding newly hatched chicks the kind of bacteria that naturally live in the digestive tract of an adult chicken. The beneficial immunity-enhancing microflora then have a chance to get established before the chicks come into contact with pathogens. You can give chicks a boost in the right direction by occasionally feeding them a tiny amount of yogurt, but take care — it doesn't take much yogurt to cause diarrhea.

Treating Wounds

Any injury in a poultry flock must be treated promptly, or it will attract picking that quickly becomes cannibalism. Wounds can be caused by faulty equipment, nails protruding from walls, serious fighting, and even mating. Cocks, usually of the heavier breeds, sometimes rub the protective feathers from a hen's back during successive matings until no feathers are left to keep the cock's claws from cutting through the hen's skin.

As soon as you discover an injured bird, isolate it. Clean broken tissue from the wound by pouring hydrogen peroxide over it. As the hydrogen peroxide bubbles up, it lifts organic matter so it can be rinsed away with more hydrogen peroxide. If the injury is serious, remove feathers from around the edges so they can't stick in the wound and hinder healing.

When the wound is clean, coat it with neomycin in the form of Neo-Predef powder (for an oozing wound) or Neosporin ointment (for a dry wound). If the injury is on the bird's foot or is quite large, wrap it in a gauze bandage and tape the bandage in place. To keep pus from forming and giving bacteria a place to grow, change the dressing daily, clean the injury with hydrogen peroxide, and reapply neomycin.

Treating Shock

Shock is a condition brought on by a serious wound or other severe stress, such as an allergic reaction to antibiotics or being chased and caught by a dog and shaken in the dog's mouth. Shock causes pale skin, reduced circulation, rapid weak pulse, rapid breathing, subnormal body temperature, weakness, and sometimes prostration and death. If the bird is valuable enough to warrant the expense, and a vet is close enough at hand, the bird may recover after veterinary treatment with steroids and fluids. Otherwise, all you can do is keep the bird warm and calm until it either recovers or dies.

Surgery

Surgery is rarely performed on chickens, due to their relatively low economic value. On those rare occasions when surgery is performed, it is done to:

- caponize broiler cocks (no longer necessary, with today's improved strains that grow bigger and faster on less feed);
- decrow a valuable breeder cock (requires the services of a skilled veterinarian);
- debeak birds to prevent cannibalism (see "Debeaking," page 138);
- dub and crop fighting cocks and chickens raised in cold climates (see "Dubbing and Cropping," page 133);
- clean out an impacted crop (see "Crop Impaction," page 264).

Following surgery, treat the surgical wound as you would any other wound, as described above.

What Went Wrong?

If, despite your best efforts, sick chickens don't get better, one or more of the following may be the cause.

- **The diagnosis was wrong.**
- **The organism causing the disease is resistant to the drug used.**
- **An inadequate dose of the drug was used.**
- **The drug was administered improperly (reread the label).**
- **The drug's expiration date has long since passed (try a fresh batch).**
- **An incompatible combination of drugs was used.**
- **The drug caused adverse side effects.**
- **The bird was reinfected (medication was discontinued too soon).**
- **An inflammation, abscess, or other condition interfered with drug action.**
- **The bird has more than one infection and not all of them were treated.**
- **Disease was caused by a nutritional deficiency that was not corrected.**
- **The bird's defense mechanism is too low (due to the disease, drug use, or poor nutrition).**
- **Supportive therapy was inadequate.**
- **Biosecurity breach was not corrected (look for ways to improve management).**

Reportable Diseases

Some diseases are so serious they must be reported either to the federal Animal and Plant Health Inspection Service or to your state pathology laboratory. Each state has its own regulations as to which diseases are reportable. Diseases that are designated as reportable are a serious threat either to the poultry industry or to public (human) health. If your flock experiences a sudden, high death rate (over 50 percent in a short time), you would do well to report it to your state veterinarian.

If a veterinary or pathology lab diagnoses a reportable disease in your flock, they are bound by law to report it. The immediate result will be quarantine of your flock to keep the disease from spreading. In some cases, you may be allowed to treat your birds under strict supervision. In other cases, you may be required to depopulate — a polite way of saying your entire flock will be destroyed. If you keep chickens for commercial purposes, you *may* be reimbursed for your loss.

Even when your flock is not involved, if a reportable disease occurs in your area, the movement of all birds may be restricted. Restriction of movement does not occur as often with birds as it does with larger livestock, especially cattle, horses, and hogs. Exactly how a particular reportable disease is handled depends on the nature and scope of the outbreak and on the virulence and contagiousness of the pathogen involved.

CHART 11-1

Reportable Diseases

Governing Body	*Disease*	*Threat To*
Federal*	chlamydiosis	public health
	Newcastle (exotic)	poultry industry
	influenza (lethal form)	poultry industry
	paratyphoid (*Salmonella enteritidis*)	public health
	spirochetosis	poultry industry
Most states	pullorum	poultry industry
	typhoid	poultry industry
Many states	chronic respiratory disease	poultry industry
	infectious laryngotracheitis	poultry industry

*United States Department of Agriculture, Animal and Plant Health Inspection Service, Federal Building, Hyattsville, MD 20782.

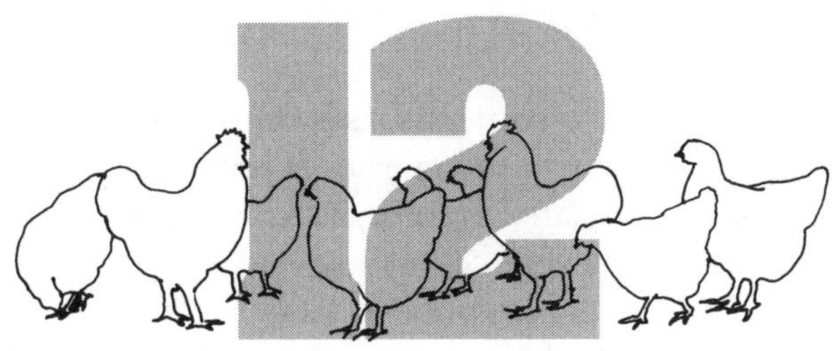

Enhancing Immunity

IMMUNITY IS THE ABILITY OF THE BODY TO RESIST INFECTION. Another word for immunity is resistance; the opposite of immunity is susceptibility. A chick hatches with a certain amount of innate immunity and acquires new immunities as it grows, but may need your help to develop additional immunity against diseases in its environment.

Immunity

Immunity can be broken down into two categories:

1. Inherited — which may be:
   a. complete (all chickens are resistant)
   b. partial (some breeds, strains, or individuals are resistant)
2. Acquired — which may be:
   a. passive, in which antibodies are transferred:
      - naturally, from hen to chick
      - artificially, by an antitoxin
   b. active, in which the production of antibodies is stimulated:
      - naturally, by disease
      - artificially, by vaccination

Inherited Immunity

Chickens are immune to some diseases due to inherited or genetically controlled factors. When the entire species is resistant, immunity is "complete." Chickens have complete immunity to a long list of diseases that infect other birds or animals but never infect chickens.

As a species, chickens are immune to some pathogens they commonly carry in their bodies, but that make them sick if their resistance is broken down. The protozoan *Histomonas meleagridis* is a classic example. It commonly lives in the poultry environment, causing chickens to get blackhead only when their resistance is drastically reduced by a massive infestation. (Turkeys, on the other hand, are highly susceptible to blackhead and often get it from chickens that carry the protozoa without being infected.)

When only certain breeds, strains, or individuals are resistant to a disease, immunity is "partial." Chickens have partial immunity to Marek's disease, since some strains never succumb to the otherwise common killer. In nearly every disease outbreak, some individuals do not become infected due to inherited immunity. Those are the birds you'll want in your breeder flock if you wish to breed for resistance, as described in chapter 1.

Passive Acquired Immunity

Acquired immunity is any resistance to disease that is not inherited, but instead is conferred by antibodies. Passive acquired immunity is resistance due to antibodies produced in the body of one bird or animal and passed on to the body of another. Passive immunity provides immediate but temporary resistance — since the antibodies are not produced within the chicken's own body, immunity is short-term, lasting only about 4 weeks.

Passive immunity may be acquired naturally or artificially. Natural passive immunity is acquired by a chick from a hen via the egg. The source of maternal antibodies is immaterial — they may result from a disease the hen once had or from a vaccination designed specifically to build up her antibodies so she can pass immunity along to her chicks.

Artificial passive immunity is acquired by a chicken when it is given an injection containing antibodies against toxin-producing bacteria. Botulism is an example of a disease caused by bacteria that produce toxins. An antibody that fights a toxin is called an "antitoxin." Fluid taken from the blood of an animal that has been immunized and therefore has antitoxins against a disease such as botulism is also called "antitoxin." An injection of antitoxin confers immediate immunity, and can therefore be used to treat disease. The immunity is only temporary, however, since it is passively acquired.

Active Acquired Immunity

Active immunity differs from passive immunity in three important ways:

- It is caused by antibodies produced within a bird's own body.
- It is not immediate but takes time, usually measured in weeks.
- It is long-term.

Although active immunity is always longer term than passive immunity, it may be temporary (as in the case of staphylococcal and streptococcal infections), it may be permanent (as in the case of typhoid), or it may be permanent *unless* stress weakens the bird's resistance. As a general rule, immunity to viruses is absolute and long lasting, while immunity to bacteria is relative (dependent on stress avoidance) and usually temporary.

Like passive immunity, active immunity can be acquired naturally or artificially. Natural acquired active immunity occurs when a chicken's body produces antibodies to fight a particular disease (see "Immune System," page 44). If the chicken recovers, its body continues to contain antibodies specific to that disease — they confer immunity only to that one disease. A bird can acquire active immunity as an embryo during incubation or at any point after it hatches.

Artificial active immunity is acquired from a vaccination containing antigens that cause a chicken's body to produce antibodies against those particular antigens. Active immunity resulting from vaccination takes about 2 weeks to develop and can be renewed through one or more booster shots to keep the level of antibodies high enough to ward off disease. The booster dose, which is usually smaller than the original vaccination dose, must be administered at a specified time following the original vaccination.

Acquired Immunity

ACTIVE		PASSIVE
NATURAL	ARTIFICIAL	EXPOSURE TO BACTERIA OR VIRUS
INVASION BY BACTERIA OR VIRUS	VACCINATION	

IMMUNE SYSTEM STIMULATED TO FORM ANTIBODIES THAT CAUSE FUTURE IMMUNITY

Vaccines

Although vaccines, like antibiotics, are used to control disease, they differ from antibiotics in two important ways.

- They are used to prevent rather than treat disease.
- They do not cause resistant strains of microbes to develop.

Since viral diseases have defied a cure, vaccines were originally developed to trigger immunity against viruses. Although most bacterial diseases can be successfully treated with antibiotics, some are so devastating that bacterial vaccines, called "bacterins", have also been developed. Few people make any distinction between vaccines and bacterins, but call them all "vaccines."

Successful vaccines against some diseases have not yet been developed because the viruses keep changing (as in the case with influenza), too many different viruses cause the disease (as in infectious bronchitis), or the virus causing the disease hasn't yet been identified (as in infectious anemia).

In addition, not all vaccines are created equal. Some trigger a good immune response, others confer only a low level of immunity. Some produce a reaction that can be as serious as the disease itself. Live virus vaccines and contaminated vaccines sometimes actually transmit disease.

A good vaccine has these five properties:

- It contains enough antigens to protect chickens against infection by a specific pathogen.
- It contains antigens from all strains of the pathogen that cause the disease.
- It is not contaminated with additional antigens.
- It is not too toxic to chickens (therefore causes no serious reaction).
- It will not cause disease.

Some state governments would like to restrict the use of vaccines to licensed veterinarians and others who hold a permit. Their reasons are that mishandled vaccines lose effectiveness and that bootleg vaccines occasionally appear having little or no effect to begin with. Purchase vaccines only from licensed, registered manufacturers, as evidenced by an assigned code number stamped on the bottle.

Vaccine Types

A vaccine derived from viruses or bacteria is used to trigger a chicken's immune response against the viruses or bacteria from which it was derived. When a vaccine is administered, a chicken's body responds by producing antibodies just as it would in a natural infection by the virus or bacteria.

The difference between an infection and a vaccination is that the pathogens in a vaccine either cause a mild case of disease or have been intentionally altered so they cannot cause disease at all. A chicken's antibody-producing tissue cannot tell the difference between the three basic vaccine forms:

- live
- modified live
- inactivated

Live vaccines are the most effective. They are used to induce infection, but to be safe they must be made from harmless microbes closely related to pathogenic microbes. Live vaccines are relatively inexpensive and easy to use, especially for mass application to large flocks, and can be applied to birds at a younger age than can inactivated vaccines. They cause immunity to develop rapidly and to spread via shedding of live viruses from successfully vaccinated birds to unsuccessfully vaccinated birds.

A live vaccine has several disadvantages. It can be easily killed by heat and chemicals (such as alcohol used to sterilize a needle). It may be contaminated with other viruses during manufacture, spreading unintended diseases. Just as the virus can spread from successfully to unsuccessfully vaccinated birds, so can it spread to susceptible nearby unvaccinated flocks. The vaccine produces some of the symptoms of the disease being vaccinated against and, if chickens are stressed or infected with some other microbe, it can cause serious disease.

Because of these dangers, only mild viruses are used in a live vaccine, and multiple application is required. Live vaccines should be used only to prevent a serious disease already present in the yard that cannot be controlled any other way. Live virus vaccines are available against epidemic tremor, infectious bronchitis, infectious bursal disease, infectious laryngotracheitis, Marek's disease, Newcastle, pox, and viral arthritis.

Live Virus Danger

Vaccines containing live viruses are supposed to give birds a mild case of disease, but they can cause serious disease if they are not used properly. The disease will remain mild if:

- **the vaccinated birds are healthy**
- **they are the right age for vaccination**
- **the vaccine is properly administered**
- **the birds are kept warm**
- **their housing is clean and dry**
- **weather conditions remain steady**

Modified live vaccines contain pathogenic organisms that have been genetically altered to make them less infectious so they can no longer cause disease, but can continue to replicate and trigger the production of antibodies. The process of genetically altering pathogens is called "attenuation," and modified live vaccines are sometimes called "attenuated" vaccines.

A modified live vaccine is more potent than a live vaccine and is therefore cheaper to use, since you need less per dose. Like a live vaccine, a modified live vaccine must be handled carefully to avoid killing the viruses or bacteria, thus destroying their ability to trigger immunity.

Like live vaccines, modified live vaccines cause shedding to unvaccinated birds. In addition, if attenuation is incorrectly done, the vaccine may cause disease rather than immunity. Even if attenuation is correct, the vaccine may cause disease as a result of contamination with other pathogens or by interfering with the bird's immune response (making it susceptible to other diseases).

Inactivated vaccines contain bacteria or viruses that have been killed by chemicals or heat. While most virus vaccines are live or modified live, bacterins are always inactivated. Inactivated vaccines are both expensive to produce and time-consuming to administer, since they require multiple doses and must be injected. Unlike other vaccines, some inactivated vaccines have a 21-day withdrawal time. In addition, they may confer only short-term, low-level immunity. To produce a higher, more uniform response, birds are often primed with live vaccine first.

On the other hand, inactivated vaccines are the easiest to store and safest to use. They do not cause disease in stressed or infected birds, as live and modified live vaccines can. They produce few adverse reactions — most commonly stress due to handling and/or a lump at the site of injection, caused by the fluid in which the killed pathogens are suspended.

New technologies under investigation that may one day offer terrific breakthroughs in disease control include biogenetically engineered recombinant DNA vaccine, for which large quantities of pure viruses can be produced at a relatively low cost, and synthetic vaccines that eliminate the risks inherent in working with genetically modified microorganisms (such as the possibility that genetically altered pathogens may mutate and cause new diseases).

Vaccination Procedure

Vaccines come in bottles containing enough for 500 or 1,000 birds. Even if you can't use it all, the cost is usually still low in relation to the cost of losing birds in a disease outbreak.

Some vaccines (such as those against Marek's disease and pox) come in two vials, one filled with powder and one with liquid. Once the two are mixed together, the vaccine is good for only about an hour, so you can't save it. Destroy unused vaccine and empty containers by burning or deep burial.

The age at which birds should be vaccinated and the precise vaccination procedure you use depend on your purpose in keeping chickens and the disease you are vaccinating against. Vaccines against some diseases come in more than one form and can therefore be administered by more than one method. Some methods of application are more suitable for flock-wide application involving large numbers of birds, others require handling individual birds to ensure that each gets an even dose.

Water vaccination is the most popular mass method. It involves withholding drinking water overnight, then adding vaccine to the water in a measured amount calculated to deliver an adequate dose, based on the amount of water an average bird drinks within a 3-hour period. Since water consumption varies with age, feed, and weather, determine the exact amount of water your flock needs by measuring how much your birds drink the day before.

A vaccine may be inactivated if the temperature is high or the water contains impurities, including sanitizers such as chlorine used to control bacteria or fungi. Do not use water sanitizers within 48 hours of vaccinating. Clean waterers and rinse them well, leaving no disinfectant residue to inactivate the vaccine.

Methods of Vaccine Application

Flock application
- **drinking water**
- **feed additive**
- **aerosol (dust or spray)**

Individual application
- **beak dip**
- **drop in eye (intraocular)**
- **drop in nose (intranasal)**
- **injection (intramuscular or subcutaneous)**
- **vent brush**
- **wing-web stab**

The vaccine can be somewhat stabilized by adding powdered milk to the water. Milk protein neutralizes sanitizers and protects a vaccine from the shock of dilution. Before adding the vaccine, stir in skim milk powder at the rate of 50 grams or ⅝ cup per 5 gallons (45 g/20 liter) of cool water. (You can find a ⅛ cup measure in the canning section of nearly any discount department store; an equivalent measure to ⅝ cup is 10 tablespoons.)

Remove drinking water the night before vaccinating. Provide vaccine-laden water in the morning, right after mixing it. If you're treating a large flock, ensure that birds low in peck order get a drink by adding only half the vaccine to as much water as the flock will drink in about 2 hours. Then add the other half to as much water as the flock will drink in another 2 hours.

Coated, pelleted feed containing vaccine, designed in Australia, is used in tropical countries, where high water temperatures inactivate vaccines.

Spray or aerosol vaccination offers an easy way to vaccinate large numbers of birds in a short time. It is most commonly used for infectious bronchitis and infectious bursal vaccines, to give boosters, and to prime a flock with live vaccine prior to administering an inactivated vaccine.

Aerosol vaccination is tricky because it can induce a severe vaccine reaction and because it requires special equipment to get the droplets just the right size. A fine mist penetrates deeply into the respiratory tract, a coarse spray not so deeply. A fine mist is used for adult birds, while a coarse spray is used to induce a milder reaction in chicks.

Since birds must be confined to a small area for the aerosol method to work, it is most often applied in brooder housing. A hand pump may be used for occasional application; a coarse-spray cabinet is used by those who regularly vaccinate large numbers of chicks.

Applying a vaccine dust by aerosol is similar, except that the powder is puffed dry rather than diluted and sprayed as a liquid.

Wing-web vaccination involves the use of a two-prong stabber. The stabber is dipped into vaccine, then used to pierce the unfeathered skin of the wing-web, or the chicken's "armpit." When vaccinating chickens of various ages, start with the oldest birds, then break off one prong to immunize chicks.

The wing-web method won't work if you stab feathers instead of skin, or if the stabber isn't adequately immersed in vaccine. When you use a live virus vaccine, you can tell if the vaccination takes by watching for slight swelling and scabbing in 1 to 2 weeks.

Injected vaccines may be administered intramuscularly (into the muscle of the breast) or subcutaneously (under loose skin of the breast or neck). Some vaccines can be applied either way. Others (such as those against cholera and erysipelas) can only be administered by subcutaneous injection; a serious reaction will occur if they are injected into the muscle or bone. Follow instructions carefully as to needle size and injection site.

Subcutaneous injection is currently the only way to administer Marek's vaccine to newly hatched chicks. Take a pinch of skin from the back of the chick's neck between your thumb and forefinger. Stick the needle into the skin and inject the vaccine, taking care to neither poke the needle out the other side nor stab your fingers.

Eye or intraocular vaccination comes in a kit with a vial of vaccine and a vial of dyed mixing solution, called diluent, with an eye dropper in the cap. Colored diluent is used to verify proper vaccine placement in the eye — color appears on a bird's tongue when the procedure is correct.

Beak dip vaccines are administered by dipping each chick's beak into the vaccine.

Vent brush vaccination requires the use of a brush to apply vaccine to the mucous membrane of the cloaca. This was once a standard vaccination method, but because it involves application of especially virulent viruses, it is no longer legal in most states.

Chart 12-1

Vaccination Methods*

METHODS
DE = drop in eye
DW = drinking water
IM = intramuscular injection
SC = subcutaneous injection
S = spray
WW = wing web

VACCINE TYPES
L - live vaccine
M = modified live vaccine
I = inactivated vaccine

Disease	DE	DW	IM	SC	S	WW
Cholera			I			
Chronic respiratory disease			I	I		
Coccidiosis		L				
Epidemic tremor		L				L
Erysipelas				I		
Infectious bronchitis	L	L	I	I	L	
Infectious bursal disease		M	I	I		
Infectious coryza			I	I		
Infectious laryngotracheitis	M					
Infectious synovitis			I	I		
Marek's disease			L	L		
Newcastle	L	L	I	I	L	
Pox						L/M
Viral arthritis			I	M/I		M

*Age of birds at application, method of application, and need for repeat application depends on the vaccine source and form — follow instructions on label.

Vaccination Programs

Your veterinarian or state poultry specialist can help you work out a vaccination program based on disease problems occurring in your area and your purpose in keeping chickens. For each vaccine you consider, take into account:

- its availability
- its cost in relation to the worth of your birds
- the size of your flock
- your flock's expected lifespan
- maternal immunity your chicks may inherit from your breeder flock
- the presence of infection in your flock, your yard, and your area
- your need for other vaccines
- your flock's past vaccination history
- state laws

Establish a vaccination program *only* to solve specific problems — past problems your flock has experienced or the serious threat of a new problem. Vaccinate against diseases your flock has a reasonable risk of getting. Do not vaccinate against diseases that do not endanger your flock. If you show your birds, if serious diseases have occurred on your place (in your own flock or in the previous owner's flock), or if serious diseases infect nearby flocks (particularly if you live near a high concentration of commercial chickens), you may have good reason to vaccinate. To learn about diseases that occur in your area, ask your veterinarian, county Extension agent, state poultry specialist, or the avian pathologist at your state diagnostic lab. In some states, it is illegal to use certain live virus vaccines or to introduce viruses by bringing in birds from another state that have been vaccinated with a live virus vaccine.

Several vaccines come in combinations that trigger immunity against more than one disease at a time. If your vaccination plan requires the use of several vaccines, a combination vaccine may save you time and money. On the other hand, sometimes a chicken's response to one vaccine interferes with development of immunity to another. Furthermore, if your birds have an adverse reaction, you may have trouble determining which vaccine in the combination caused the reaction. Whenever you use a vaccine, record the vaccine's name, manufacturer, and serial number in your flock history.

Vaccine Failures

Vaccine failures usually result from improperly storing or handling a vaccine or from using improper vaccinating procedures. Whenever you use a vaccine, read and follow instructions regarding storage and handling, method of application, dosage, recommended age of birds at the time of first vaccination, and the timing of revaccinations (boosters). All these factors affect the level, quality, and duration of immunity.

If your birds are in poor health, the results of vaccinating may be worse than not vaccinating at all. Unless you deliberately use vaccine to slow the spread of pox or infectious laryngotracheitis, do not vaccinate chickens that have symptoms of the disease you're vaccinating against.

Some diseases, including infectious bursal disease, reduce resistance to other diseases. Chicks that hatch with a good level of maternal antibodies against infectious bursal disease are protected against early damage to their immune system, but the same antibodies that confer immunity also interfere with the desired immune response to vaccines.

If vaccination fails, consider these possible causes:

- Vaccine was not stored in the refrigerator or otherwise as directed (improperly stored vaccines decay rapidly).

- Vaccine's expiration date long since passed.
- Vaccine was not handled in a hygienic manner.
- Wrong vaccine was used (not all vaccines protect against all strains).
- Wrong dosage was used (underdosing is more common than overdosing).
- Vaccine was administered incorrectly.
- Housing sanitation is poor.
- Flock was exposed to pathogens before immunity took effect.
- Flock's immune response was suppressed (due to heat stress, feed contaminated with mycotoxins, poor health, etc.).

No vaccine will protect your flock 100 percent — every vaccine has at least a 5 percent failure rate. In addition, disease can occur if you bring in new birds that are not on the same vaccination program as your old ones (a vaccine may cause your old birds or your new birds to shed pathogens). Then, too, you never know what disease may turn up next. Good management with an eye toward disease prevention remains your best defense.

Natural Vaccination

Before commercial vaccines became widely available, farmers practiced natural immunization by mixing young birds with older ones, thus exposing the young ones to any diseases the older ones were exposed to. Genetically resistant flocks were developed by culling birds that did not fully recover and keeping (immunized) survivors as breeders.

Chicks may be naturally vaccinated for a variety of respiratory diseases, most notably infectious bronchitis and mild Newcastle disease. Signs that natural vaccination may be occurring include mild wheezing and watery eyes. Cull birds that do not recover within a week so they don't have a chance to reproduce more weaklings.

Other diseases for which natural vaccination commonly occurs through gradual exposure include chronic respiratory disease, infectious coryza, and infectious bursal disease. Chicks exposed to infectious bursal disease (IBD) before the age of 14 days rarely develop noticeable symptoms.

Natural vaccination can backfire if chicks are exposed to massive amounts of microbes before immunity is complete. In at least one disease, Marek's, there is an alternative to gradual exposure — raise a few turkeys with your chickens. Turkeys carry a related though harmless virus that keeps the Marek's virus from causing tumors.

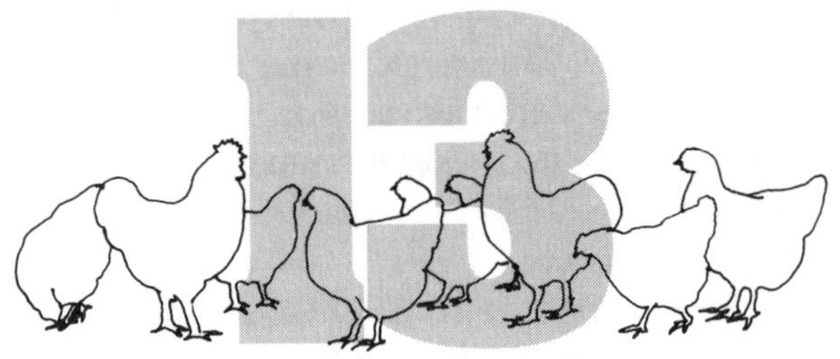

Incubation and Brooding

CHICKENS ARE MORE LIKELY TO REMAIN HEALTHY if they have a healthy start from the time they hatch. Modern practices of selective breeding and artificial incubation have minimized some problems that occurred in the past, but along the way new ones have been introduced. Good hatchability and strong, healthy chicks result from:

- proper egg collection and storage
- correct operation of incubator
- good incubator sanitation
- healthy, well conditioned breeders
- proper feeding of breeders
- hereditary vigor

Hatching Egg Care

Collect hatching eggs several times a day so they will neither heat nor chill. To help you track hereditary and/or egg-transmitted problems, identify the eggs from each breeder or breeder group by writing a code on each egg with a grease pencil or China marker. If you trapnest hens to identify their eggs, check nests often, especially in warm weather. Hens can suffer from being enclosed in a small, hot space, and may soil their eggs if confined in the nest too long.

Eggs laid in floor litter have twenty to thirty times more bacteria on their shells than eggs laid in cages. The eggs of floor-reared hens are therefore 3 percent lower in hatchability and result in more rough red navels in newly hatched chicks. In addition, contaminated eggs may explode during incubation, contaminating other eggs and causing them to subsequently explode.

Bacteria on the shell, from feces or contaminated dust and nest litter, is more likely to get into the egg if the shell is porous. Older hens lay eggs that are more porous than pullets' eggs. Vitamin or mineral deficiency or imbalance in the breeder flock, or a respiratory virus, can also cause shells to be more porous than otherwise.

Manage your flock so that eggs will be clean when you collect them, which includes keeping litter dry so hens won't track mud into nests. Minimize bacterial contamination by dry cleaning slightly soiled eggs with fine sandpaper. Avoid saving heavily soiled eggs for hatching. If valuable eggs become soiled and must be washed, use water warmer than the eggs (but not over 140°F, 60°C), otherwise bacteria may be forced through the shell.

Household detergent combined with a dash of chlorine bleach (Clorox) serves as both sanitizer and cleaning agent. Other ways to thoroughly sanitize eggs: dip them for 1 minute in a chlorine compound, quaternary ammonia product (such as Germex), 1 percent iodine solution, or other sanitizer designed specifically for use on hatching eggs.

Store eggs in clean cartons to avoid introducing contamination during storage.

Egg Storage

Hatching problems can occur due to storing eggs for too long or at the wrong storage temperature. The storage temperature must be below "physiological zero," the temperature above which development (however erratic) begins to take place. The optimum storage temperature for hatching eggs is 55°F (13°C). The storage area should have low enough humidity not to attract mold, but should not be so dry that moisture is rapidly drawn from the eggs.

The less moisture that evaporates from eggs during storage, the greater their hatching rate will be. Speed of evaporation varies from one strain to another. Small eggs, such as those laid by bantams and jungle fowl, have a relatively large surface-to-volume ratio, so they evaporate more quickly than large eggs. Early season eggs of any size evaporate more slowly than late summer eggs.

Eggs have a built-in ability to remain hatchable after several days of storage, otherwise a hen could not collect a batch of eggs to hatch all at one time. Even under the best storage conditions, hatchability drops after 6 days. You can increase storage time to as long as 3 weeks, while maintaining reasonable hatchability, by wrapping each egg in plastic wrap.

Incubation

Temperature, relative humidity, ventilation, and turning during incubation all affect the hatch. Eggs must be turned at least three times a day at regularly spaced intervals, as close to 8 hours apart as possible. Fairly inexpensive incubators are available that improve the hatching rate by automatically turning eggs every hour.

Ventilation is necessary to bring in oxygen and remove carbon dioxide generated by developing embryos. Most incubators have either adjustable vents you can open or plugs you can remove as the hatch progresses.

Operating an incubator at the correct temperature can be tricky. Unless the incubator is extremely well insulated, temperature fluctuations in the room where the incubator is set up can affect the hatch. Sunlight falling on the incubator can cause its temperature to rise. A thermometer that isn't properly positioned according to the incubator manufacturer's instructions can give a false temperature reading. Even if the thermometer is properly placed, incubation temperature can't be accurately set if the numbers are too close together, as is often the case. The thermometer itself may be inaccurate — it's always wise to check a new thermometer against a second or even third thermometer whose accuracy you are sure of.

When incubation temperature is too low, chicks take longer than 21 days to hatch. They will tend to be big and soft with unhealed navels, crooked toes, and thin legs. They may grow slowly or may not learn to eat and drink at all.

When the temperature is too high, chicks hatch before 21 days. They tend to have splayed legs and can't properly walk, a problem that does not improve as the chicks grow. These chicks should be culled.

No matter what combination of temperature and humidity is suggested by the manufacturer, you'll have to make minor adjustments depending on your location and the eggs you hatch. Keep accurate records as you make adjustments, and after a few hatches you will hit on the optimum combination for your particular situation.

Whether your incubator is still-air (no fan) or a forced-air (has a fan), its optimum temperature and humidity are interrelated. As the temperature goes down, relative humidity must go up to maintain the same hatching rate. Here are some likely combinations:

still-air: 102°F (38.9°C) at 58 percent
100°F (37.8°C) at 61 percent

forced-air: 99°F (37.2°C) at 56 percent
98°F (36.7°C) at 70 percent

For a successful hatch, moisture must evaporate from eggs at just the right rate. Small eggs, such as those laid by bantams and jungle fowl, evaporate more rapidly than larger eggs. Small eggs therefore hatch better at a higher humidity or lower temperature than regular-sized eggs.

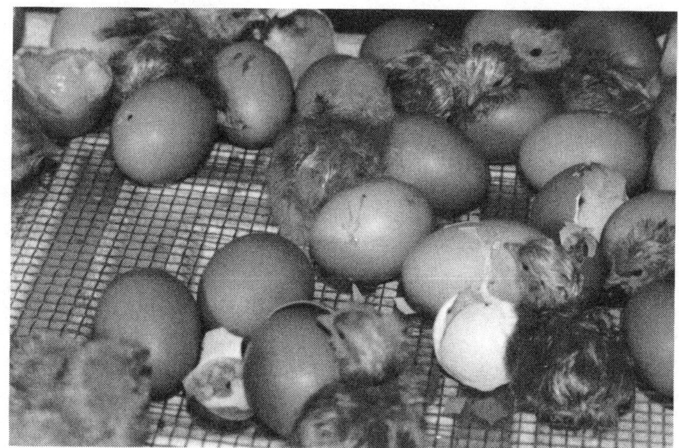

Good incubator sanitation ensures a healthy hatch.

Incorrect humidity can cause embryos to die in the shell or chicks to be small. Too-high humidity can lead to omphalitis, otherwise known as "mushy chick disease." In high humidity the yolk sac does not absorb completely and the navel therefore cannot heal properly. Bacteria in the incubator invade through the unhealed navels, causing deaths for up to 14 days after the hatch.

Incubator Sanitation

Bringing eggs together from various sources is a sure way to introduce disease-causing organisms into your incubator. For healthier chicks, hatch only your own eggs. If you must bring in eggs from other sources, fumigate them (see page 213). If you sell hatching eggs to a custom hatchery, do not bring chicks home from one.

Good incubator sanitation improves hatching success and gives chicks a healthy start in life. It also offers an important way to break the disease cycle in a flock. Another way to break the disease cycle is to avoid hatching year-round.

Hatching itself is a major source of incubator contamination. By the time the hatch is over, the incubator is littered with organic debris that provides an ideal environment for disease-causing organisms. If you practice continuous hatching (continuously adding new settings of eggs as previous settings hatch), keep a separate small incubator to use for hatching. Thoroughly clean the hatcher after each hatch.

Begin by vacuuming out loose down. Then wipe out hatching debris with a damp sponge, or the debris will protect disease-causing organisms from the disinfectant. Scrub the hatcher with detergent and hot water, followed by a good disinfectant such as Germex or chlorine bleach (¼ cup bleach per gallon of hot water, or 30 ml/l). If possible, let the incubator dry in the sun.

Styrofoam Incubators

Although no one has formally studied the difficulty of cleaning styrofoam incubators, people using them have experienced hatching difficulties in successive years in spite of sanitation practices that would be adequate for a wooden incubator. Since disinfectants may not adequately penetrate the porous styrofoam, fumigation may be the only option.

Clean your hatcher at the end of each hatching season. Cleaning and disinfecting does not destroy all disease-causing organisms, but it does make the environment less favorable for the survival of any microorganisms that remain. If you let cleanup go until the beginning of the next season, you'll have more microbes to contend with, harbored all that time in fluff and droppings.

Fumigation

Commercial and custom hatcheries routinely fumigate their incubators to minimize the spread of salmonella and other bacteria. Small home incubators rarely need fumigation, except after a serious disease outbreak. Fumigation rids an incubator of disease-causing organisms by means of gas that penetrates cracks and other areas you can't reach with a brush or spray. Prior to fumigation, thoroughly clean hatching debris from the incubator.

For the fumigant, you will need formaldehyde (CH_2O), the most effective disinfectant against viruses, but one that works only in an enclosed space. It is a toxic, volatile chemical that has a strong odor, is caustic, and irritates the eyes. A common brand name is Formalin, formaldehyde mixed with water in a 40 percent solution (37 percent by weight). You will also need potassium permanganate ($KMnO_4$), a poison that comes in the form of a dry powder.

These two chemicals are available from drugstores and veterinarians, but their safe use requires knowledge and care. Wear plastic gloves while handling them. If you get any on yourself, flush your skin with plenty of water. If you normally keep your incubator in the house, move it to an outbuilding for fumigation. Due to the danger of inhaling the gas, this is *not* a safe procedure to carry out in your living room.

For mixing the chemicals, you'll need a tall earthenware or enamel container. **Do not use metal** — the chemicals may eat right through it. **Do not use glass unless it's Pyrex** — the chemical reaction will generate heat that might crack regular glass. **Use a container ten times larger than the combined volume of the chemicals,** so none can splash out during the chemical reaction that will cause the mixture to bubble up.

Close all vents to make the incubator airtight. Holding your breath to avoid inhaling poisonous gas, combine the chemicals in the earthenware or enamel container and place the container in the incubator, off the floor somewhere near the center. Quickly close the incubator door.

Run the incubator at normal temperature and humidity for at least 30 minutes, preferably overnight. At the end of the fumigation period, open the incubator and all the vents to let the gas escape. Also ventilate the room or outbuilding in which the incubator is located.

Determining Chemical Amounts for Fumigation

To figure out how much of each chemical you need, determine the cubic footage of your incubator by multiplying its length times its width times its height. As a general rule, use twice as much Formalin by liquid measure (ml or cc) as potassium permanganate in dry measure (g). For each cubic foot, measure out 1.2 cc Formalin and 0.6 g potassium permanganate (per cubic meter, 40 cc Formalin and 20 g potassium permanganate). ***Do not*** **mix them together until you're ready to fumigate.**

Fumigating Eggs

Fumigation of hatching eggs is an effective method of controlling diseases when eggs are brought together from varying sources (a common way to spread disease from flock to flock) or where valuable hatching eggs become dirty.

Fumigating eggs before hatching destroys organisms on the outside of the shell. The procedure is the same as for fumigating an empty incubator. If you are making only one setting at a time, you can place the eggs in the incubator and fumigate both at the same time. If you make weekly settings, fumigate eggs before placing them in the incubator, which means keeping a separate incubator just for fumigation. If you use a separate hatcher, time your settings so you can fumigate new eggs right after the previous hatch.

If you fumigate eggs during incubation, do so either within 12 hours after setting them or after the fourth day. Otherwise, the fumigant may harm embryos during the early days of development. Commercial and custom hatcheries often fumigate again after moving eggs to the hatching incubator (but never after eggs have pipped, or chicks may be injured). Fumigate eggs for 20 minutes using 0.8 cc Formalin and 0.4 g potassium permanganate per cubic foot (26 cc Formalin and 13 g potassium permanganate per cubic meter).

Fertility

During incubation, remove eggs that are not developing properly to eliminate a potential source of incubator contamination. The first eggs that can be identified as developing improperly are infertiles, which look clear during candling.

The cause of infertility may be easy or difficult to identify. Sometimes the germinal disc or "zygote" dies between the time an egg leaves a hen's ovary and the time incubation begins — a phenomenon known as "weak fertility." Since weak fertility is indistinguishable from infertility, the cause is impossible to trace.

One cause of infertility may be an incorrect ratio of cocks to hens. The optimum mating ratio for lightweight laying breeds is one cock for up to one dozen hens; the optimum ratio for heavier meat breeds is one cock per eight hens. More hens than that, and the cocks may not get around to all of them; more cocks than that, and the cocks will be so busy fighting among themselves that they won't have time to get around to all the hens.

Even if the mating ratio is right, fertility will be low in a breeding flock that's too closely confined. In a small flock with only one cock, the cock may prefer some hens and ignore the others. Hens that are high in the peck order tend to be mated less often than hens lower in peck order. The answer is to either disrupt the order by rotating cocks or identify and artificially inseminating the infertile hens.

A cock that's too old or too fat may have fertility problems. Frozen combs and wattles can also cause infertility (see "Frostbite," page 132). A cock with a leg or foot injury may have trouble breeding. Never catch a rooster by one leg, or you may permanently damage a joint. Excessively showing breeders, cocks or hens, can cause stress that leads to infertility. During hatching season, keep valuable show birds in the breeding pen.

Nutrition can affect fertility. Vitamin E deficiency causes a cock's testes to degenerate, resulting in reduced fertility or even sterility. Vitamin A deficiency also causes reduced fertility in cocks. Cocks with large combs that interfere at the feed trough may have low fertility. Eggs laid by hens that are underweight or overweight may be infertile. Supplementing lay ration with grains during the breeding season interferes with vitamin, mineral, and protein balance.

Diseases that affect fertility include chronic respiratory disease, infectious coryza, infectious bronchitis, and Newcastle. Eggs from breeders that have recovered from any of these diseases may be infertile. Marek's disease can cause permanent ovary damage that leads to infertility. Parasite problems, internal or external, can interfere with fertility.

Infertility problems may be breed-related. A classic example is low fertility caused by the abnormal semen of white Wyandotte cocks with rose or pea combs. Heavily feathered breeds such as Brahma, Cochin, Orpington, and Wyandotte may have fertility problems unless the feathers are clipped from around their vents. Cocks with crests, such as Houdan or Polish, may not see well enough to catch wily hens unless their crests are clipped back.

Season can affect fertility, which tends to be low during times of year when daylight hours are fewer than 14. Just as lighting keeps hens laying during short winter days, it also improves the fertility of cocks. Fertility is highest in spring and drops during the heat of summer.

Hatchability

Just because a fertile egg contains a sperm cell, making it potentially capable of development during incubation, doesn't mean the egg will survive the 21 days of incubation and hatch into a healthy chick. Many things can happen to affect the egg's hatchability.

On average, even a hen hatches only 89 percent of her fertile eggs. Not many years ago, 60 percent was considered a reasonable rate for artificial incubation. Today's improved incubators average 85 percent. By conventional definition, anything more than 75 percent of fertiles hatched is considered a high rate; less than 50 percent is low.

If you are hatching in the mid to high range, you can probably improve your rate by fine-tuning the way you run your incubator. If your hatches fall in the low range, look for other causes.

The age of your hens may be a factor. The small eggs with small yolks laid by pullets are low in hatchability and produce a high percentage of deformed embryos. Hatchability rises as eggs reach full size, but drops again by 3 to 4 percent between a hen's first and second year. Whether hatchability continues to drop thereafter is a matter of contention, but hatchability is certainly likely to go down in hens that are out of condition, parasitized, or diseased. Hatchability is especially affected by salmonellosis, which is transmitted through the egg and causes embryo or early chick death.

Salmonellosis and other diseases are transmitted from infected breeders to their offspring through hatching eggs in one of two ways:

- The infectious organism may enter the egg as it is being formed within an infected hen.
- Bacteria may get on the shell as the egg is laid or when it lands in a contaminated nest. Bacteria then enter the egg through the shell, which occurs more readily if the shell cracks or gets wet (for example, during improper washing).

Diseases Transmitted Through Hatching Eggs

Colibacillosis
- Air-sac disease
- Chronic respiratory disease
- Omphalitis

Egg drop syndrome

Epidemic tremor

Infectious anemia

Infectious stunting syndrome

Infectious synovitis

Lymphoid/Sarcoma
- Lymphoid leukosis
- Osteopetrosis

Pseudomonas

Rotaviral enteritis

Runting syndrome

Salmonellosis
- Arizonosis
- Paratyphoid
- Pullorum
- Typhoid

Viral arthritis

Egg-transmitted Disease Cycle

INFECTED EGGS SPREAD DISEASE IN INCUBATOR
INFECTED BREEDERS MAY LAY INFECTED EGGS
INFECTED CHICKS SPREAD DISEASE IN BROODER
INFECTED BIRDS SPREAD DISEASE TO OTHERS IN FLOCK

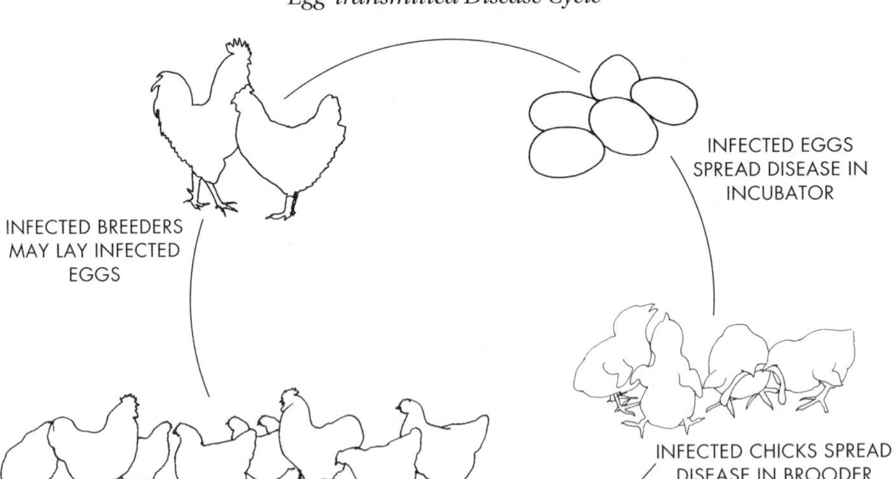

Diseases then spread from infected chicks to healthy chicks in the incubator (often inhaled in fluff) or in the brooder (usually through ingested droppings in feed or water).

Hatchability and Nutrition

Nutritional deficiency is one of the most common causes of poor hatchability. Lay ration contains less protein, vitamins, and minerals than a breeder flock needs, affecting egg composition and resulting in poor hatchability. The older the breeders are, the worse the problem becomes.

In some areas, feed stores carry breeder ration. In other areas, the closest thing is gamebird ration. If you can find neither, feed your flock a handful of dry catfood two or three times a week and either add a vitamin/mineral supplement to the drinking water or give each bird ½ cc vitamin AD&E injectable every 3 weeks. Start this regime 6 weeks before you plan to start collecting hatching eggs.

An embryo's appearance, combined with the day on which it died, provides a clue regarding which nutrient might be lacking. For example, in riboflavin deficiency, deaths peak at three points: the fourth, tenth, and fourteenth day of incubation. Embryos may be dwarfed, have beaks that look like a parrot's, have unusually short wings and legs, and have clubbed down — a condition, seen most often in black breeds, in which the down is clumpy, and curls in a characteristic way because the down sheaths fail to rupture.

CHART 13-1

Nutrition-Related Hatching Problems

Symptom	*Deficiency*
Day of Death:	
Early incubation	vitamin A
1-7th day	biotin
4th day	riboflavin vitamin E
10th day	riboflavin
10th – 21st day	magnesium
14th day	riboflavin
17th day	vitamin B12
18th – 19th day	vitamin D
19th – 21st day	biotin
20th & 21st day	manganese
Late incubation	folic acid pantothenic acid vitamin E vitamin K selenium excess
At pipping	folic acid selenium excess
Soon after hatch	vitamin E
Embryonic Appearance:	
Beak/head abnormal	zinc
Beak, short	vitamin B12
upper/lower beak short	vitamin D
crooked (parrot beak)	riboflavin manganese
Embryonic Appearance (cont.):	
Bones/beak soft & rubbery	vitamin D
Clubbed down	riboflavin
Eyes pale	vitamins A & D
small	zinc
Feathers, abnormal	pantothenic acid
black in ermine pattern	vitamin D
Fluid in body	vitamin B12
Growth, dwarfed	riboflavin
stunted	vitamin D
Legs/feet/wings twisted	biotin
Legs, bowed	vitamins A & D
short	riboflavin manganese
undeveloped	vitamin B12
missing	zinc
Perosis	vitamin B12 manganese
Navel not closed	iodine
Skull deformed	biotin manganese
Spine poorly developed	zinc
Incubation time too long	iodine

Inbreeding

Inbreeding is a sure way to reduce hatchability. Continuous, close inbreeding causes a phenomenon known as "inbreeding depression," for which low hatchability is usually the first sign. Later signs are fewer and fewer eggs laid, and chicks lacking in "constitutional vigor," meaning they're droopy and unthrifty, and may or may not die soon after hatching.

Inbreeding is unavoidable if you raise an exhibition strain or you're trying to preserve one of the fast-disappearing classic breeds. For every 10 percent increase in inbreeding, however, you can expect a 2.6 percent reduction in hatchability. A flock that reaches 30 percent hatchability is nearing extinction

CHART 13-2

Incubation Trouble-Shooting

Problem	*Cause*	*Solution*
Eggs:		
infertile	too many or too few cocks	1 cock/12 light breed hens 1 cock/8 heavy breed hens
	cock too old	use younger cock
	cock too fat	condition cock
	cocks have foot/leg injuries	treat injuries
	frozen combs and wattles	treat for frostbite
	excessive showing of breeders	keep breeders home
	eggs stored too long	store 6 days or less
	wrong storage temperature	store eggs at 55°F (13°C)
	hens too fat or too thin	condition hens
	flock too closely confined	give breeders more room
blood ring	breeder flock unhealthy	check for parasites and diseases
	breeder ration low in vitamins	feed alfalfa meal and cod liver oil
	eggs chilled or heated	collect hatching eggs often
	improper fumigation	do not fumigate between 12th and 96th hour
	irregular incubator temperature	control temperature
green appearance	aspergillosis	do not hatch eggs with cracked or poor shells; clean and disinfect incubator between hatches
Embryos:		
die day 1–2	eggs stored too long	store 6 days or less
	irregular incubator temperature	control temperature
	improper turning	turn eggs at 8-hour intervals
	deficient breeder rations	vitamin-mineral supplement
	inbreeding	obtain new cock
die day 1–7	aflatoxicosis	avoid feeding breeders moldy grain
die at 12–18 days	temperature too high or low	control temperature
	poor ventilation	open vents or remove plug
	incorrect breeder ration	feed milk, yellow corn, alfalfa meal, cod liver oil
die at 19–21 days (yellowish brown fluid in eggs)	colibacillosis	hatch only clean, sanitized eggs
die at 21 days (without pipping)	eggs not turned properly	turn at least 3 times/day
	hereditary weakness	use stock with high hatchability
	wrong temperature	control hatching temperature
	pseudomonas	improve incubator sanitation
die at 21 days (pipped)	humidity too low	increase humidity
	temperature too low	increase temperature
	temporary temperature surge	control temperature

Problem	Cause	Solution
Embryos (cont.):		
die at 21 days (pipped and unpipped)	omphalitis paratyphoid	hatch only clean, sanitized eggs hatch eggs only from typhoid-clean breeders
die at 21 days (pipped, but chicks too big to work out of shell)	poor hatching ventilation	open vents or remove plug
Hatch:		
early	high incubation temperature	decrease temperature ½°
slow	low incubation temperature	increase temperature ¼°
late	temperature too low power outage eggs stored too long	increase temperature cover incubator during power outages store 6 days or less
Chicks:		
can't get free of shell	hatching humidity too low hatching temperature too high too much hatching ventilation	increase hatching humidity decrease temperature ½° at hatching time reduce vent openings
sticky, shells clinging	hatching humidity too low	increase hatching humidity
sticky, smeared with yolk	hatching temperature too low hatching humidity too high	increase hatching temperature open vents or remove plug
rough navels	hatching temperature too high temperature fluctuation hatching humidity too low	decrease hatching temperature check wafer in incubator increase hatching humidity
small	eggs too small humidity too low temperature too high	hatch only normal-sized eggs increase humidity decrease temperature
short down	temperature too high humidity too low	decrease temperature increase humidity
splayed legs	temperature too high	decrease temperature
crooked toes	temperature too low	increase temperature
big, soft, weak	temperature too low poor ventilation	increase temperature open vents or remove plug
unabsorbed yolk sac	hatching humidity too high	decrease humidity
mushy and smell bad	omphalitis	sanitize incubator
crossed beaks	hereditary	cull breeders

due to failure to reproduce. A flock can become extinct after only six to eight generations of brother-sister matings.

Inbreeding depression has two distinct causes: concentration of genetic factors and the inbreeding itself. You can therefore slow the decline and improve reproduction in two ways. First, by selecting and culling for number of eggs laid, hatchability of the eggs, and vigor of the resulting offspring. Second, by using less close matings that result in more gradual inbreeding — making fifty birds the minimum size for an inbred flock.

Better yet, occasionally introduce birds from a different strain. Mating birds from different strains invariably results in hybrid vigor. The opposite of inbreeding depression, hybrid vigor causes more rapid growth, larger size, increased viability, and improved productivity.

Lethal Genes

One result of inbreeding is concentration of lethal genes — recessive genes that show up only when two birds with the same trait are mated. Many lethals are related to specific breeds.

Japanese chickens carry the most widely studied lethal, the creeper gene, a trait that was once valued in broody hens because it causes short legs and therefore keeps the hen's body close to her chicks. When a creeper hen is mated to a cock carrying the creeper gene, one-quarter of the chicks die during the first week of incubation.

Dark Cornish carry a similar short-leg gene that causes death at the time of hatch. Signs of "Cornish lethal" include short beaks and wings, and bulging eyes.

New Hampshires carry a lethal that causes death in the twentieth and twenty-first day of hatch. Signs are crooked necks, short upper beaks, and shriveled leg muscles.

The silver gray Dorking has a lethal that causes death in the ninth day of incubation. Embryos have short necks and beaks.

A Barnvelder lethal causes "Donald Duck syndrome," in which the upper beak curls upward, the lower beak curls downward, and death occurs in the last days of incubation.

Congenital tremor is a lethal gene found in a number of breeds including Ancona, Plymouth Rock, Rhode Island Red, white Leghorn, and white Wyandotte. Chicks hatch but can't control their neck muscles. When a chick tries to stand, its head falls over and the bird falls down. Unable to eat or drink, it dies soon after hatching.

This is by no means a complete list of all the possible lethal genes. Among other lethals are those found in the black Minorca (short legs with extra toes), Rhode Island Red (short legs, wings, and beaks), white Leghorn (short legs and parrot-like beaks), and white Wyandotte (early embryonic death). Two common genetic factors that don't qualify as lethal genes, but that do reduce hatchability, are frizzledness and rumplessness.

One way to avoid the effects of lethal genes is to avoid mating closely related birds. Another way is to deliberately mate related birds and try to ferret out and cull breeders carrying lethal genes.

Genetic Defects

Two common hereditary defects, wry neck and wry tail, are caused by recessive genes, meaning they show up only when two birds are mated that carry the same gene.

Wry or twisted neck, resulting from curvature of the spine or "scoliosis," occurs as birds grow, and is particularly common among brown Leghorns. It usually happens to a group of related birds and does not affect their ability to drink.

Wry or twisted tail is a condition in which the tail feathers lean or twist to one side due to weakness in the vertebrae that hold the tail. Wry tail usually shows up as the tail feathers grow and become heavy.

Do not use birds with either of these defects as breeders. Cull breeders you can identify as carrying these recessive genes.

Chick Identification

You can't identify problem breeders unless you have some way to track their offspring. Chicks can be tracked in one of two ways: embryo dyeing and toe-punching. Embryo dyeing works best on chicks with white or light-colored down, and wears off as soon as the chicks grow their first feathers. Toe-punching works for all chicks and is permanent. You might want to combine the two techniques, dyeing embryos so you can toe-punch chicks that get mixed up during the hatch.

Embryo Dyeing

Injecting dye into eggs before they hatch lets you color-identify chicks from different matings. Dyeing in no way affects a chick's health or growth rate, provided you handle the eggs carefully and use only clean materials.

You will need a 20-gauge, 1-inch (25mm) long hypodermic needle, a sharp sewing needle of the same size or a little bit bigger, and a set of food dyes in 2 or 3 percent concentration (sold at most grocery stores). Among the primary colors, red, green, and blue show up best. Purple, made by combining red and blue, also works well. Yellow and orange don't show up well at all, since chick down is often yellowish to start with.

Embryos dye best during the eleventh to fourteenth day of incubation. To avoid chilling the eggs, remove no more eggs from the incubator than you can dye within 30 minutes.

About ½ inch (13 mm) from the pointed end, disinfect an area about the size of a quarter by wiping it with 95 percent rubbing alcohol or 2 percent tincture of iodine. Dip the sharp needle into the alcohol or iodine. Cushioning the egg in one hand, make a tiny hole in the center of the disinfected area by pressing against it with the needle, twisting the needle back and forth until it just penetrates the shell and membranes. Take care to make only a tiny hole that does not go deeper than necessary to pierce the inside membrane (no more than ⅛ inch or 3mm).

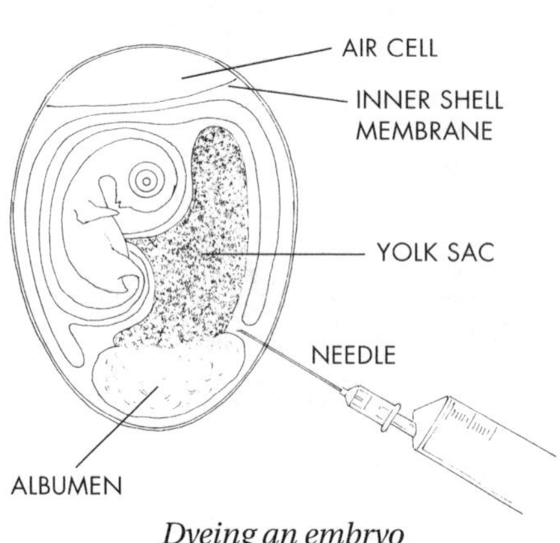

Dyeing an embryo

Dip the hypodermic needle into the alcohol or iodine and fill it with ½ cc of dye. Insert it into the hole so the tip is just beneath the inner shell membrane. *Very* slowly depress the plunger to release the dye without letting it overflow. To avoid mixing two colors, use a clean needle if you change dyes.

Seal the hole with a drop of melted paraffin or a tiny piece of adhesive bandage (Sheer Strip sticks best). Return the eggs to the incubator.

Toe-Punching

A toe-punch, available from many poultry supply catalogs, is about the size of fingernail clippers. It functions like a paper-hole punch and is used to remove the web between the toes of a newly hatched chick. As the chick grows, you can identify its parentage by the pattern of its punched-out webs.

When chicks are dry and ready to come out of the incubator, hold each gently but securely in one hand with one foot extended. Carefully position the punch over the web. With one firm stroke, punch away the web. Don't just punch a hole through the web, or the web may eventually grow back.

The pattern of removed webs lets you identify chicks from up to sixteen different matings. Here's how it works: on each foot, a chick has three main toes and therefore two webs — the outer web (between the middle and outside toe) and the inner web (between the middle and inside toe).

Starting at the chick's left side, the first web (left outer) stands for 1; the next web (left inner) stands for 2; the next web (right inner) stands for 4; the far right-hand web (right outer) stands for 8. Assign each mating a number from 1 to 15 and identify chicks from each mating by adding up the numbers corresponding to the punched webs. (For a sixteenth mating, leave the chicks unpunched.)

Chicks in batch number 1 have the left outer web punched. Chicks in batch number 2 have the left inner web punched. Chicks in batch number 3 have both the left outer and left inner webs punched (1 + 2 = 3). Chicks in batch number 5 have the left outer and right inner webs punched (1 + 4 = 5). And so forth.

Toe-punching works only if you know when you open the incubator which chicks came from which mating. You can identify chicks by:

- dyeing embryos
- hatching different matings at different times
- keeping eggs from different matings on different hatching trays
- enclosing small groups of eggs in upside-down baskets (pedigree baskets) such as plastic pint-size fruit baskets.

Toe punch patterns

Left Foot		*Right Foot*
\o¦ /	1	\ ¦ /
\ ¦o/	2	\ ¦ /
\o¦o/	3	\ ¦ /
\ ¦ /	4	\o¦ /
\o¦ /	5	\o¦ /
\ ¦o/	6	\o¦ /
\o¦o/	7	\o¦ /
\ ¦ /	8	\ ¦o/
\o¦ /	9	\ ¦o/
\ ¦o/	10	\ ¦o/
\o¦o/	11	\ ¦o/
\ ¦ /	12	\o¦o/
\o¦ /	13	\o¦o/
\ ¦o/	14	\o¦o/
\o¦o/	15	\o¦o/
\ ¦ /	16	\ ¦ /

Brooding

The typical death rate among chicks is 5 percent or less during the first 7 weeks, up to half of which usually occurs during the first 2 weeks. As distressing as occasional deaths among chicks can be, they're nothing to be concerned about.

On the other hand, stress caused by chilling, overheating, dehydration, or starvation, or any combination thereof, can drastically reduce the immunity of newly hatched chicks, making them susceptible to diseases they might otherwise resist. As soon as you remove chicks from the incubator, place them in a clean carton or disinfected brooder.

Chilling or overheating can occur if the brooder is too cool or too warm. You can tell chicks are comfortable when they are evenly distributed in the brooder. If they crowd to the corners, they are too warm. If they crowd beneath the heat source, they are cold. Brooding chicks at too cool a temperature increases their susceptibility to salmonella infections. Start the brooding temperature at approximately 95°F (35°C) and reduce it 5°F (3°C) each week until you reach room temperature.

Smothering can occur if chicks don't get enough heat or are placed in a draft, causing them to pile on top of each other to stay warm. As a result, the chicks on the bottom may be smothered. Smothering due to drafts or insufficient heat usually occurs at night. It can be prevented by placing a cardboard ring around the chicks during their first week of life, which keeps them near the source of heat and out of corners. Smothering also occurs when chicks are transported in stacked boxes with too few ventilation holes, or in the trunk of a car where air circulation is poor. In older chicks, piling may be caused by fright, especially if they've been moved to unfamiliar housing. When you move chicks to new housing, keep on dim lights and check the chicks often during the first few nights.

Crowding causes litter to become hard-packed and caked with droppings. Pads of litter and droppings may stick to the chicks' feet, causing crippling and/or infection. In crowded conditions, litter may have a strong odor, usually of ammonia. Severe ammonia fumes cause chicks to sit around with their eyes closed. If crowding is not corrected, chicks' eyes may become inflamed.

Feather- and toe-picking may result from crowding or from a diet too low in protein. Commercial chick starter usually contains enough protein to prevent picking. For more details, see "Cannibalism," page 135.

Brooder Diseases

Disease is usually not a problem in newly hatched chicks unless either they contract an egg-transmitted disease during incubation or the brooder environment is contaminated. The brooder may become contaminated either because it was not thoroughly cleaned after the last batch of chicks or because disease-causing organisms are being shed by chicks with an egg-transmitted disease, passing the disease on to other chicks in the brooder.

Since adult birds are reservoirs of infection (whether or not the adult birds themselves are sick), brood chicks away from older birds to give them time to develop natural immunities. Natural immunity is the result of gradual exposure to infectious organisms, rather than exposure to a high concentration that can cause disease instead of immunity.

The age at which chicks first show symptoms gives you a clue as to what disease might be involved. The diagnostic charts in chapter 9 list diseases by

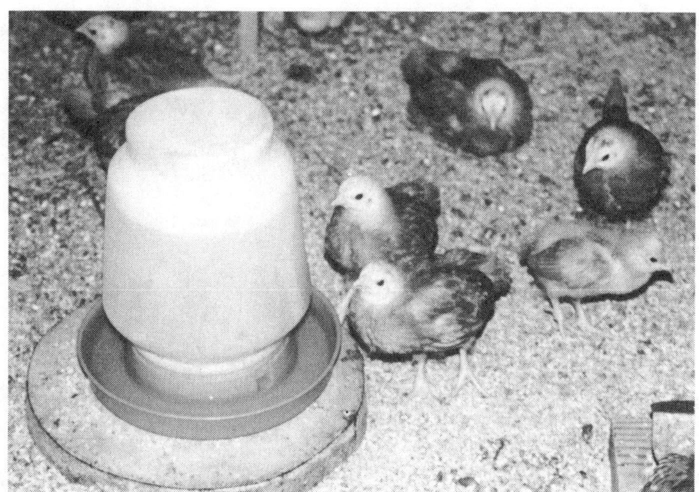
ALLAN DAMEROW

Chicks up to three weeks old benefit from a vitamin supplement in their drinking water.

age group. If your chicks get sick, look for a disease in their age group that most closely matches their symptoms. If you can't find a good match, consider diseases that are common in chicks slightly younger or older than yours.

The most common brooder disease, especially in warm humid weather, is coccidiosis. If you brood chicks in a temperate climate, or you hatch late in the season, prevent coccidiosis by using medicated starter ration containing a coccidiostat from day 1 to 16 weeks.

Brooder Nutrition

Slow growth in chicks can result from nutritional deficiencies that are all too common in breeder-flock diets. General signs of deficiency are poor growth and lack of vigor. All chicks up to 3 weeks old, especially chicks that have been shipped, benefit from the addition of a vitamin supplement in their drinking water.

Starve-Out

Starvation or "starve-out" results when chicks don't start eating within 2 to 3 days of hatch, causing them to get too weak to actively seek food. Starve-out can occur when shipped chicks are in transit for too long, so that they become weak before they are offered feed. It can also be caused by feeders that are placed where chicks can't find them or by feeders that are so high chicks can't reach them.

Other causes are excessive heat over feeders that drives chicks away, and using sand or sawdust as litter for newly hatched chicks. To keep chicks from eating litter instead of feed, cover the litter with paper toweling or burlap until chicks start eating well.

ALLAN DAMEROW

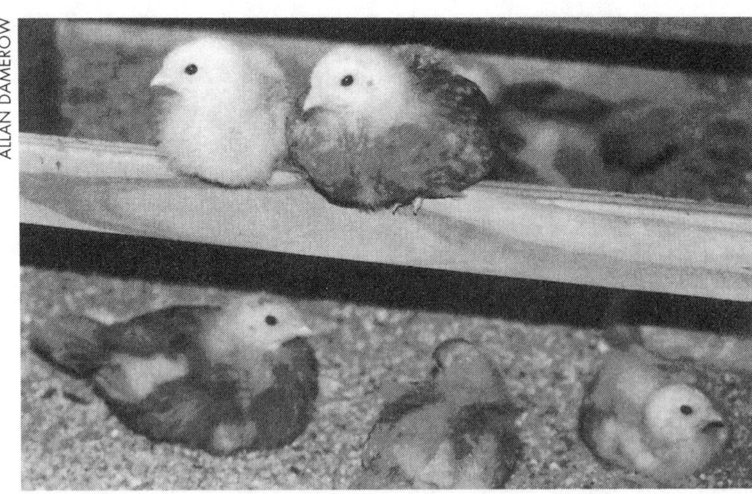

Healthy chicks are bright-eyed and perky.

Dehydration

Chicks will die if they do not start drinking by the time they are 4 days old. Chicks that can't find water don't grow at the proper rate, develop bluish beaks, and stop peeping. Deaths start occurring on the fourth day and continue until the sixth day. If water is available, but some chicks can't find it, the ones surviving after the sixth day are those that found the water.

If chicks have been shipped, make sure they know where to find water by dipping each beak into the fount as you transfer birds from the shipping carton to the brooder. Do not place the waterer on a platform where chicks can't reach it. If you switch from one waterer to another, leave the old waterer in place for a few days until the chicks get used to the new one. Stick your finger into the water to make sure a bad electrical connection isn't causing chicks to get a shock each time they try to drink.

Slipped Tendon

Slipped tendon, properly known as "perosis," may result from brooding chicks on paper or other slick surfaces. It occurs most often in heavy and fast-growing breeds, and may be caused either by hereditary factors or improper nutrition. If the cause is manganese deficiency, the problem should clear up after 1 month of feeding the chicks a supplement containing manganese. (Slipped tendon is described more fully in chapter 15).

Crooked Toes

A chick with crooked toes walks on the sides of its feet, causing the toes to accumulate manure clumps and/or develop sores. Chicks can have crooked toes if humidity was low during incubation or the brooder floor is cold. For unknown reasons, crooked toes have been associated with infrared brooding and wire floors. They may also be hereditary, occurring most often in heavy breeds, especially in males. If you can't identify a cause, don't keep crooked-toed chickens as breeders.

Crooked toes can be easily distinguished from curled-toe paralysis caused by riboflavin deficiency. In the former condition, toes twist to the side but the chick can still walk fine. In curled-toe paralysis, the toes curl under, causing the chick to walk on the tops of its toes. Because walking is difficult, the chick spends a lot of time resting on its hocks.

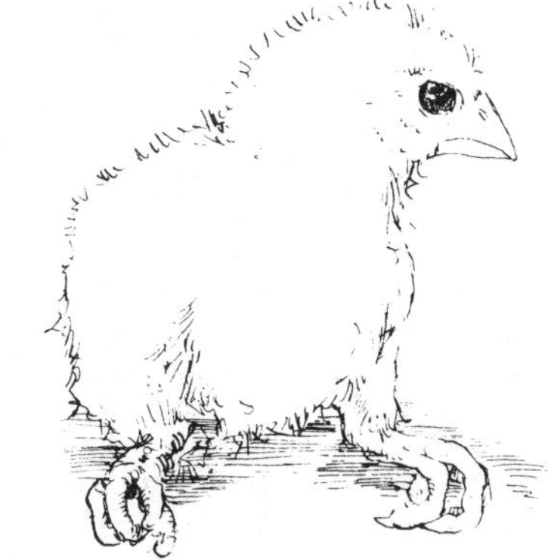

Chick with curled toe paralysis

Curled-toe paralysis can occur where breeder hens are fed unsupplemented lay ration. The chicks grow slowly and may have diarrhea during their first week or two of life. In a severe case, the toes curl completely back and the legs become so weak the chicks walk on their hocks. Deaths occur after about 3 weeks.

If the starter ration (rather than breeder ration) lacks sufficient riboflavin, symptoms will occur when chicks are 10 to 14 days old. An early warning sign is alert chicks that can't stand up. If you supply a multivitamin supplement in the chicks' water before their feet are permanently damaged, they should recover in 2 to 3 days.

Crooked toes can also be caused by flexing of the toes due to vitamin E deficiency, a condition known as "encephalomalacia" (sometimes called "crazy chick disease"), described fully in chapter 15.

Brooding Deficiencies

When *vitamin A* is deficient in the chicks' ration, the birds won't grow and will appear drowsy, weak, uncoordinated, and emaciated. They will have ruffled feathers, will stumble and stagger when they try to walk, and may have dry, dull eyes.

Thiamin (vitamin B1) deficiency in starter ration shows up suddenly when chicks are 2 weeks old and lose their appetites. As they lose weight, their feathers ruffle, they develop weak legs, and they become unsteady on their feet. Progressive paralysis starts at the feet and works upward, until chicks sit back on their hocks with their heads pointed upward (the so-called "star gazing" posture). Chicks given an oral thiamin supplement may recover.

In *riboflavin* (vitamin B2) deficiency, chicks continue to have good appetites but grow slowly and become weak and emaciated. They may have diarrhea, droopy wings, and dry skin. They are reluctant to move, doing so by walking on their hocks with the help of their wings.

Pyridoxine (vitamin B6) deficiency causes chicks to walk with jerky move-

CHART 13-3

Nutritional Problems in Chicks

Sign	Deficiency/ Imbalance
Beak, crusty	biotin pantothenic acid
Blood, hemorrhage	copper vitamin K vitamin B12
clots slowly	vitamin K
Bones, soft (rickets)	calcium phosphorus vitamin D
Breast, muscles, degenerated (white muscle disease)	selenium & vitamin E biotin
Droppings, soft	niacin riboflavin
Eyes, dry/dull	vitamin A
scabby or crusty	biotin pantothenic acid
stuck together	vitamin A
pointed upward (star gazing)	thiamin
Feathers, black in brown or red breed	vitamin D
lack color	copper folic acid iron
long or uneven	amino acid protein
rough and frizzled	folic acid niacin pantothenic acid zinc
ruffled	vitamin A thiamin
Feet, bottoms rough and cracked	biotin pantothenic acid niacin
scaly	riboflavin
toes curl	zinc

Sign	Deficiency/ Imbalance
Legs, short/thick	manganese zinc
twisted (slipped tendon)	biotin choline folic acid manganese nicotinic acid pyridoxine zinc
hocks enlarged	niacin zinc
muscles degenerated (white muscle disease)	selenium & vitamin E
paralyzed	thiamin
weak	thiamin
Mouth, inflamed (black tongue)	niacin
Nervous disorders, excessive fright	chloride
jerky movements	pyridoxine
trembling (encephalomalacia)	vitamin E
uncoordinated	vitamin A vitamin E
Parasites (coccidia, roundworm)	vitamin A
Skin, dry	riboflavin
pale	folic acid copper iron pyridoxine
greenish fluid beneath	selenium & vitamin E
Wings, droopy	riboflavin

ments. They may run around flapping their wings, then fall onto their sides backs, jerking their heads and legs. Pyridoxine deficiency is similar to encephalomalacia, except that here the nervous activity is much more intense and ends in exhaustion and death.

Folic acid deficiency causes poor growth, anemia (skin appears pale), and slipped tendon. It can cause lack of feather color in Rhode Island Red and black Leghorn chicks and poor feathering in any breed.

Vitamin E deficiency causes chicks to stumble and stagger when they walk. A serious deficiency may result in encephalomalacia, exudative diathesis, or white muscle disease (all described in chapter 15).

Vitamin K deficiency causes a chick's blood to clot slowly, so the chick may bleed to death from a relatively minor wound. Chicks will be deficient in vitamin K if the breeder-flock diet was deficient.

14

Chickens and Human Health

THE CHANCE THAT YOU WILL GET A DISEASE from your chickens is pretty slim, especially if you practice common sense hygiene that includes washing your hands after working in or around your hen house. Many of the organisms that cause the diseases described in this chapter are fairly common in the human environment, whether or not that environment includes chickens. Ordinarily, those organisms cause no problems. Exceptions are in people with impaired immune systems or low resistance due to systemic therapy (immunosuppressive or antibacterial therapy, for example), pregnancy, obesity, diabetes, or some disease unrelated to chickens.

The low risk of getting any of these diseases is no consolation to those few who might be infected. This chapter, then, is offered in the spirit of helpfulness — physicians tend to overlook or misdiagnose diseases they don't often see. If you visit your doctor about a condition you suspect might be related to your chickens, mention your concern to your doctor.

Although many of these diseases have sources other than the poultry environment, the focus here is on their relationship with chickens. Diseases that humans can get, directly or indirectly, from chickens can be broken down into four categories: environmental, parasitic, zoonotic, and toxic.

CHART 14-1

Poultry-Related Human Diseases

Category	*Chicken Disease*	*Risk of Human Infection*
ENVIRONMENTAL		
Aspergillosis	Aspergillosis	low
Candidiasis	Thrush	moderate
Cryptococcosis	none	very low
Farmer's Lung	none	low
Hen Worker's Lung	none	low
Histoplasmosis	Histoplasmosis	very low
Pseudomonas	Pseudomonas	extremely low
PARASITIC		
Mites	Mites	low
Ticks	Ticks	low
Toxoplasmosis	Toxoplasmosis	extremely low
Worms	Worms	extremely low
ZOONOTIC		
Chlamydiosis	Chlamydiosis	low
Conjunctivitis	Newcastle	moderate
Erysipeloid	Erysipelas	low
Listeriosis	Listeriosis	extremely low
MEAT/EGG-BORNE TOXINS		
Campylobacter	Campylobacteriosis	moderate
Clostridium	Botulism	extremely low
	Necrotic enteritis	moderate
Colitis	Colibacillosis	moderate
Salmonella	Paratyphoid (*E. enteritidis*)	moderate
Staph poisoning	Staphylococcosis	extremely low

Environmental Diseases

It is possible for humans to contract some infections from the same sources as chickens, the result of environmental exposure rather than inter-species contagion. Most human diseases caused by the poultry environment are mycoses or fungal infections.

Aspergillosis

Aspergillus fumigatus fungus is quite common in both poultry and human environments, but infection is more common in chickens than in humans. Humans get infected by inhaling spores from decaying litter. It is a rare disease that affects primarily people with low resistance or compromised immune systems, in whom the infection can be serious and occasionally fatal. In others, the usual result is allergic bronchitis (a respiratory disease characterized by coughing), usually successfully treated with anti-asthmatic drugs.

Aspergillus flavus, found in moldy grains, peanuts, and manioc (fed to both chickens and humans), produces a poison that has been implicated as the cause of human liver cancer in tropical Africa and Asia, where the fungus is common.

Candidiasis

Candida albicans yeast commonly lives in the bowels of humans, chickens, and many other animals. Infection is transmitted by direct contact with yeast in droppings and is usually superficial, except in people with low resistance or compromised immunity. Infection may involve the mouth (children), the genitals (adults), or the skin under fingernails (all ages), resulting in an itchy rash that eventually swells with pus. It can be treated with an anti-fungal powder or cream (such as nystatin) and corticosteroid cream (such as hydrocortisone).

Cryptococcosis

Cryptococcocus neoformans is a fungus found worldwide in bird environments (more commonly birds other than chickens). The fungus is not known to infect chickens, but on rare occasions does cause infection in humans. It inflicts primarily men between the ages of 40 and 60, particularly those who use steroids, have Hodgkin's disease, or otherwise have suppressed immune systems.

Infection can be acute or chronic and may affect the brain or lungs, or become systemic and affect the entire body. The most likely result of inhaling the fungus is meningitis or inflammation of the brain covering. Symptoms include headache, stiff neck, blurred vision, and confusion, leading to coma and death if not treated with anti-fungal drugs. Inhaling the fungus may cause growths in the lungs. Symptoms of lung infection are chest pain and coughing, sometimes involving phlegm. Lung cases usually clear up on their own.

Hen Worker's Lung

Hen worker's lung is an allergic reaction to blood protein and droppings inhaled in poultry dust. Few people develop this disorder, which usually requires prolonged exposure such as a professional poultry worker might experience. Symptoms may come on suddenly, approximately 6 hours after exposure. They include difficult or painful breathing, cough, fever, chills, and sometimes loss of appetite, nausea, and vomiting. The symptoms, easily mistaken for flu, may last several hours or up to 2 days, although complete recovery may take weeks.

The allergy sometimes develops gradually, starting with bouts of breathing difficulties and coughing that increase in frequency and severity. The allergy occasionally takes a chronic form, resulting in difficult or painful breathing brought on by physical activity, accompanied by the coughing up of phlegm, extreme fatigue, and gradual weight loss. If corrective measures are not taken, the end result may be respiratory failure.

This disease is difficult to diagnose. The primary clue is the relationship of symptoms to exposure — for example, professional workers who experience relief during their days off. Backyard keepers may experience symptoms 4 to 8 hours after exposure, something that can be hard to determine if you visit your coop two or more times a day. Although frequent attacks reduce the lung's elasticity and eventually cause scar tissue, an early chest x-ray may appear normal, leading to a possible misdiagnosis of heart condition.

Hen worker's lung can usually be cleared up by avoiding the poultry environment. Complete recovery is possible if avoidance occurs before lung tissue becomes scarred. Whether or not you suffer from hen worker's lung, it makes good health sense to wear a dust mask when you work in the coop, particularly during cleanup, and to install a fan to remove floating dust particles from the air.

Farmer's Lung

Farmer's lung is an allergic reaction similar to hen worker's lung, but caused by the spores of *Micropolyspora faeni* or *Thermoactinomyces vulgaris* inhaled from moldy grains or litter. The allergy typically occurs in areas of high rainfall, usually toward the end of winter following a wet summer. Symptoms are nearly identical to those of hen worker's lung. Prevention involves wearing a face mask when working in dusty areas and avoiding the storage of moist litter or grain over winter.

Histoplasmosis

Inhaled *Histoplasma capsulatum* spores from old, dry chicken droppings while cleaning or dismantling an old chicken house (or while working in infected garden soil) can cause a rare though potentially serious infectious fungal disease. Histoplasmosis occurs mainly in the Ohio and central Mississippi river valleys where the altitude is low, rainfall is 35 to 50 inches a year, and temperatures remain even. Infection does not spread from birds to humans. It usually occurs only in someone who inhales large numbers of spores or who has an immunodeficiency disorder.

Histoplasmosis settles first in the respiratory system and may produce no symptoms (other than an abnormal chest x-ray) or may cause symptoms virtually identical to those of flu — fever, coughing, joint pains, and general discomfort. In patients with suppressed immunity, the disease may spread throughout the body, requiring treatment with anti-fungal drugs to prevent a fatal outcome.

Most cases require no treatment — the disease usually clears up on its own. Avoid infection by misting litter to control dust before cleaning your coop and by wearing a respirator or a dampened handkerchief over your mouth and nose while you work.

Pseudomonas

Pseudomonas aeruginosa bacteria are commonly found in soil, particularly in humid environments. In the rare case where chickens become infected, their contaminated meat decays rapidly. Human infection is extremely rare and most likely to occur through an open wound or a deep puncture, typically to the foot. The puncture turns purplish-black toward the center with a reddened area around the outside, and requires antibiotic treatment.

Parasitic Diseases

Parasitic diseases are among the most unlikely diseases a human can get from a chicken.

Mites and Ticks

Mites may crawl onto your body if you handle infested chickens, but they usually won't stay long. Minimize discomfort by taking a shower and washing your clothing.

A tick can also get on you from a chicken. If the tick bites, it might possibly transmit a disease such as tick paralysis (characterized by loss of appetite, weakness, lack of coordination, and gradual paralysis) or Rocky Mountain spotted fever (characterized by severe headache, chills, muscle pains, and prostration).

If you find a tick trying to burrow into your skin, grasp it with a pair of tweezers and pull until it releases its hold — pull gently but firmly so you neither crush the tick nor break its body away while its head remains in your skin. Disinfect the bite with rubbing alcohol. See your doctor if you experience any symptoms of a tick-borne disease.

Worms

You aren't likely to get infested by worms from your chickens, since most worms that prefer poultry do not invade humans. You can, however, accidentally ingest worm eggs if you eat without washing your hands after handling contaminated soil or litter. Such an infestation causes few or no symptoms and is easy to treat with an appropriate anthelmintic.

Toxoplasmosis

Toxoplasma gondii protozoa rarely infect chickens and even more rarely infect humans. Toxoplasmosis results from eating raw or undercooked meat of infected chickens (or other animals). Infection usually causes no ill effect, except in people with immunodeficiency disorders and in unborn children. One-third of the pregnant women who get toxoplasmosis during pregnancy pass it to their unborn children, resulting in serious damage (such as blindness or retardation), miscarriage, or stillbirth.

The most common symptoms of toxoplasmosis are fatigue, low fever, and muscle pains. The disease is self-limiting and usually goes away on its own. Extremely rare are serious cases involving vital organs (eye, brain, or heart), which may be diagnosed through blood tests and treated with antimalarial and sulfa drugs.

Zoonoses

Many diseases are species specific, meaning they affect only one species, whether it be chickens, humans, or some other animal. A few diseases, called "zoonoses," are shared by animals and humans. Some chicken diseases are caused by zoonotic organisms — creatures so flexible that they can adapt to the human species. Don't be too quick to suspect you have a zoonosis unless your chickens have been positively diagnosed as having the disease.

Chlamydiosis

Humans can contract chlamydiosis, a rare form of pneumonia, by inhaling dust from feathers or dried droppings of infected birds. The disease was first recognized in psittacine birds (parrots), and so was called "psittacosis" or "parrot fever." The same disease, when transmitted from chickens to humans, is sometimes called "ornithosis."

Virulent strains appear in cyclic fashion, but not every avian outbreak causes human illness. The two most likely causes of chlamydiosis in humans are heavy exposure while dressing birds, more often turkeys than chickens (solution: wet feathers before plucking), and exposure to dusty, crowded facilities (improve ventilation and wear a dust mask and gloves).

The incubation period (time between exposure and first symptoms) is 1 to 2 weeks. Symptoms include loss of appetite, fever, chills, severe headache, dry cough, constipation, muscle stiffness, and sensitivity to light; sometimes rash, diarrhea, and vomiting. Early symptoms may be easily confused with flu or other forms of pneumonia. Left untreated, chlamydiosis can be fatal, especially in those over the age of 50, but usually clears up after 10 days of antibiotic treatment.

Conjunctivitis

Humans who handle vaccine for Newcastle disease often suffer from conjunctivitis (eye inflammation) within 1 to 4 days. Conjunctivitis can also occur in those who butcher infected birds and, much less likely, those who treat sick chickens. The virulence of Newcastle disease in chickens has no bearing on whether or not humans become infected. Symptoms are itchy, red, watery, sometimes swollen eye (usually only one). No treatment is known. Recovery is spontaneous and complete, usually in 4 days, but may take as long as 3 weeks.

Erysipeloid

Erysipeloid is a bacterial skin infection that invades through a cut or other wound on a person who handles or slaughters infected birds. Infection usually appears within a week as an itchy, burning, raised and hardened purplish-red patch on the hand that may gradually grow larger.

Infection is most likely to occur in butchers, kitchen workers, veterinarians, and artificial inseminators — more often those handling fish, pork, and turkey than chickens. The infection is self-limiting. Treated with penicillin, it usually clears up within 2 to 3 weeks.

Listeriosis

Listeriosis is more common in animals other than chickens, and is even rarer in humans. It is, however, life threatening to senior citizens over the age of 70 and to unborn children infected through their mother's blood. The disease spreads to humans who handle or butcher infected birds or who eat improperly cooked infected meat.

Symptoms range from mild skin irritation, to fever and muscle aches, to meningitis (inflammation of the brain covering) or blood poisoning. The most likely result of infection in humans, primarily those who process the meat of infected birds, is conjunctivitis (eye inflammation).

Diagnosis requires blood tests — be sure to tell your doctor you suspect listeriosis, or the lab won't think of looking for *Listeria.* The disease is easily treated with antibiotics.

Meat and Egg Contamination

One of the reasons people raise their own chickens, even though doing so costs more than purchasing store-bought meat and eggs, is due to concerns about pesticide and herbicide residues, bacterial contaminants, and antibiotics in commercial poultry products. Sadly, no one is seriously guarding the safety of our meat and egg supply. Even the physician who oversees the food-borne-diseases branch of the Centers for Disease Control and Prevention, Dr. James Hughes, has been quoted as saying, "We've got the most rudimentary surveillance of food-borne diseases you can imagine." The CDC tracks and reports on food-borne illnesses, but does little to control them.

Pesticides and herbicides are used on most feed crops that make up chicken rations. Unless you have a source of so-called organic rations, your eggs and chicken meat will contain no less residue from pesticides and herbicides than commercial meat, which in any case is extremely low.

Antibiotics at low levels, along with growth-promoting hormones, are used commercially to make chickens reach market weights faster and with lower feed costs. You can easily avoid antibiotics and hormones in homegrown meat by not making them part of your management routine and by observing the withdrawal period for any drug you use for therapeutic purposes.

Bacteria pose the greatest threat among contaminants in poultry meat or eggs, especially those that are commercially produced, since large-scale production lends itself to unsanitary practices. Homegrown meat birds, by contrast, are usually killed and cleaned individually, are rinsed under a running faucet (rather than in a vat of rapidly contaminated water), and are refrigerated promptly; similarly, homegrown eggs are exposed to fewer sources of contamination. Nonetheless, remaining aware of the dangers of bacterial contamination is the first step toward avoiding them.

Food-Borne Bacteria

If meat or eggs are held at room temperature for too long, any bacteria present will proliferate. Some multiply more rapidly than others. Since there's no way to tell whether or not bacteria are present, you can't go wrong if you always handle meat and eggs as if they are contaminated.

In a healthy adult, bacterial food poisoning is usually little more than an

CHART 14-2

Food-Borne Bacteria

	Infective	*Toxic*
Campylobacter jejuni		x
Clostridium botulinum		x
C. perfringens		x
Escherichia coli	x	x
Salmonella enteritidis	x	
Staphyloccus aureus		x

annoyance. In the very young, the aged, or someone with a weakened immune system, however, bacterial food poisoning can be serious or even fatal. General symptoms are loss of appetite, nausea, vomiting, abdominal cramps, and diarrhea that comes on suddenly. In many cases, illness strikes a group of people who have shared a tainted meal.

Most cases are resolved with bed rest and plenty of fluids. For most people, the most serious consequence is loss of body fluids and salts (electrolytes). Since symptoms resemble the flu, most cases go untreated and end in spontaneous recovery. Unless the illness is complicated by other factors, antibiotics may be of little help and may actually make matters worse.

The most common causes of bacterial food poisoning are *Campylobacter, E. coli,* and *Salmonella.* Some food-borne bacteria are infective — they cause disease by invading the intestine wall. Others produce toxins that inhibit nutrient absorption. Some work both ways.

Egg Sanitation

A freshly laid egg is warm and moist, and therefore attracts bacteria and molds that exist in the poultry environment. After leaving a hen's warm body, the egg immediately starts to cool. As its contents contract, a vacuum is created that can draw bacteria and molds through the 6,000-plus pores in the shell, potentially causing egg spoilage and human illness.

Eggs produced at home in a clean environment, collected often and promptly placed under refrigeration (after cracked or seriously soiled eggs are discarded), rarely pose a health problem. Eggs that are slightly soiled with dirt or dried droppings should be dry cleaned with fine sandpaper. Improperly washing them can do more harm than good.

Eggs produced in a not-so-clean environment and those destined for market may need to be washed. Market eggs are often subjected to storage temperatures that are higher than desirable (causing bacteria and mold on the shell to multiply) and to repeated warming and cooling (drawing more microorganisms through the shell each time).

If you wash eggs, use water that is 20°F (11°C) warmer than the eggs are, otherwise vacuum action may draw microorganisms through the shell or tiny cracks may develop in the shell that expose eggs to invasion by bacteria and molds. Wash eggs with detergent (not soap) to remove soil. Rinse them in water of the same temperature as the wash water, adding a sanitizer to reduce the number of microorganisms on the shell (the sanitizer won't eliminate *all* bacteria and mold). If you wash a large number of eggs, change the wash and rinse solution often, since both rapidly become contaminated.

Sanitizers that will not introduce off odors, colors, or flavors include chlorine solution (such as Clorox bleach) and quaternary ammonium compounds or "quats," used at the rate of 100 to 200 parts per million. Don't get carried away and combine chlorine and a quat, or they'll counteract each other.

Dry eggs thoroughly before placing them in cartons, since wet shells more readily pick up bacteria.

Salmonellosis

Salmonella bacteria can be found almost everywhere. You would have a hard time finding meat, eggs, or any other food that did not harbor one of the 2,200 salmonella strains. An estimated 3 to 4 million cases of salmonellosis occur each year. No one knows the exact number, since not all cases are reported. Only about 5 percent of all cases can be traced to chickens.

Over 150 different salmonella strains that produce paratyphoid infections in chickens cause serious illness in humans. In the 1960s, outbreaks of salmonella poisoning from bacteria in eggs resulted in institution of the Egg Products Inspection Act in the United States. Among other things, the Act removed substandard non-Grade A (cracked or "check") eggs from the marketplace. For a time, fewer incidence of salmonellosis in humans were reported.

Since the 1960s, however, an especially virulent, antibiotic-resistant strain of *S. enteritidis* has appeared in commercial poultry flocks, and incidents of salmonella poisoning have doubled.

Until a few years ago, experts believed that *S. enteritidis* infected an egg through the shell, after the egg was laid, and that frequent egg collection and disinfection would minimize contamination. In the 1980s, a new outbreak of salmonellosis in the Northeast led to the discovery of salmonella bacteria in hens' ovaries, infecting eggs before they were laid. The bacteria have since spread to regions outside the Northeast and are becoming antibiotic resistant, possibly due to drug overuse by commercial producers.

An infected hen won't always lay salmonella-contaminated eggs, and a hen that usually lays normal eggs may occasionally produce a contaminated egg. According to the Centers for Disease Control, only about 1 in 5,000 to 10,000 eggs is contaminated. The problem is compounded, however, when one contaminated egg is added to a recipe along with several good eggs, or foods are served that contain raw eggs. The concentration of bacteria increases when egg-rich foods — quiche, homemade eggnog or mayonnaise, custard pie, hollandaise and bernaise sauce, and the like — are held at room temperature before they are served.

Despite all the press coverage of salmonella poisoning, experts claim your chance of getting salmonellosis from eggs is only about 1 in 2 million. In a healthy person, poisoning requires eating a large number of bacteria. Most cases occur not in homes but in restaurants, schools, hospitals, and other institutions where fresh eggs may not be cooked long enough or may sit on a counter too long, allowing any bacteria present to rapidly multiply. Most of the 500 deaths per year occur in nursing homes.

Salmonella bacteria, when present, are concentrated in an egg's yolk, since the white has antibacterial properties. They may also be present in undercooked meat. Although salmonella poisoning from eating chicken gets a lot of publicity, rare beef is a more common cause, since most people cook their chicken thoroughly. Chicken is thoroughly cooked at 180°F (82°C); salmonella bacteria are killed at any temperature above 142°F (61°C).

CHART 14-3

Bacterial Food Poisoning Quick-Check

Bacteria	*Incubation*	*Symptoms*	*Duration*
Campylobacter jejuni	2-5 days	cramps diarrhea fever headache	2-7 days
Clostridium botulinum	18-36 hours	difficulty: breathing seeing speaking swallowing constipation no fever	fatal without care
C. perfringens	8-24 hours	diarrhea gas pains no fever	24 hours
Escherichia coli	3-4 days	cramps watery or bloody diarrhea no or low fever	1-8 days
Salmonella spp.	12-72 hours	diarrhea fever vomiting	2-7 days
Staphylococcus aureus	2-8 hours	diarrhea vomiting headache fever	3-6 hours

Many people who have salmonellosis never know it, believing instead that they have an upset stomach or a mild case of flu. The illness usually runs its course in a week or less. Symptoms begin 12 to 72 hours after eating contaminated food, which tastes and smells normal. Symptoms include nausea, fever, abdominal cramps, and diarrhea.

A serious infection can spread from the intestines to the bloodstream and other body sites, causing death, especially among: infants, the elderly, anyone with an impaired immune system, a patient undergoing treatment with antibiotics (which remove beneficial bacteria from the intestines, clearing the way for disease-causing bacteria), an ulcer patient taking antacids (which reduce bacteria-killing stomach acids).

Most infections are relatively mild and most people recover without treatment, as long as they avoid dehydration by drinking lots of fluids. Hospitalization and antibiotic treatment are needed if symptoms persist or the diarrhea is severe and/or accompanied by high fever, weakness, or disorientation.

Campylobacteriosis

Although campylobacteriosis gets less press than salmonellosis, it is the world's leading food-borne pathogen, the most common cause of diarrheal illness in humans, and of growing concern to chicken keepers because of its prevalence in commercially produced poultry. Of the three species that cause human disease, *Campylobacter jejuni* — which causes campylobacteriosis in chickens — has been identified more than 90 percent of the time.

Campylobacteriosis is an occupational hazard in poultry processing plants. Humans become infected by handling infected birds or by eating undercooked infected poultry. (Unlike salmonellosis, campylobacteriosis does not infect humans through raw or undercooked eggs.)

The bacteria produce a toxin that irritates the lining of the intestine, causing abdominal pain and watery, sometimes bloody diarrhea, occasionally accompanied by a fever ranging from 100° to 104°F (38-40°C). Campylobacteriosis can be prevented by observing the same precautions that prevent salmonellosis, as outlined on page 242.

Clostridium Poisoning

Clostridium perfringens is called the "buffet germ" because it proliferates and creates toxins in slowly cooling foods and in foods kept at low holding temperatures. Prevent it by keeping cooked meat and eggs at 140°F (60°C) or by cooling them quickly to less than 40°F (5°C). When you cook for a crowd, divide large amounts of food to speed cooling. Separate chicken from gravy or stuffing before you store them in the refrigerator. Most strains of *C. perfringens* cause a mild, self-limiting illness, but some can be serious to fatal. See a doctor

Cooking Poultry

Follow these precautions whenever you handle poultry meat and eggs.

Handling Poultry

When you butcher chickens, avoid feather and fecal contamination; rinse meat thoroughly in clear water.

Thaw frozen poultry thoroughly before cooking it.

Thaw raw meat in the refrigerator (or in a plastic bag under cold running water), never on the counter top.

Wash hands, knife, cutting board, and other utensils after contact with raw meat.

Sanitize counters by wiping them with 2 teaspoons of chlorine bleach in a quart of warm water.

Wipe counters with either paper towels or a dish cloth washed in soap and chlorine bleach after each use.

Don't let cooked meat (such as chicken barbecue) come into contact with raw meat or the plate it was carried on.

Before storing cooked meat, cool it quickly to slow the multiplication of bacteria.

Cooking Poultry

Heat poultry meat to 185°F (85°C).

Reheat leftovers to 165°F (74°C).

Cook casseroles and other combination foods to 160°F (71°C).

Barbecue until no red shows at the joints.

Hold cooked poultry above 140°F (60°C) for no longer than 2 hours.

Handling Eggs

Collect eggs often and refrigerate them promptly.

Don't use cracked or dirty eggs.

Wash hands and utensils after contact with raw eggs.

Don't serve foods containing uncooked eggs.

Don't hold foods prepared with raw or undercooked eggs at room temperature.

Promptly refrigerate leftovers.

Cooking Eggs

Heat eggs and egg-rich foods to 160°F (71°C).

Poach eggs for 5 minutes in boiling water.

Boil eggs in shells for 7 minutes.

Fry eggs (in an electric frying pan set at 250°F, 121°C) as follows:

Scrambled, 1 minute;
Sunnyside up, uncovered, 7 minutes;
Sunnyside, covered or basted, 4 minutes;
Over easy, 3 minutes one side, then 2 minutes.

Hold cooked eggs between 40° and 140°F (5-60°C) for no longer than 2 hours.

When in Doubt: **Call the toll-free USDA meat and poultry hotline:**

1-800-535-4555

if you experience cramps, severe diarrhea, and bloating gas.

Clostridium botulinum is usually associated with improperly canned low-acid foods. Home-canned vegetables are the most common source, but unconfirmed reports have implicated canned chicken meat. Botulinum-laden food may or may not appear cloudy, contents may swell causing jars to crack or lids to become loose. Do not use any canned food that smells improper or that sprays out when you open the container. Never test suspect foods by tasting them. Cook home-canned chicken to 176°F (80°C) for at least 30 minutes — the toxin is readily destroyed by heat.

The botulinum toxin affects the nervous system, causing double vision, slurred speech, and difficulty breathing and swallowing. Symptoms may occur any time from 4 hours to 8 days after eating poisoned food, but usually appear within 18 to 36 hours. Botulism affects everyone who shares a poisoned meal. If you suspect botulism poisoning, get immediate medical attention. Nerve damage is irreversible. Untreated botulism poisoning can cause death due to paralysis of the respiratory system.

Colitis

E. coli from poultry droppings may contaminate meat during butchering, although avian strains are not a significant cause of infection in humans. Of the 3 percent of commercial meat contaminated with *E. coli,* beef is more likely than chicken to carry it. Coliform bacteria invade the intestine wall and also produce toxins, causing severe cramps and watery diarrhea that soon turns bloody. Prevention and treatment is the same as for salmonellosis.

Staphylococcal Food Poisoning

Staphylococcus aureus bacteria are present wherever there are chickens. About 50 percent of the strains generate toxins that cause food poisoning in mishandled poultry meat. Symptoms are nausea, vomiting, cramps, diarrhea, and sometimes headache, fever, and prostration. Recovery is usually spontaneous and occurs in about a day. Typically, several people get ill after sharing a meal together. Staph bacteria can't be destroyed by heat, making sanitary butchering especially important.

Humans can potentially get a superficial staph infection (impetigo) while treating chickens for bumblefoot or an infected breast blister. Although there has never been a proven case of a chicken infecting a person, wear plastic gloves during treatment and thoroughly wash your hands afterward.

15

Diseases and Disorders

This alphabetic listing is designed to serve as a quick reference to the most critical information surrounding common diseases and disorders. The information is organized and cross-referenced for easy retrieval. Unless otherwise noted, cross references are found within this chapter. Following are explanations of the categories used in each disease and disorder entry.

Sample Listing

Common Name

ALSO CALLED — alternative names, scientific names (for the benefit of specialists and readers who consult technical works), and names no longer in vogue (for readers who peruse old poultry books)

INCIDENCE — how common the disease is and the geographic area in which it is likely to be found

SYSTEM/ORGAN AFFECTED — primary body part or system the disease affects

INCUBATION PERIOD — amount of time from exposure to the first sign of infection (helps diagnose the disease based on past contacts or identify the source of infection once the disease has been diagnosed)

PROGRESSION — how hard the disease hits a flock, how fast it spreads, and whether it is acute (short-term, ending in recovery or death) or chronic (long-term)

SYMPTOMS — most likely symptoms or combinations of symptoms; since no two cases are ever exactly alike, not all symptoms will always appear; age groups are approximations only

PERCENTAGE AFFECTED — proportion of an affected flock likely to be involved

MORTALITY — percentage of affected birds likely to die from the disease

POSTMORTEM FINDINGS — changes that occur within a diseased bird's body (for details on postmortem examination, see chapter 10)

RESEMBLES — diseases with similar symptoms and, when possible, how to tell them apart

DIAGNOSIS — best way to identify the disease through a combination of flock history, symptoms, and postmortem findings; some diseases are so similar to others that laboratory tests are required for a positive diagnosis, some can *only* be identified by laboratory tests (for diagnostic guidelines, see chapter 9)

CAUSE — primary cause of the disease (for information on the causes of infectious diseases, see chapter 7)

TRANSMISSION — how the disease spreads

PREVENTION — steps for preventing the disease (for information on immunity, see chapter 12)

TREATMENT — approaches toward dealing with the diseases (for information on therapy, see chapter 11)

HUMAN HEALTH RISK — any potential risk this disease poses for humans (additional information can be found in chapter 14)

- A -

A-avitaminosis. *See* Roup (nutritional)
Acariasis. *See* "Mites," page 67
Acute Death Syndrome. *See* Sudden Death Syndrome
Acute Heart Failure. *See* Sudden Death Syndrome
Adenoviral Infection. *See* Infectious Anemia
AE. *See* Epidemic Tremor

Aflatoxicosis

Also Called — aspergillus toxicosis, x disease
Incidence — rare but increasingly more common worldwide
System/Organ Affected — entire body
Incubation Period — up to 2 weeks, depending on amount of toxin ingested
Progression — usually acute, sometimes chronic
Symptoms — in incubated eggs from poisoned hens: embryo death during first week
— in young birds: loss of appetite, slow growth, weakness, increased susceptibility to bruising and heat stress, sudden death
— in hens: reduced egg production, smaller eggs with decreased hatchability, increased susceptibility to infection (especially cecal coccidiosis and Marek's disease)
— in cocks: weight loss, reduced fertility
Percentage Affected — 100 percent of those consuming contaminated feed
Mortality — none in adult chickens
Postmortem Findings — none or light-colored muscles; sometimes swollen kidneys and enlarged liver with pale yellowish areas that are white at the center
Resembles — fatty liver syndrome, lymphoid leukosis; infectious anemia, except that infectious anemia affects only growing birds
Diagnosis — difficult: symptoms, feed analysis, microscopic examination of liver tissue
Cause — toxins produced by *Aspergillus flavus, A. parasiticus,* and *Penicillium puberulum* mold in litter and in corn and other grain (especially grain that's insect damaged, drought stressed, or broken into pieces); increases susceptibility to infectious diseases and often found in combination with infectious anemia and/or fatty liver syndrome
Transmission — eating moldy grain
Prevention — avoid moldy grain; use only fresh feed (most commercial feeds contain mold inhibitors); store feed in plastic bin (metal sweats) in cool, dry place
Treatment — remove and deeply bury moldy grain; minimize stress; boost dietary energy and protein and offer a vitamin supplement until recovery
Human Health Risk — aflatoxin (a poison and a carcinogen) is rapidly excreted in droppings so there is little danger of residue in meat; residue may appear in yolks of eggs up to 10 days after contaminated rations are withdrawn; humans may get food poisoning from eating moldy grain

AI. *See* Influenza
Airsacculitis. *See* Air-Sac Disease

Air-Sac Disease

Also Called — airsacculitis, air-sac infection, air-sac syndrome (one form of colibacillosis and/or mycoplasmosis)

Incidence — common worldwide

System/Organ Affected — respiratory

Incubation Period — 6 to 21 days

Progression — acute to chronic

Symptoms — in young birds, 5 to 12 weeks old (most commonly 6 to 9 weeks old): coughing, rattling, nasal discharge, breathing difficulty, loss of appetite, rapid weight loss, standing around with eyes closed, stunted growth

Percentage Affected — 100 percent

Mortality — up to 30 percent

Postmortem Findings — thick mucus in nasal passages and throat; cloudy air sacs containing cheesy material; transparent film covering liver and heart

Resembles — chronic respiratory disease, except that CRD affects older birds and is usually milder

Diagnosis — flock history, symptoms, postmortem findings, confirmed by laboratory identification of bacteria

Cause — *Escherichia coli* and *Mycoplasma gallisepticum* (sometimes *M. synoviae)* bacteria; often occurs in combination with or following vaccination for chronic respiratory disease, infectious bronchitis, infectious laryngotracheitis, Newcastle

Transmission — contact with infected or carrier birds; inhaling contaminated dust or respiratory droplets; spread from breeders to chicks through hatching eggs

Prevention — avoid dusty litter; provide good ventilation; avoid chilling and other forms of stress; buy mycoplasma-free birds

Treatment — keep birds warm and well fed with high protein rations and a vitamin E supplement; treatment with antibiotics such as tylosin (trade name Tylan) or erythromycin (trade name Gallimycin) is effective *if* started early *and* bacteria are identified so ineffective drugs can be avoided, otherwise results may be variable and disappointing; survivors continue to carry and transmit *M. gallisepticum*

Human Health Risk — none known

Algae Poisoning

Incidence — West and Midwest, rare in chickens

System/Organ Affected — nervous system or liver and other internal organs

Incubation Period — minutes

Progression — acute

Symptoms — in all ages: weakness, staggering, collapse, convulsions, lying on breast with legs extended toward rear, neck extended and curved backward until head almost touches back, paralysis, rapid death

Percentage Affected — 100 percent of those drinking toxic water

Mortality — 100 percent

Postmortem Findings — swollen liver

Resembles — botulism

DIAGNOSIS — identification of toxins in water (turns dark green, bluish green, or brownish green)

CAUSE — two different kinds of toxins in "bloom" or "waterbloom" produced by blue green algae (cyanobacteria) growing in shallow inland lakes, ponds, or sloughs in warm (72-80°F, 22-27°C), dry, low-wind days of summer and fall

TRANSMISSION — drinking surface water containing concentrated toxins

PREVENTION — keep chickens away from shallow inland water; apply 3/4 pound (12 ounces) copper sulfate (powdered bluestone) per acre of water as bloom is forming, repeat every 2 to 3 weeks throughout bloom season

TREATMENT — restrict birds' activity; offer vitamin-electrolyte supplement

HUMAN HEALTH RISK — none

Ammonia Blindness. *See* Conjunctivitis

Anaphylactic Shock. *See* "Antibiotic Reactions," page 190.

Aplastic Anemia. *See* Infectious Anemia

Arizona Infection. *See* Arizonosis

Arizonosis

ALSO CALLED — avian arizonosis, AA, Arizona infection, paracolon (one form of salmonellosis)

INCIDENCE — worldwide but rare in chickens

SYSTEM/ORGAN AFFECTED — digestive

INCUBATION PERIOD — 5 days

PROGRESSION — acute in chicks, chronic in mature birds

SYMPTOMS — in chicks up to 3 weeks old: droopiness, closed eyes, diarrhea with vent pasting, weakness, twisted neck, resting on hocks, difficulty walking, leg paralysis, blindness; sometimes trembling

PERCENTAGE AFFECTED — 100 percent

MORTALITY — up to 50 percent, starting at 1 week of age

POSTMORTEM FINDINGS — retained yolk sac; yellowish, mottled, swollen liver; discolored heart; ceca or abdominal cavity filled with cheesy material

RESEMBLES — paratyphoid; nervous symptoms resemble those of Newcastle and other nerve diseases

DIAGNOSIS — laboratory identification of bacteria

CAUSE — *Salmonella arizonae* bacteria that persist in the environment for months and affect turkey poults more often than chicks

TRANSMISSION — contaminated droppings in soil, litter, feed, or water; contaminated feathers, dust, hatchery fluff; spread from infected breeders to chicks through hatching eggs (eggs can blow up during incubation, further spreading bacteria); spread by infected eggs and chicks in incubator and brooder; spread on dirty equipment, boots, feet of insects and rodents, droppings of infected reptiles (especially lizards), rodents, and other animals

PREVENTION — keep breeders on wire flooring; collect hatching eggs often; hatch only eggs from *S. arizonae*-free breeders; hatch only clean eggs; clean and disinfect incubator and brooder after each hatch; in chicks, minimize chilling, overheating, parasitism, withholding of water or feed; keep water free of droppings; control reptiles, rodents, cockroaches, beetles, fleas, and flies

TREATMENT — none effective, survivors are carriers
HUMAN HEALTH RISK — diarrhea may result from lack of sanitation after handling infected chicks

Arthritis, Staphylococcic. *See* Staphylococcic Arthritis
Arthritis/synovitis. *See* Staphylococcic Arthritis
Arthritis, Viral. *See* Viral Arthritis
Ascaridiasis. *See* "Large Roundworm," page 83
Ascites. *See* Broiler Ascites
Asiatic Newcastle Disease. *See* Newcastle Disease (exotic)

Aspergillosis (acute)

ALSO CALLED — *Aspergillus* infection, brooder pneumonia, mycotic pneumonia, pneumomycosis, pulmonary aspergillosis
INCIDENCE — worldwide but rare
SYSTEM/ORGAN AFFECTED — respiratory; sometimes liver or brain
INCUBATION PERIOD — up to 2 weeks
PROGRESSION — acute
SYMPTOMS — in hatching eggs: green appearance when candled
— in chicks, usually under 3 weeks of age: gasping, sleepiness, swollen eyes, yellow cheesy material in eye, loss of appetite; sometimes nasal discharge, diarrhea, twisted neck, paralysis; convulsions, death
PERCENTAGE AFFECTED — high
MORTALITY — up to 10 percent
POSTMORTEM FINDINGS — grayish yellow lungs
RESEMBLES — dactylariosis; infectious bronchitis, infectious laryngotracheitis, and Newcastle, except that acute aspergillosis seldom infects chicks over 40 days old
DIAGNOSIS — flock history, symptoms, postmortem findings
CAUSE — spores of *Aspergillus fumigatus* fungus and other molds commonly found in the poultry environment that multiply readily at normal incubation temperature and humidity
TRANSMISSION — through the shells of hatching eggs, spreads in incubator if infected eggs break; inhaled from contaminated air, feed, or brooder litter
PREVENTION — do not hatch eggs with cracked or poor shells; thoroughly clean and disinfect incubator and brooder between hatches; clean and disinfect feeders and waterers daily; avoid stress, moldy litter, moldy feed, dusty conditions
TREATMENT — none, cull (try thiabendazole at the rate of 10 mg/lb or 22 mg/kg every 12 hours); prevent reinfection by replacing litter and disinfecting incubator and brooder with copper sulfate (powdered bluestone)
HUMAN HEALTH RISK — the same fungus that affects chicks can affect a human with reduced resistance; see "Aspergillosis," page 231

Aspergillosis (chronic)

ALSO CALLED —*Aspergillus* infection, mycotic pneumonia, pneumomycosis, pulmonary aspergillosis
Incidence — worldwide but rare
System/Organ Affected — respiratory; sometimes liver or brain
INCUBATION PERIOD — 2 weeks or more
PROGRESSION -- chronic

Symptoms — in mature birds: gasping, coughing, bluish comb, loss of appetite, rapid weight loss

Percentage Affected — few at a time

Mortality — few (higher in confined than in free-ranged birds; highest after birds have been handled, especially carried by legs)

Postmortem Findings — numerous small, yellowish or cream-colored pearl-shaped cheesy nodules in lungs (nodules turn green and furry in advanced stages); circular, yellow, dished-out nodules attached to air sacs in chest and abdomen

Resembles — infectious bronchitis, infectious laryngotracheitis, and Newcastle, except that aspergillosis usually does not cause gurgling, rattling, or other respiratory sounds

Diagnosis — flock history, symptoms, postmortem findings

Cause — spores of *Aspergillus fumigatus* fungus and other molds found in the environment of all poultry, especially in areas surrounding feeders and waterers (appear blue green and can easily be seen while growing); infects confined flocks (especially in winter) where stress is high, nutrition is poor, immunity has been reduced by another disease, and/or exposure is heavy from seriously moldy litter or grain

Transmission — inhaled from contaminated air, feed, or litter, particularly where temperature and humidity are high

Prevention — avoid alternating conditions of wet (when fungi multiply) and dry (when fungi spread by blowing in dust); avoid stress, damp or moldy litter, moldy feed, dusty conditions; periodically move feeders and waterers or place them on platforms; spray litter with copper sulfate (powdered bluestone); control humidity and dust by providing good ventilation (opened windows work better than fans)

Treatment — none, cull; control spread of disease by adding ½ teaspoon copper sulfate (powdered bluestone) per gallon of drinking water served in a non-metal waterer for 5 days; prevent reinfection by cleaning facilities, disinfecting with copper sulfate solution (½ teaspoon per gallon of water), and replacing litter

Human Health Risk — the same fungus that affects chickens can affect humans with reduced resistance; see "Aspergillosis," page 231

***Aspergillus* Infection.** *See* Aspergillosis (acute); Aspergillosis (chronic)

***Aspergillus* Toxicosis.** *See* Aflatoxicosis

Avian Arizonosis. *See* Arizonosis

Avian Chlamydiosis. *See* Chlamydiosis

Avian Cholera. *See* Cholera (acute), Cholera (chronic)

Avian Diphtheria. *See* Infectious Laryngotracheitis

Avian Distemper. *See* Newcastle Disease

Avian Encephalomyelitis. *See* Epidemic Tremor

Avian Hemorrhagic Septicemia. *See* Cholera (acute)

Avian Infectious Bronchitis. *See* Infectious Bronchitis

Avian Influenza. *See* Influenza

Avian Leukosis. *See* Lymphoid Leukosis, Marek's Disease, Osteopetrosis

Avian Malaria. *See* Malaria
Avian Malignant Edema. *See* Necrotic Dermatitis
Avian Monocytosis. *See* Bluecomb
Avian Pasteurellosis. *See* Cholera (acute), Cholera (chronic)
Avian Plasmodia. *See* Malaria
Avian Pox. *See* Pox (dry), Pox (wet)
Avian Tuberculosis. *See* Tuberculosis
Avian Vibrionic Hepatitis. *See* Campylobacteriosis

- B -

Bacillary White Diarrhea. *See* Pullorum
Big Liver Disease. *See* Lymphoid Leukosis

Blackhead

ALSO CALLED —histomoniasis, infectious enterohepatitis
INCIDENCE —throughout North American but rare in chickens
SYSTEM/ORGAN AFFECTED — ceca and liver
INCUBATION PERIOD — 7 to 12 days
PROGRESSION — acute or chronic
SYMPTOMS — in young birds 4 to 6 weeks old: no symptoms or droopiness, drowsiness, weakness, ruffled feathers, increased thirst, loss of appetite, weight loss, darkened face; sometimes bloody cecal discharge
PERCENTAGE AFFECTED — 25 to 50 percent
MORTALITY — limited to exceeding 30 percent, peaks at 17 days, subsides by 28th day
POSTMORTEM FINDINGS — thickened ceca filled with grayish yellow cheesy, sometimes blood-tinged, material adhering to the lining; sometimes liver mottled with circular, dished-out spots, dark at the center and grayish white or yellowish green at the rim (differing from spots due to leukosis, mycosis, trichomoniasis, and tuberculosis, which are raised and yellowish gray)
RESEMBLES — cecal coccidiosis, salmonellosis
DIAGNOSIS — symptoms, postmortem findings (spots on liver), laboratory identification of protozoa required when postmortem findings are insignificant
CAUSE — *Histomonas meleagridis* protozoan present wherever poultry occur except where soil is dry, loose, and sandy; free-living forms do not live long, but may survive for years in cecal worm eggs; tends to affect turkeys more often than chickens
TRANSMISSION — eating droppings from infected chickens, earthworms containing infective cecal worm eggs, or protozoa attached to flies, sowbugs, grasshoppers, or crickets; carried by cecal worms *(Heterakis gallinarum);* spread by wild birds
PREVENTION — easy, with good management and sanitation; worm regularly against cecal worms; place feeders and waterers on wire platforms; low-level drugs in feed may be the only preventive in contaminated housing (due to longevity of infectious cecal worm eggs, range rotation of free-ranged flocks is ineffective)
TREATMENT — none effective; recovered birds are carriers
HUMAN HEALTH RISK — none known

Bluecomb

ALSO CALLED — avian monocytosis, the greens, mud fever, new wheat disease, nonspecific infectious enteritis, pullet disease, summer disease, X disease

INCIDENCE —rare in chickens

SYSTEM/ORGAN AFFECTED — digestive

INCUBATION PERIOD — unknown

PROGRESSION — spreads extremely slowly

SYMPTOMS — in pullets approaching maturity: depression, hunching up, loss of appetite, weight loss, distended sour-smelling crop, bluish comb, greenish watery or pasty bad-smelling diarrhea, dehydration, sunken eyes, shriveled shanks, cold-feeling body

PERCENTAGE AFFECTED — low

MORTALITY — up to 50 percent

POSTMORTEM FINDINGS — white streaks in breast muscles; sometimes yolk in abdominal cavity, mucus-filled intestines, dark liver, swollen kidneys

RESEMBLES — any acute septicemia

DIAGNOSIS — difficult

CAUSE — unknown (chickens are resistant to the coronavirus that causes bluecomb in turkeys), possibly a virus combined with stress induced by hot or rainy weather, lack of drinking water, lack of shade, or change in feed; sometimes follows the feeding of immature oat or wheat grains

TRANSMISSION — unknown

PREVENTION — practice good sanitation; breed for resistance

TREATMENT — none known, cull; affected birds may respond to molasses flush (see page 192) or ½ teaspoon copper sulfate (powdered bluestone) per gallon of drinking water served in a non-metal waterer for 2 days

HUMAN HEALTH RISK — none known

Botulism

ALSO CALLED — food poisoning, limberneck, toxicoinfection, Western duck sickness

INCIDENCE —rare

SYSTEM/ORGAN AFFECTED — nerves

INCUBATION PERIOD — high dose of toxin produces symptoms within hours, low dose takes up to 2 days

PROGRESSION — acute

SYMPTOMS — in birds of all ages: sudden death or leg weakness and drowsiness followed by progressive flaccid (not rigid) paralysis of legs, wings, and neck, difficulty swallowing, ruffled, loose feathers (raised hackles on cocks), lying on side with outstretched neck and eyes partly closed; sometimes trembling, diarrhea; coma and death due to heart and/or respiratory paralysis

PERCENTAGE AFFECTED — depends on how many eat the toxin

MORTALITY — usually less than 100 percent, depending on amount of toxin consumed

POSTMORTEM FINDINGS — none obvious; sometimes mouth fills with mucus and dirt, or crop and intestines contain suspicious organic matter or maggots

RESEMBLES — castor-bean poisoning (see page 142); tick paralysis (see "Soft Ticks," page 73); lameness caused by mild botulism resembles Marek's disease (pseudo-botulism form), except that in pseudo-botulism birds recover quickly, usually within 24 hours

DIAGNOSIS — flock history (birds ate rotted organic matter), symptoms (progressive flaccid paralysis, loose feathers, mucus and dirt in mouth), absence of postmortem findings, laboratory identification of bacteria (if Marek's disease or castor-bean poisoning is suspected)

CAUSE — *Clostridium botulinum,* soil-borne bacteria commonly found in the poultry environment that produce toxins when they multiply in warm, moist, decaying vegetable or animal matter (including dead chickens)

TRANSMISSION — consuming decayed organic matter, maggots feeding on rotting animal tissue, or beetles (in litter) that contain toxin; drinking water containing contaminated organic matter

PREVENTION — do not feed spoiled food to chickens; burn or deeply bury dead rodents, chickens, or other animal carcasses, and rotting, solid vegetables such as cabbages; control flies; acidify soil with ammonium sulfate fertilizer; avoid wet spots in litter; keep birds away from marshy or swampy areas where vegetation rots in water; keep chickens from scratching in compost piles; immunize flock with type C toxoid

TREATMENT — remove source of poisoning from yard; move bird to cool environment; squirt cool water into crop twice daily; flush with molasses or Epsom salts (see "Flushes," page 192); inject intravenously with antitoxin (expensive, if available); remove contaminated litter and disinfect with calcium hypochlorite or iodine-based disinfectant

HUMAN HEALTH RISK — humans are poisoned by toxin types A, B, E, and F; chickens are poisoned by type C, rarely by types A and E; chickens and humans can be poisoned by the same contaminated food or water; reports of human poisoning from eating contaminated chicken meat are unconfirmed (see "Clostridium Poisoning," page 241)

Breast Blister

ALSO CALLED — keel cyst, keel bursitis, sternal bursitis

INCIDENCE —common

SYSTEM/ORGAN AFFECTED — keel

PROGRESSION — chronic

SYMPTOMS — in growing or mature cocks, particularly of the heavy breeds: large blister on keel that eventually becomes a callus or thick scar

PERCENTAGE AFFECTED — up to 10 percent

MORTALITY — low

RESEMBLES — infectious synovitis, except an uninfected blister is filled with clear or bloody fluid, an infected blister contains creamy or cheesy material

DIAGNOSIS — flock history (breed and sex), symptoms

CAUSE — irritation and inflammation due to pressure of breast bone against roost or wire floor

TRANSMISSION — not contagious; occurs in birds with weak legs or with poor feather development offering no breast protection; most likely where floor is wire, roosts have sharp corners, or litter is wet or hard-packed

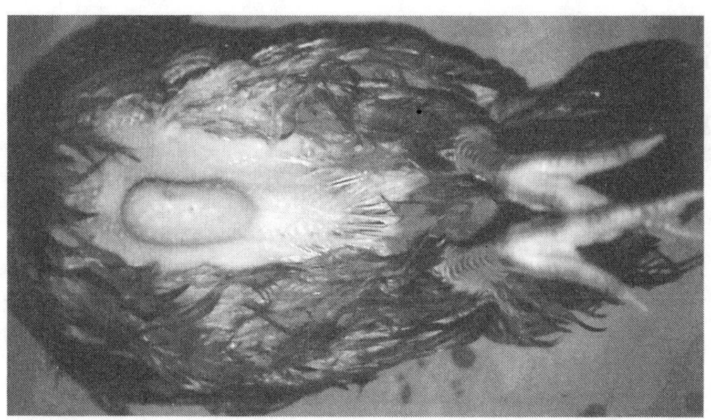
ALLAN DAMEROW

Breast blister

PREVENTION — wrap roosts in something soft to cushion the breast bone or do not provide a roost for cocks

TREATMENT — open and drain blister, clean with iodine, and pack with Neosporin; antibiotic treatment in drinking water or by injection may be necessary if blister becomes infected with *Mycoplasma synoviae* (infectious synovitis) or *Staphylococcus aureus* (necrotic dermatitis)

HUMAN HEALTH RISK — none, as long as blister is not infected

Broiler Ascites

ALSO CALLED — ascites with right ventral failure, ARVF, dropsy, water belly

INCIDENCE — common worldwide, especially in winter at high altitudes

SYSTEM/ORGAN AFFECTED — heart

INCUBATION PERIOD — unknown

PROGRESSION — acute

SYMPTOMS — in male broilers 4 to 7 weeks old: ruffled feathers, slow growth, reluctance to move; sometimes sudden death

PERCENTAGE AFFECTED — low

MORTALITY — up to 30 percent

POSTMORTEM FINDINGS — dark red muscles; thick, straw-colored fluid in abdominal cavity; liver swollen, discolored, and sometimes mottled or pimpled (early stage) or small and pale with rounded edges (later stage); bloody lungs; distended right side of heart

RESEMBLES — salt poisoning (see page 31)

DIAGNOSIS — symptoms, postmortem findings

CAUSE — unknown, may be due to genetically inadequate respiratory system failing to draw in enough oxygen; may be nutritionally related (e.g., excess salt in rations); in newly hatched chicks, may be caused by putting chicks into brooder too soon after using volatile disinfectant

TRANSMISSION — unknown

PREVENTION — none known; may help to provide good air circulation and avoid ammonia fumes

TREATMENT — none known

HUMAN HEALTH RISK — none known

Broiler Runting Syndrome. *See* Infectious Stunting Syndrome
Bronchitis. *See* Infectious Bronchitis
Brooder Pneumonia. *See* Aspergillosis (acute); Aspergillosis (chronic)

Bumblefoot

ALSO CALLED — staphylococcosis, plantar pododermatitis

INCIDENCE — common

SYSTEM/ORGAN AFFECTED — foot pad

PROGRESSION — chronic

SYMPTOMS — in maturing birds, especially in males of heavy breeds: lameness, reluctance to walk, inflamed foot (one or both), hot, hard, swollen, or pus-filled abscess or dark black scab on bottom of foot, resting on hocks; sometimes sores appear on hocks and bottoms of toes

PERCENTAGE AFFECTED — 1 to 2 percent

MORTALITY — usually low; up to 50 percent if untreated

POSTMORTEM FINDINGS — pus or cheesy material in foot pad; sometimes hock joints filled with grayish white fluid

DIAGNOSIS — symptoms (abscess in foot pad)

CAUSE — *Staphylococcus aureus* bacteria, present wherever there are chickens

TRANSMISSION — contaminated hatching eggs; bacteria enters foot through injury caused by splinters, sharp roosts, jumping from roost on to hard or rocky ground, housing on wire, irritation due to improper litter management

PREVENTION — practice good sanitation; provide deep, dry litter that does not pack; avoid high perches; round off edges of perch and sand off splinters; feed vitamin supplement (especially vitamin A); do not breed susceptible chickens to avoid getting more of the same

TREATMENT — difficult to cure; inject swollen area with ½ cc penicillin/streptomycin (Combiotic); if abscess is large, wash foot, cut open abscess, squeeze out cheesy core, rinse well with hydrogen peroxide, pack with Neosporin, wrap foot with gauze bandage or strip of clean cloth, and tape; confine bird on deep litter and dress foot every 2 or 3 days

HUMAN HEALTH RISK — superficial skin infection (impetigo); wear plastic gloves when treating a bird, wash hands afterward, gather blister contents in paper towel and dispose by burning or deep burial

ALLAN DAMEROW

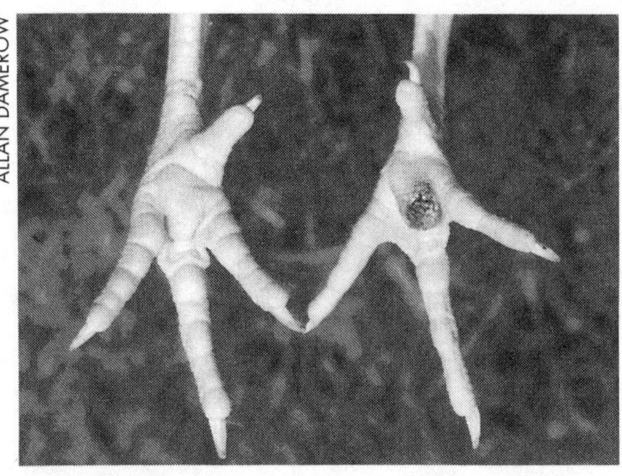

Healthy foot (left) compared to bumblefoot (right).

- C -

Cage Fatigue

ALSO CALLED — cage layer fatigue, cage layer osteoporosis, cage layer paralysis, osteoporosis

INCIDENCE — no longer common

SYSTEM/ORGAN AFFECTED — bones

PROGRESSION — usually chronic but can be acute

SYMPTOMS — in caged pullets, usually high-production commercial strains in summer: weakness, squatting, inability to stand (but will continue to eat and drink if feed and water are within reach)

— in laying hens: thin-shelled eggs with low hatchability followed by cessation of laying, paralysis, death due to dehydration

PERCENTAGE AFFECTED — depends on duration of dietary deficiency

MORTALITY — depends on duration of dietary deficiency

POSTMORTEM FINDINGS — deformed or collapsed rib cage; soft, thin, or fragile bones that break easily

RESEMBLES — Marek's disease and other paralytic conditions; rickets

DIAGNOSIS — flock history (age, sex, and housing method), symptoms, postmortem findings

CAUSE — low calcium or phosphorus diet or disturbance in the metabolism of dietary minerals, particularly calcium (causing hen to draw calcium from her own bones)

TRANSMISSION — nutritional, does not spread from bird to bird

PREVENTION — house hens on litter; feed properly balanced diet supplemented with ground oyster shell or limestone; allow birds out into the sunshine

TREATMENT — calcium phosphate supplement; if hen can't get up, give 1 gram calcium carbonate in a gelatin capsule daily for 1 week, cover wire cage bottom with solid boards or move pullets to floor, pullets should recover within a week

HUMAN HEALTH RISK — none

Cage Layer Fatigue/Osteoporosis/Paralysis. *See* Cage Fatigue

Campylobacteriosis

ALSO CALLED — avian vibrionic hepatitis, campylobacter hepatitis, enteric campylobacteriosis, infectious hepatitis, liver disease

INCIDENCE — common worldwide, especially in floor-reared flocks

SYSTEM/ORGAN AFFECTED — intestines

INCUBATION PERIOD — 24 hours

PROGRESSION — sometimes acute, usually chronic, spreads slowly

SYMPTOMS — in chicks up to 4 weeks old: depression, watery diarrhea, slow growth (chronic), death (acute)

— in growing or mature birds: sudden death of apparently healthy birds (acute) or listlessness, scaly shrunken comb, weight loss, unthriftiness, sometimes mucousy, bloody diarrhea (chronic)

— in hens: 35 percent drop in egg production (may be only sign)

PERCENTAGE AFFECTED — few at a time totaling 30 to 100 percent

MORTALITY — 10 to 15 percent

POSTMORTEM FINDINGS — intestine filled with mucus and watery fluid; pale, watery bone marrow; sometimes green- or brown-stained liver with characteristic yellow star-shaped patches

RESEMBLES — blackhead, bluecomb, infectious anemia, cholera, typhoid, lymphoid leukosis, pullorum, ulcerative enteritis

DIAGNOSIS — symptoms (thin birds), postmortem findings (stars on liver, when present), laboratory fecal examination to identify bacteria (since campylobacters are sensitive to drying, ask veterinarian or pathologist for a suitable collection container)

CAUSE — *Campylobacter fetus jejuni* bacteria that among birds affect only chickens, survive well in the environment, and resist disinfectants; often occurs in combination with another infection such as Marek's disease, pox, or parasites

TRANSMISSION — droppings of infected or carrier birds in feed or water; spread by flies, cockroaches, and rodents; spread on contaminated equipment and soles of shoes; may spread from breeders to chicks through hatching eggs

PREVENTION — good management and sanitation; do not combine birds from different sources; keep birds free of internal parasites, coccidia, and other stress-inducing infections; house chickens on wire to keep them from picking in droppings; control flies, cockroaches, rodents; cull weak, unthrifty birds; remove infected flock, disinfect, and leave housing vacant for 4 weeks before introducing new birds

TREATMENT — none effective

HUMAN HEALTH RISK — eating undercooked meat of infected birds can cause serious diarrhea, see "Campylobacteriosis," page 241

Candidiasis. *See* Thrush

Canker

ALSO CALLED — roup, trichomoniasis

INCIDENCE — worldwide, especially in warm climates or during warm weather, but rare in chickens

SYSTEM/ORGAN AFFECTED — mouth, throat, and crop

INCUBATION PERIOD — 2 weeks

PROGRESSION — acute or chronic

SYMPTOMS — usually in young or growing birds: loss of appetite, rapid weight loss, weakness, darkened head, extended neck, frequent swallowing, sunken breast (due to empty crop), watery eyes, foul-smelling discharge from mouth, white or yellow sores in mouth and throat, inability to close mouth or swallow due to massive sores

PERCENTAGE AFFECTED — high

MORTALITY — limited, usually within 8 to 10 days due to suffocation

POSTMORTEM FINDINGS — cheesy white or yellowish raised buttons on throat walls; sometimes crop filled with foul-smelling fluid

RESEMBLES — capillary worms (see page 84), thrush, pox (wet)

DIAGNOSIS — flock history (drinking from stagnant water), symptoms, laboratory identification of protozoa from throat scrapings

CAUSE — *Trichomonas gallinae* protozoan parasite that infects a variety of birds, primarily pigeons

TRANSMISSION — stagnant drinking water or feed contaminated with discharge from infected bird's mouth; spread by wild birds and pigeons

PREVENTION — good sanitation; keep pigeons away from chickens; avoid bringing in new birds that may be carriers

TREATMENT — move unaffected birds to sanitary surroundings; isolate infected birds; combine 1 pound copper sulfate (powdered bluestone) with 1 cup vinegar and 1 gallon water, mix well, add 1 tablespoon (½ ounce) solution per gallon drinking water for 4 to 7 days, served in a non-metal waterer; non-meat birds may be treated with metronidazole (trade name Flagyl) injections or pills or with carnidazole (Spartrix) pills for 5 days; recovered birds are carriers

HUMAN HEALTH RISK — none known; not the same as trichomoniasis in humans

Cannibalism. *See* page 135

Capillariasis. *See* "Capillary Worm," page 84

Cauliflower Gut. *See* Necrotic Enteritis

Cestodiasis. *See* "Tapeworm," page 89

Chicken Anemia Agent Infection. *See* Infectious Anemia

Chicken Pox. *See* Pox (dry)

Chlamydiosis

ALSO CALLED — avian chlamydiosis, AC, ornithosis, parrot fever, psittacosis

INCIDENCE — worldwide but rare in chickens

SYSTEM/ORGAN AFFECTED — respiratory, entire body

INCUBATION PERIOD — 5 to 9 days

PROGRESSION — acute or chronic, spreads slowly

SYMPTOMS — in all ages: no recognizable symptoms or droopiness, nasal discharge, greenish yellow diarrhea, loss of appetite, weakness, weight loss

PERCENTAGE AFFECTED — 100 percent

MORTALITY — mostly in younger birds

POSTMORTEM FINDINGS — not always obvious; enlarged discolored liver; dark, soft, enlarged spleen; sometimes enlarged heart

Do not post birds you suspect have chlamydiosis

RESEMBLES — aspergillosis, cholera, colibacillosis, influenza, mycoplasmosis, pasteurellosis

DIAGNOSIS — history (contact with infected birds), symptoms, postmortem findings, laboratory identification of chlamydia

CAUSE — *Chlamydia psittaci,* a bacteria-like organism that affects many species of bird but cannot survive long off birds; often found in combination with salmonellosis

TRANSMISSION — contagious; contact with infected birds and their droppings or inhaled dust; spread by wild birds

PREVENTION — control wild birds; blood test periodically and cull reactors where outbreaks occur; keep chickens away from ponds, lakes, and other surface water frequented by wild birds; after an outbreak, disinfect with quaternary ammonium compound or an alcohol-iodine solution

TREATMENT — none effective, relapse is likely, survivors may be carriers; this is a **reportable disease,** see "Reportable Diseases" page 196

HUMAN HEALTH RISK — high chance of lung infection, see "Chlamydiosis," page 235

Cholera (acute)

Also Called — avian cholera, avian hemorrhagic septicemia, avian pasteurellosis, fowl cholera

Incidence — relatively common worldwide; more likely in warm climates and in free-ranged birds; more prevalent in late summer, fall, and winter

System/Organ Affected — entire body (septicemic)

Incubation Period — 4 to 9 days

Progression — acute, spreads rapidly, kills quickly

Symptoms — in mature birds or those approaching maturity: sudden death (hens dead in nests) or fever, loss of appetite, increased thirst, depression, drowsiness, ruffled feathers, head pale and drawn back, increased respiratory rate, mucous discharge from mouth and nose, watery white diarrhea later becoming thick and greenish yellow, bluish comb and wattles, death within hours of first symptoms; survivors may recover and either eventually die from emaciation and dehydration or develop chronic cholera

Percentage Affected — high

Mortality — 10 to 20 percent among mature birds, can be as high as 45 percent; rare in birds under 16 weeks old

Postmortem Findings — none in case of sudden death, otherwise blood in lungs and in fatty tissue of abdomen; heart surrounded by fluid containing cheesy flakes; swollen, grayish liver (looks cooked) with small grayish white spots (resembles cornmeal); sticky mucus in digestive tract, especially in the crop and intestine

— in hens: yolk in abdominal cavity

Resembles — erysipelas, septicemic colibacillosis, poisoning (see page 139), typhoid

Diagnosis — symptoms, postmortem findings, laboratory identification of bacteria

Cause — *Pasteurella multocida* bacteria that affect a variety of birds and increase in virulence as disease spreads; bacteria survive for 1 month in manure, 3 months in moist soil; destroyed in 10 minutes by sunlight, also easily destroyed by disinfectants, drying, heat

Transmission — contagious; contact with mucus from the nose, mouth, or eyes of birds or animals with chronic infection; mucus contaminating feed or drinking water; mucus on feed sacks, shoes, and used equipment; picking at carcasses of dead birds

Prevention — vaccination is not effective; purchase only cholera-free birds; avoid purchasing growing or mature birds, which may be carriers; avoid stress due to heat, rough handling, parasites, abrupt change in rations, poor nutrition, and poor sanitation; provide clean, safe drinking water; do not mix birds of different ages; control wild birds, rodents, and other animals; keep pets away from chickens; burn or deeply bury carcasses of dead chickens

Treatment — none effective, disease recurs when medication is discontinued and survivors may be carriers; isolate and dispose of infected flock, thoroughly disinfect and dry housing, leave it vacant at least 3 months before introducing new birds

Human Health Risk — in poorly ventilated housing, possible upper respiratory tract infection (which can in turn infect chickens through mucus discharged from human's mouth or nose); wear protective mask

Cholera (chronic)

Also Called — avian cholera, avian pasteurellosis, endemic fowl cholera, roup

Incidence — worldwide but less common than acute cholera

System/Organ Affected — primarily respiratory

Incubation Period — weeks to months

Progression — chronic

Symptoms — in birds at least 6 weeks old: cheesy nasal discharge, loss of appetite, rapid weight loss, increased thirst; lameness or swelling of leg joints, wing joints, foot pads, wattles, and sinuses; swollen, sticky eyes; sometimes bluish, hot comb; sometimes breathing difficulties, rattling, and sneezing

— in hens: drop in egg production, increased blood spotting in eggs

— in cocks: loss of aggressive behavior and desire to crow

Percentage Affected — limited

Mortality — limited

Postmortem Findings — sinuses filled with yellow cheesy material; white cheesy matter along breast bone; wrinkled, bloody and/or off-colored yolks

Resembles — bluecomb, which is even less common than chronic cholera; infectious coryza, except that coryza is associated with a foul odor; Newcastle, except that Newcastle often includes nervous symptoms

Diagnosis — symptoms, postmortem findings, laboratory identification of bacteria

Cause — *Pasteurella multocida* (also called *P. septica)* bacteria of low virulence or lingering after an acute cholera infection

Transmission — contagious; contact with mucus from the nose, mouth, or eyes of carriers, including wild birds, wild animals (opossums, rodents, raccoons), domestic animals (dogs, pigs); feed or drinking water contaminated with mucus; mucus on feed sacks, shoes, and used equipment; picking at the carcasses of dead birds

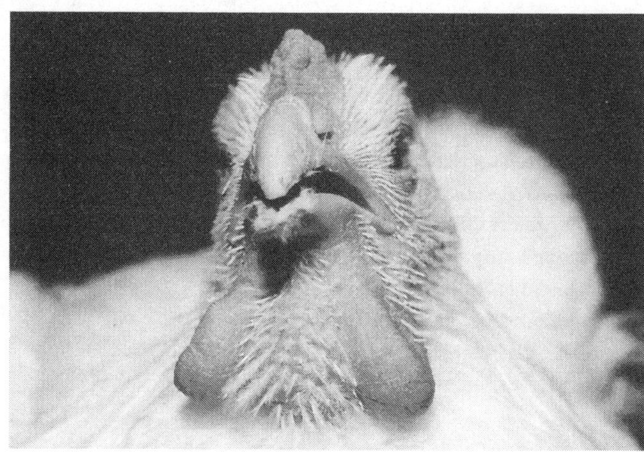

ARTHUR A. BICKFORD, DVM, U. CAL. DAVIS

Face swollen with cholera

PREVENTION — same as for acute cholera
TREATMENT — same as for acute cholera
HUMAN HEALTH RISK — same as for acute cholera

Chondrodystrophy. *See* Slipped Tendon

Chronic Respiratory Disease

ALSO CALLED — CRD, MG, PPLO (pleuropneumonialike organism) infection, stress disease (one form of mycoplasmosis) (the same disease in turkeys is called "infectious sinusitis")
INCIDENCE — common worldwide, primarily in winter in large commercial flocks
SYSTEM/ORGAN AFFECTED — respiratory, sometimes entire body
INCUBATION PERIOD — 6 to 21 days
PROGRESSION — chronic, spreads slowly, lasts longer in colder weather
SYMPTOMS — in broilers, 3 to 8 weeks old: drop in feed consumption, slow growth
— in growing or mature birds: no symptoms or droopiness, coughing, sneezing, rattling, gurgling, swollen face, nasal discharge, ruffled feathers, frothy eyes, squeaky crow, drop in laying; sometimes darkened head, loss of appetite, weight loss, yellowish droppings
PERCENTAGE AFFECTED — nearly 100 percent
MORTALITY — usually low except in young birds
POSTMORTEM FINDINGS — thick mucus in nasal passages and throat; cheesy material in air sacs; thickened heart sac; transparent film covering liver
RESEMBLES — other respiratory diseases (infectious coryza, cholera, infectious bronchitis, Newcastle), except that CRD spreads more slowly than most
DIAGNOSIS — flock history (time of year, age, potential contact with carriers), symptoms (respiratory distress, weight loss, drop in laying), postmortem findings, laboratory identification of bacteria
CAUSE — *Mycoplasma gallisepticum* bacteria, often aided by *Escherichia coli* and/or a reovirus; often seen in combination with cholera, infectious bronchitis, infectious coryza, Newcastle; often follows vaccination for infectious bronchitis or Newcastle
TRANSMISSION — contagious; contact with infected or carrier birds and their respiratory discharges; inhaling contaminated dust; spread from breeders through hatching eggs; spreads on shoes, crates, etc.
PREVENTION — purchase mycoplasma-free stock; minimize stress due to sudden weather changes, feed changes, drafts, chilling, crowding, transporting, showing, worming, vaccinating, dust, and ammonia fumes; vaccinate; after outbreak, clean and disinfect housing and leave empty for a few weeks
TREATMENT — none effective; tylosin (Tylan) or erythromycin (Gallimycin) will reduce death rate but survivors are carriers; this is a **reportable disease** in many states, see "Reportable Diseases" page 196
HUMAN HEALTH RISK — none known

Circling Disease. *See* Listeriosis
Cloacitis. *See* Pasted Vent
Clostridial Dermatomyositis. *See* Necrotic Dermatitis

Coccidiosis (cecal)

ALSO CALLED — cocci (coxy)
INCIDENCE — common worldwide, especially in warm, humid weather
SYSTEM/ORGAN AFFECTED — cecum
INCUBATION PERIOD — 5 to 6 days
PROGRESSION — usually acute, spreads rapidly, survivors recover in 10 to 14 days
SYMPTOMS — in chicks or young birds: droopiness, huddling with ruffled feathers, loss of appetite, retarded growth, bloody diarrhea in early stages
PERCENTAGE AFFECTED — 80 to 100 percent
MORTALITY — high
POSTMORTEM FINDINGS — pale breast muscles, swollen cecal pouches filled with bloody or cheesy material
RESEMBLES — blackhead, necrotic enteritis, salmonellosis
DIAGNOSIS — flock history, postmortem findings, fecal test (see page 92)
CAUSE — *Eimeria tenella* coccidial protozoan parasites
TRANSMISSION — contact with droppings of infected birds; spread on used equipment, feed sacks, feet of humans and wild birds, etc.
PREVENTION — defies good sanitation; breed for resistance; hatch and brood chicks early in the season; raise chicks on clean, dry litter to expose them gradually and let them develop resistance; avoid crowded, damp conditions; in warm, damp weather, treat chicks to 16 weeks of age with medicated starter or coccidiostat in drinking water, according to directions on label *(excessive use of coccidiostat can be toxic);* most adults are immune
TREATMENT — 1 teaspoon amprolium (20 percent) per gallon drinking water for 5 days; antibiotic treatment guards against secondary infection; follow treatment with a vitamin supplement (especially A and K); survivors are immune, but may never be as productive as uninfected birds
HUMAN HEALTH RISK — none known

Coccidiosis (intestinal)

ALSO CALLED — cocci (coxy)
INCIDENCE — common worldwide, especially in warm, humid weather
SYSTEM/ORGAN AFFECTED — intestinal tract
INCUBATION PERIOD — 5 days
PROGRESSION — usually chronic
SYMPTOMS — in growing or semi-mature birds: droopiness, huddling with ruffled feathers, loss of interest in water and feed, retarded growth or weight loss, watery, mucousy, or pasty, tan or blood-tinged diarrhea (see chart 6-2 page 100); sometimes emaciation and dehydration
— in mature birds: thin breast, weak legs, drop in laying; sometimes diarrhea
— in yellow-skinned breeds of all ages: pale comb, skin, and shanks
PERCENTAGE AFFECTED — 80 to 100 percent
MORTALITY — limited to high
POSTMORTEM FINDINGS — vary with *Eimeria* species (see chart 6-2 page 100)
RESEMBLES — infectious anemia, ulcerative enteritis, salmonellosis, worms, and other enteritic diseases

DIAGNOSIS — flock history (exposure to large number of oocysts), symptoms, postmortem findings, fecal test (see page 92)

CAUSE — several different species of coccidial protozoan parasites (see chart 6-2 page 100) that flourish in warm, humid environments and survive for long periods outside a bird's body; more than one species may infect a bird at one time; the presence of coccidia does not always cause infection

TRANSMISSION — droppings of infected birds; spread on used equipment, feed sacks, feet of humans and wild birds, etc.

PREVENTION — same as for cecal coccidiosis; not all coccidiostats are effective against all coccidial species

TREATMENT — same as for cecal coccidiosis (except that choice of drugs depends on identification of species involved); survivors are immune to the coccidial species causing the infection, but may not be as productive as uninfected birds

HUMAN HEALTH RISK — none known

Coccidiosis (respiratory). *See* Cryptosporidiosis

Cold. *See* Infectious Coryza, Infectious Bronchitis

Colibacillosis. (*See also* Air-Sac Disease, Chronic Respiratory Disease, Infectious Synovitis, Omphalitis, Swollen Head Disease)

ALSO CALLED — coliform infection, *E. coli* infection

INCIDENCE — common worldwide

SYSTEM/ORGAN AFFECTED — various

PROGRESSION — severe and acute to mild and chronic; spreads rapidly

SYMPTOMS — in incubated eggs: dead embryos late in incubation with watery yellowish brown yolk sacs, instead of normal thick yellowish green (yolk sac infection)

— in newly hatched chicks: swollen, inflamed navel, death within 6 days of hatching (omphalitis)

— in growing birds: lameness, listlessness, ruffled feathers, fever, swollen joints, recovery in about a week or emaciation (infectious synovitis)

— in growing or mature birds: sudden numerous deaths of apparently healthy birds with full crops (acute septicemia)

— in mature birds: clear eye that becomes blind, swollen leg joint filled with golden-colored fluid (infectious synovitis), yellow, watery, or foamy diarrhea (enteritis)

— in hens: cessation of laying, upright penguin-like posture, death within 6 months (salpingitis)

PERCENTAGE AFFECTED — varies

MORTALITY — varies

POSTMORTEM FINDINGS — vary with location of infection, may include: dehydration; greenish liver; swollen liver, spleen, and kidneys with grayish dots; cheesy or fibrous material covering heart; thick, inflamed intestines filled with mucus and blood

— in hens: yellowish fluid or yolk-like material in body cavity or distended oviduct filled with whitish curdy or yellowish cheesy material (salpingitis, see page 53)

RESEMBLES — many other diseases; acute septicemia resembles cholera and typhoid

DIAGNOSIS — flock history, symptoms, postmortem findings, laboratory identification of bacteria

CAUSE — many strains of *Escherichia coli* bacteria commonly found in the poultry environment that infect birds with impaired resistance; often occurs as a secondary infection to chronic respiratory disease or infectious coryza

TRANSMISSION — ingested droppings of infected birds or mammals in feed or water; spread by infected breeders to chicks through hatching eggs

PREVENTION — good sanitation and ventilation; avoid stress; keep drinking water free of droppings; control rodents; practice good incubator sanitation and hatch only clean eggs

TREATMENT — keep birds warm and well fed with high protein rations and a vitamin E supplement; antibiotic treatment is effective only if started early and *E. coli* strain is identified in order to avoid ineffective drugs, otherwise results of treatment can be variable and disappointing

HUMAN HEALTH RISK — minimal (see "Escherichia Coli", page 243)

Coliform Infection. *See* Colibacillosis

Congenital Loco. *See* Congenital Tremor

Congenital Tremor

ALSO CALLED — congenital loco, jittery chicks, crazy chick disease (not the same as encephalomalacia, which is also called crazy chick disease)

INCIDENCE — rare

SYSTEM/ORGAN AFFECTED — nervous system

SYMPTOMS — in newly hatched chicks: uncontrolled movements, head tremors, sagging of head until beak touches floor, standing only a short time before falling over backward (somersaulting), death due to inability to eat or drink

PERCENTAGE AFFECTED — low

MORTALITY — 100 percent

POSTMORTEM FINDINGS — irregularities in muscle, bone, and/or brain

RESEMBLES — epidemic tremor and encephalomalacia, except that congenital tremor starts at the time of hatch

DIAGNOSIS — symptoms

CAUSE — injury during hatching or hereditary defect caused by a recessive genetic trait

TRANSMISSION — does not spread

PREVENTION — cull breeders whose chicks are affected

TREATMENT — none; cull

HUMAN HEALTH RISK — none

Conjunctivitis

ALSO CALLED — ammonia blindness, keratoconjunctivitis

INCIDENCE — common in flocks raised on deep litter, especially in winter

SYSTEM/ORGAN AFFECTED — eyes

INCUBATION PERIOD — hours

PROGRESSION — acute

Symptoms — in all ages: rubbing eyes with wings, reluctance to move, avoiding sunlight, one or both eyes cloudy (in case of vitamin A deficiency, nose and eyes water, later become encrusted with white cheesy material), blindness

Percentage Affected — 80 to 100 percent

Mortality — varies

Postmortem Findings — none significant

Resembles — any mild respiratory disease

Diagnosis — history (detection of ammonia fumes), symptoms (eye and eyelid damage)

Cause — ammonia fumes from accumulated droppings, vitamin A deficiency, infection

Transmission — environmental, does not spread from bird to bird

Prevention — provide proper nutrition and good ventilation; avoid wet litter

Treatment — replacing wet litter or correcting vitamin A deficiency in early stages leads to recovery in about 2 months, but won't reverse blindness

Human Health Risk — squinting in ammonia fumes is no less unpleasant for humans than it is for chickens

Contagious Catarrh. *See* Infectious Coryza

Coryza. *See* Infectious Coryza

Crazy Chick Disease. *See* Encephalomalacia, Congenital Tremor

CRD. *See* Chronic Respiratory Disease

Crooked Legs. *See* Twisted Leg

Crop Binding. *See* Crop Impaction

Crop Impaction

Also Called — crop binding, pendulous crop

Incidence — rare

System/Organ Affected — crop

Symptoms — in mature birds: distended, sour-smelling crop filled with feed and roughage (crop feels hard when pressed between fingers), emaciation

Percentage Affected — up to 5 percent

Mortality — limited, deaths due to impaired digestion

Postmortem Findings — sometimes sores in crop lining

Resembles — thrush, except that in crop impaction birds appear otherwise healthy

Diagnosis — symptoms

Cause — unknown, possibly genetic susceptibility, injury, fungal infection, improper fermentation of crop contents, or insufficient rations forcing birds to eat litter or fibrous vegetation that pack the crop until it loses muscle tone and cannot empty itself

Transmission — does not spread from bird to bird

Prevention — provide proper rations and plenty of clean, fresh water; if feed is withheld preparatory to worming, offer a moistened ration 1 hour after worming

Treatment — disinfect skin, slit through skin with very sharp blade, pull skin aside and slit through crop, clean out crop, isolate bird and keep wound clean until it heals

Human Health Risk — none

Crop Mycosis. *See* Thrush
Crud. *See* Necrotic Enteritis

Cryptosporidiosis

ALSO CALLED — coccidiosis
INCIDENCE — not common
SYSTEM/ORGAN AFFECTED — respiratory (lungs, air sacs), cloaca, cloacal bursa
PROGRESSION — acute (lasting 2 to 3 weeks) or chronic
SYMPTOMS — in birds 4 to 17 weeks old: no symptoms or pale skin, coughing, sneezing, swollen sinuses, nose and eye discharge, extending neck to breath, sitting with weight on keel, reluctance to move, slow growth; sometimes diarrhea
PERCENTAGE AFFECTED — 5 to 25 percent
MORTALITY — high
POSTMORTEM FINDINGS — air sacs contain clear, foamy, white, or gray fluid or thick, white, cheesy material; ceca filled with foamy fluid
RESEMBLES — any mild respiratory disease
DIAGNOSIS — laboratory identification of oocysts from moist cotton swab vigorously rubbed against windpipe
CAUSE — *Cryptosporidium baileyi* protozoa; usually infect in combination with other respiratory diseases including cholera, chronic respiratory disease, infectious bronchitis, Newcastle, and others
TRANSMISSION — inhaled oocysts from respiratory discharges and droppings of infected birds
PREVENTION — none known other than meticulous sanitation
TREATMENT — none known; reduce mortality with supportive therapy (see page 192) and treatment of concurrent infection(s); survivors are immune
HUMAN HEALTH RISK — none known

Curled-Toe Paralysis. *See* "Crooked Toes," page 226
Cutaneous Pox. *See* Pox (dry)

- D -

Dactylariosis

ALSO CALLED — dactylaria
INCIDENCE — rare
SYSTEM/ORGAN AFFECTED — brain, lungs
INCUBATION PERIOD — 6 to 10 days
PROGRESSION — acute
SYMPTOMS — in chicks 1 to 6 weeks of age: tremors, circling, incoordination
PERCENTAGE AFFECTED — up to 5 percent
MORTALITY — up to 100 percent
POSTMORTEM FINDINGS — granular tumors in brain
RESEMBLES — aspergillosis, encephalomalacia
DIAGNOSIS — flock history (age of birds, litter derived from wood), symptoms, postmortem findings
CAUSE — *Dactylaria gallopava* fungus contaminating sawdust or shredded tree bark used as litter

Transmission — inhaled from moldy litter
Prevention — avoid moldy litter
Treatment — cull affected birds and replace litter
Human Health Risk — none known

Dikkop. *See* Swollen Head Syndrome
Diphtheritic Pox. *See* Pox (wet)
Dermatitis, Necrotic. *See* Necrotic Dermatitis
Dermatitis, Vesicular. *See* Ergotism
Dropsy. *See* Broiler Ascites

- E -

Egg Binding. *See* page 54

Egg Drop Syndrome

Also Called — EDS
Incidence — sporadic worldwide, except in North America
System/Organ Affected — reproductive
Incubation Period — 7 to 17 days
Progression — spreads slowly, lasts 4 to 10 weeks
Symptoms — in mature hens, especially broiler-breeders and brown-egg layers: gradual drop in laying up to 40 percent lasting 4 to 10 weeks, eggs with pale shells, thin gritty shells, soft shells, or no shells (hens may eat eggs, making it look like they are laying less than they actually are)
Percentage Affected — varies greatly
Mortality — low
Postmortem Findings — none obvious; inactive ovary and atrophied oviduct
Resembles — Newcastle and influenza in loss of egg quality, except that in EDS birds do not appear sick; infectious bronchitis, except bronchitis does not involve soft-shelled or shell-less eggs
Diagnosis — symptoms (pale-shelled, thin-shelled, soft-shelled, and shell-less eggs nearing peak of production); laboratory identification of virus through blood testing
Cause — adenovirus (originally introduced into chicken flocks through Marek's vaccine grown in a medium derived from duck embryos); the virus is primarily carried by ducks and geese but does not infect them
Transmission — contact with infected waterfowl or surface water contaminated by them; spread from breeders to chicks through hatching eggs; contact with infected chickens and their body discharges, especially droppings; contact with contaminated equipment, particularly cartons for hatching egg storage
Prevention — good sanitation; breed for resistance; vaccinate birds at 14 to 16 weeks of age; avoid flockwide injections or vaccinations using one needle; scrupulous sanitation limits the virus's spread
Treatment — none; discard obviously affected eggs; force molt hens to renew production
Human Health Risk — none known

Emphysema

Also Called — windpuff

Incidence — rare

System/Organ Affected — respiratory

Symptoms — bird grows large and round without associated weight gain

Percentage Affected — individual birds

Mortality — only among severely affected birds

Postmortem Findings — accumulation of air beneath the skin

Resembles — no other disease

Diagnosis — symptoms, postmortem findings

Cause — ruptured air sac due to a defect in the respiratory tract or injury due to rough handling, caponizing, crash landing while flying, heavy coughing caused by respiratory infection

Transmission — unknown; often follows brooder house fires

Prevention — unknown

Treatment — release air by puncturing skin with a large hypodermic needle or other sharp instrument

Human Health Risk — none known

Encephalomalacia

Also Called — crazy chick disease

Incidence — rare

System/Organ Affected — brain

Progression — acute

Symptoms — in chicks 1 to 8 weeks (most commonly 2 to 4 weeks) old: sudden loss of balance with legs outstretched, toes flexed, head pulled in or bent back, flapping wings and falling over, circling, moving head from side to side; sometimes trembling head and legs; paralysis, death

— in hens: 15 to 30 percent drop in laying for up to 2 weeks

Percentage Affected — 1 to 10 percent

Mortality — 100 percent in chicks

Postmortem Findings — none or softened, swollen, deteriorated brain with red, brown, or greenish yellow discoloration

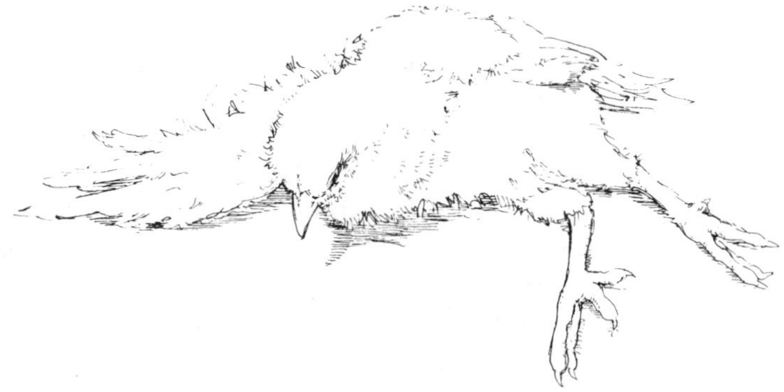

Chick suffering from encephalomalacia

RESEMBLES — curled-toe paralysis, except that in curled-toe paralysis toes curl instead of flex and chicks tend to walk on their hocks (see "Crooked Toes," page 226); pyridoxine deficiency, except that in pyridoxine deficiency the nervous activity is much more intense and often ends in death (see "Brooding Deficiencies," page 227)

DIAGNOSIS — symptoms, postmortem findings, ration evaluation

CAUSE — vitamin E deficiency, often related to selenium deficiency

TRANSMISSION — nutritional, does not spread from bird to bird

PREVENTION — use only fresh feed, fortified with vitamin E and containing antioxidants; store feed in cool dry place, use within 2 weeks of purchase; do not use expired vitamin supplements

TREATMENT — successful only if begun before brain is seriously damaged; for chicks: ½ teaspoon vitamin AD&E powder per gallon of water until symptoms disappear; for older birds: ¼ cc AD&E injected into breast (intramuscular) in addition to vitamin powder in drinking water; recovered birds may be blind in one or both eyes

HUMAN HEALTH RISK — none

Encephalomyelitis. *See* Epidemic Tremor

Endemic Fowl Cholera. *See* Cholera (chronic)

Endemic Newcastle. *See* Newcastle Disease

Enlarged Hock Disease. *See* Infectious Synovitis

Enteric Campylobacteriosis. *See* Campylobacteriosis

Enteritis. *See* Bluecomb, Colibacillosis, Infectious Stunting Syndrome, Necrotic Enteritis, Rotaviral Enteritis, Ulcerative Enteritis

Enterohepatitis. *See* Blackhead

Enterotoxemia. *See* Necrotic Enteritis

Epidemic Tremor

ALSO CALLED — avian encephalomyelitis, AE, encephalomyelitis, infectious avian encephalomyelitis, New England disease, star-gazing syndrome

INCIDENCE — worldwide but rare; more often in large commercial flocks in winter and spring

SYSTEM/ORGAN AFFECTED — nervous system

INCUBATION PERIOD — 5 to 40 days (9 to 21 average)

PROGRESSION — rapid, lasts 21 to 30 days in mature birds

SYMPTOMS — in 1- to 3-week-old chicks: dull eyes followed by lost coordination, jerky or irregular gait, inability to stand, sitting on hocks, falling over with outstretched wing, weak peeping; sometimes periodic vibration of the head and neck and "buzzing" sound when chick is held; death due to inability to eat or to being trampled by other chicks

— in mature hens (symptoms easily go unnoticed): 5 to 10 percent drop in egg production for 2 weeks, poor hatchability of eggs, poor livability of chicks

PERCENTAGE AFFECTED — 40 to 60 percent

MORTALITY — in chicks: 25 percent average, may be as high as 90 percent in mature birds: none

POSTMORTEM FINDINGS — none obvious

RESEMBLES — congenital tremor, except that congenital tremor affects chicks from the time of hatch; encephalomalacia, except that encephalomalacia usually affects older chicks; Marek's disease, except that Marek's usually affects much older birds; Newcastle, encephalitis (bacterial, fungal, or mycoplasmal), rickets, deficiency of riboflavin or vitamin A or E, salt or pesticide poisoning (see "Poisoning," page 139)

DIAGNOSIS — history (age of birds), symptoms, confirmed by laboratory procedures

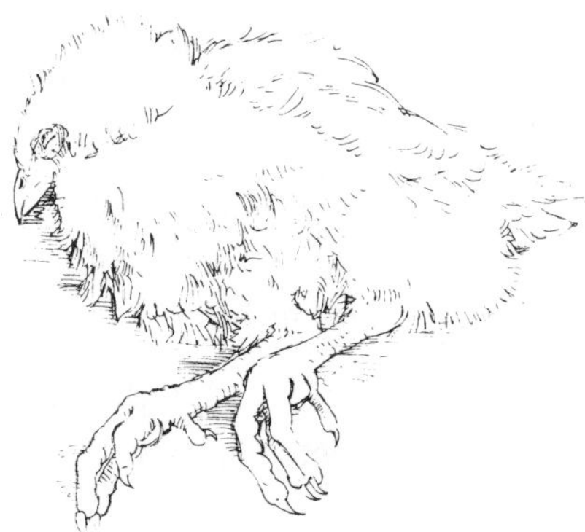
Chick dead from epidemic tremor

CAUSE — picornavirus that survives for up to 4 weeks in droppings

TRANSMISSION — contact with infected birds or their droppings; spread from infected breeders through hatching eggs; spread by turkeys, pheasants, coturnix quail; spreads on used equipment; spread by ticks

PREVENTION — cull breeders whose chicks are affected; vaccinate breeder pullets over 8 weeks of age, but at least 4 weeks before production starts

TREATMENT — none; chicks may survive but should be culled since they will never be good layers or breeders; survivors of an adult outbreak become immune and are not carriers

HUMAN HEALTH RISK — none known

Ergotism

ALSO CALLED — sod disease, vesicular dermatitis

INCIDENCE — worldwide but rare

SYSTEM/ORGAN AFFECTED — endocrine, nervous, blood vessels

SYMPTOMS — in all ages: listlessness; loss of appetite; increased thirst; diarrhea; convulsions; bluish, wilted, cold comb that eventually shrivels; abnormal feathering; sores on legs, shanks, and tops of toes; slow growth; low egg production

PERCENTAGE AFFECTED — low

MORTALITY — 25 percent

POSTMORTEM FINDINGS — inflamed intestines

RESEMBLES — mycotoxicosis resulting from trichothecene poisons generated by *Fusarium* spp in corn, barley, brewer's grains, oats, sorghum, and safflower seed

DIAGNOSIS — flock history (fed moldy grains), symptoms, feed analysis

CAUSE — toxic alkaloids produced by *Claviceps purpurea* fungus in stored wheat, rye, and other cereal grains

TRANSMISSION — contaminated grain and grass seed, particularly rye

PREVENTION — use commercially prepared, pelleted feeds

TREATMENT — replace contaminated feed

HUMAN HEALTH RISK — humans may be poisoned by eating contaminated grain

Erysipelas

ALSO CALLED — *Erysipelothrix* infection

Incidence — worldwide but rare in chickens; most likely to occur in cool months

System/Organ Affected — entire body (septicemic)

Incubation Period — short

Progression — acute, sometimes followed by chronic infection

Symptoms — usually in growing free-ranged cocks: listlessness, loss of appetite, greenish-yellow diarrhea; sometimes nasal discharge and/or breathing difficulties, lameness due to swollen joints, purple blotches on skin; sudden death

— in cocks: reduced fertility

— in hens: up to 70 percent drop in egg production

Percentage Affected — up to 40 percent

Mortality — nearly 100 percent

Postmortem Findings — none significant or small blood spots in almost any tissue or organ; swollen liver, kidney, spleen; yellow nodules in ceca; pus surrounding swollen joints

Resembles — cholera, except that cholera does not cause enlarged spleen; chlamydiosis, colibacillosis, Newcastle, salmonellosis, streptococcosis

Diagnosis — flock history (age and sex, presence of wounds, birds ranged on land that once held turkeys, pigs, or sheep), symptoms (sudden losses among apparently healthy cockerels), postmortem findings (blood-spotted breast muscle), confirmed by laboratory identification of bacteria

Cause — *Erysipelothrix rhusiopathiae* bacteria that survives for many years in alkaline soil and is resistant to disinfectants; affects turkeys more often than chickens; often follows stress due to overcrowding, dampness, bad weather, poor sanitation, ration change, vaccination

Transmission — bacteria in soil from droppings of infected chickens (or turkeys, pigs, or sheep) enters through wounds caused by fighting, cannibalism, or poorly designed equipment; bacteria ingested from soil, water, or meat (cannibalism)

Prevention — breed for genetic resistance; in erysipelas-prone areas, keep chickens away from range previously occupied by turkeys, pigs, or sheep; avoid crowding; control rodents

Treatment — since disease poses human health risk, eliminate infected flock and start over on fresh ground; otherwise, move birds to clean environment (will control losses but contaminate new ground); add sodium or potassium penicillin to drinking water at the rate of 1,000,000 IU per gallon for 5 days; survivors are resistant to future infection, but may be carriers

Human Health Risk — painful infection that can be serious to fatal without medical attention; see "Erysipeloid," page 236

Erysipelothrix Infection. *See* Erysipelas

Escherichia coli Infections. *See* Air-Sac Disease, Chronic Respiratory Disease, Colibacillosis, Omphalitis, Swollen Head Disease

European Fowl Pest. *See* Influenza

Exotic Newcastle Disease. *See* Newcastle Disease (exotic)

Exudative Diathesis

Also Called — exudate diathesis

INCIDENCE — rare
SYSTEM/ORGAN AFFECTED — skin and muscle tissue
SYMPTOMS — in chicks 1 to 4 weeks old: breast and legs look greenish blue, chicks stand with legs far apart due to fluid under skin, paralysis
PERCENTAGE AFFECTED — 1 to 5 percent
MORTALITY — 100 percent
POSTMORTEM FINDINGS — yellow or bluish green gelatinous fluid under skin; blood spots in breast and leg muscles
DIAGNOSIS — symptoms, postmortem findings, ration evaluation
CAUSE — vitamin E deficiency, usually related to selenium deficiency; sometimes occurs in combination with white muscle disease
TRANSMISSION — nutritional problem, does not spread from bird to bird
PREVENTION — use only fresh feed fortified with vitamin E and selenium; store feed in cool dry place and use within 2 weeks of purchase
TREATMENT — vitamin E and selenium supplement in feed or orally (300 IU per bird); replace old feed
HUMAN HEALTH RISK — none

- F -

Facial Cellulitis. *See* Swollen Head Syndrome
False Botulism. *See* Marek's Disease
Fatal Syncope. *See* Sudden Death Syndrome

Fatty Liver Syndrome

ALSO CALLED — fatty liver and kidney syndrome, FLKS, pink disease
INCIDENCE — sporadic worldwide
SYSTEM/ORGAN AFFECTED — liver
PROGRESSION — chronic
SYMPTOMS — in commercial broiler chicks: depression, ruffled feathers, inability to stand
— in mature hens, particularly in warm weather: sudden death (sometimes after puncture from cock's toenails) or sudden drop in laying to about 50 percent, diarrhea; sometimes overweight (25 to 35 percent above normal); enlarged, pale combs and wattles
PERCENTAGE AFFECTED — 1 to 5 percent, depending on diet
MORTALITY — less than 5 percent (dead birds have pale heads)
POSTMORTEM FINDINGS — excess body fat, often pink; mushy yellow, greasy liver; pale, yellowish heart; dark, smelly matter in small intestine; sometimes large blood clots in abdomen (called "fatty liver-hemorrhagic syndrome" or "FLHS")
RESEMBLES — campylobacteriosis
DIAGNOSIS — flock history, symptoms, postmortem findings
CAUSE — unknown; may be genetic; may be caused by molds in feed or water that damage liver; may be caused by high stress due to heat, high egg production, inapparent disease; may be due to biotin deficiency, perhaps caused by disease that increases biotin requirement; often associated with high-energy feeds combined with inactivity
TRANSMISSION — nutritional, does not spread from bird to bird

PREVENTION — avoid moldy or high-energy feeds (consisting mostly of grains), raise birds on litter with room for activity; provide good ventilation to prevent heat stress

TREATMENT — none effective; restrict feed consumption; substitute wheat bran for part of corn; feed brewer's yeast, dried molasses, or alfalfa and other green leafy plants; oral or injectable biotin supplement

HUMAN HEALTH RISK — none

Favus

ALSO CALLED — white comb

INCIDENCE — rare in North America

SYSTEM/ORGAN AFFECTED — comb

PROGRESSION — spreads slowly

SYMPTOMS — in growing and mature cocks with well-developed combs, usually of the Asiatic breeds: grayish white patches on comb that scale off (comb looks dusted with flour), thicken, and join to form a wrinkled crust that smells moldy; sometimes crust spreads to unfeathered areas creating honeycomb appearance where feathers are lost, soon followed by depression, weakness, emaciation, and death

MORTALITY — rare

POSTMORTEM FINDINGS — spots, nodules, and yellowish cheesy deposits in digestive and upper respiratory tracts

RESEMBLES — mites, skin disorders due to poor nutrition

DIAGNOSIS — symptoms

CAUSE — *Microsporum gallinae* fungus

TRANSMISSION — contact with infected birds or sloughed-off scales

PREVENTION — improve nutrition and sanitation; breed for resistance

TREATMENT — most birds recover in a few months without treatment; recovery may be hastened with daily liberal applications of anti-fungal or mange medication (for pets) until symptoms disappear

HUMAN HEALTH RISK — scalp infection

Flip-Over Disease. *See* Sudden Death Syndrome

Food Poisoning. *See* Botulism

Fowl Cholera. *See* Cholera (acute), Cholera (chronic)

Fowl Diphtheria. *See* Pox (wet)

Fowl Pest. *See* Influenza

Fowl Plague. *See* Influenza

Fowl Pox. *See* Pox (dry)

Fowl Spirochetosis. *See* Spirochetosis

Fowl Typhoid. *See* Typhoid

Fusariotoxicosis

ALSO CALLED — trichothene mycotoxicosis

INCIDENCE — worldwide in temperate zones, but rare

SYSTEM/ORGAN AFFECTED — digestive system and skin

INCUBATION PERIOD — accumulative

PROGRESSION — acute

SYMPTOMS — in birds of all ages: refusal to eat, slow growth, abnormal feathering, depression, bloody diarrhea, sores at corners of mouth and on skin, reduced resistance to respiratory diseases

— in hens: sudden drastic drop in egg production, thin shells

PERCENTAGE AFFECTED — high

MORTALITY — low

POSTMORTEM FINDINGS — sores in upper digestive tract, reddening throughout digestive tract, mottled liver, shriveled spleen

DIAGNOSIS — symptoms and feed analysis

CAUSE — trichothecene (type T-2) toxins produced by *Fusarium sporotrichioides* and other fungi in wheat, rye, millet, barley, corn, safflower seeds

TRANSMISSION — poisoning due to eating contaminated feed; burning of skin coming into contact with caustic toxins

PREVENTION — use commercially prepared pelleted feed

TREATMENT — replace moldy feed

HUMAN HEALTH RISK — serious diarrhea from eating same contaminated grains that poison chickens

- G -

Gangrenous Cellulitis/Dermatitis/Dermatomyositis. *See* Necrotic Dermatitis

Gapes. *See* "Gapeworm," page 88

Gas Edema Disease. *See* Necrotic Dermatitis

Gout (articular)

INCIDENCE — sporadic

SYSTEM/ORGAN AFFECTED — excretory system

INCUBATION PERIOD — long

PROGRESSION — chronic

SYMPTOMS — in all ages: enlarged foot joints with pasty white urate deposits easily seen through the skin

PERCENTAGE AFFECTED — individual birds only

MORTALITY — none

POSTMORTEM FINDINGS — white tissue surrounding joints, white semi-fluid deposits within joints

RESEMBLES — no other disease

DIAGNOSIS — symptoms, postmortem findings

CAUSE — abnormal accumulation of urates in the body due to kidney damage, excessive protein in diet, or hereditary susceptibility

TRANSMISSION — genetic and/or related to nutrition

PREVENTION — none known

TREATMENT — none known

HUMAN HEALTH RISK — none

Gout (visceral)

ALSO CALLED — acute gout, nephrosis, renal failure, renal gout, gout (visceral), visceral urate deposition

INCIDENCE — not common in North America

SYSTEM/ORGAN AFFECTED — kidneys

INCUBATION PERIOD — 14 days or more

PROGRESSION — acute
SYMPTOMS — in chicks: flockwide deaths soon after hatch
— in mature birds: sudden death or depression, weight loss, darkened head and shanks, white pasty diarrhea, cessation of laying, attempting to hide
PERCENTAGE AFFECTED — 1 to 5 percent
MORTALITY — 2 to 4 percent per month, usually totaling no more than 50 percent but can be up to 100 percent
POSTMORTEM FINDINGS — dry, shrunken breast muscles; both kidneys shriveled or one shriveled and one pale and swollen; chalky white needle-like crystals in kidneys and on surfaces of liver, abdominal fat, keel, and in joints
RESEMBLES — any inflammation of the kidneys
DIAGNOSIS — symptoms, postmortem findings
CAUSE — kidney failure due to inability to excrete urates for unknown reasons; possibly due to genetic defect, kidney damage from disease, water deprivation, fungal toxins, excessive dietary protein (30 to 40 percent), excess calcium (3 percent or more), excess sodium-bicarbonate, calcium-phosphorus imbalance, vitamin A deficiency; sometimes follows bluecomb; often follows kidney damage due to infectious bronchitis
TRANSMISSION — does not spread from bird to bird
PREVENTION — provide plenty of pure drinking water, cool in summer and warm in winter; feed balanced, commercially prepared rations; avoid excessively high protein rations
TREATMENT — none if problem is genetic, otherwise improve nutrition
HUMAN HEALTH RISK — none

Gray Eye. *See* Marek's Disease
The Greens. *See* Bluecomb
Gumboro Disease. *See* Infectious Bursal Disease

- H -

Heart Attack. *See* Sudden Death Syndrome
Helicopter Syndrome. *See* Infectious Stunting Syndrome
Helminthiasis. *See* "Internal Parasites: Worms" (chapter 5)
Hemophilus Infection. *See* Infectious Coryza
Hemorrhagic Anemia Syndrome. *See* Infectious Anemia
Hepatitis. *See* Blackhead, Campylobacteriosis, Infectious Anemia
Histomoniasis. *See* Blackhead

Histoplasmosis

INCIDENCE — worldwide but rare, in North America found only along Mississippi, Missouri, and Ohio rivers
SYSTEM/ORGAN AFFECTED — entire body
INCUBATION PERIOD — 2 weeks
PROGRESSION — acute or chronic
SYMPTOMS — all ages: emaciation, sometimes diarrhea
PERCENTAGE AFFECTED — low
MORTALITY — 100 percent
POSTMORTEM FINDINGS — mushy liver and spleen

DIAGNOSIS — laboratory identification of fungus

CAUSE — *Histoplasma capsulatum* fungus that proliferates in soil rich with the droppings of chickens and other birds

TRANSMISSION — inhaled fungi

PREVENTION — keep area free of dry accumulations of droppings from starlings and other birds

TREATMENT — none

HUMAN HEALTH RISK — possible respiratory infection from inhaled dust, see "Histoplasmosis," page 233

- I -

IBD. *See* Infectious Bursal Disease

Inclusion Body Hepatitis. *See* Infectious Anemia

Infectious Anemia

ALSO CALLED — adenoviral infection, aplastic anemia, chicken anemia agent infection, CAA infection, hemorrhagic anemia syndrome, HAS, hemorrhagic disease, hemorrhagic syndrome, inclusion body hepatitis, IBH

INCIDENCE — common in major chicken-producing countries, especially in commercial broiler flocks raised on reused litter

SYSTEM/ORGAN AFFECTED — blood

INCUBATION PERIOD — 3 days

PROGRESSION — acute, sudden onset with rapidly increasing deaths; lasts about 3 weeks

SYMPTOMS — in growing broilers, 3 to 20 weeks old (most often 5 to 9 weeks): sudden deaths of apparently healthy birds or depression, huddling, ruffled feathers, drawn-in head, pale comb, wattles, skin, and legs; sometimes diarrhea (may be bloody); death or recovery within 2 days

PERCENTAGE AFFECTED — usually low

MORTALITY — 5 to 10 percent average, may be up to 40 percent during first 5 days

POSTMORTEM FINDINGS — enlarged, pale, dull greenish, yellow, or tan liver mottled with red spots; bright red, watery blood; pale, yellow, fatty bone marrow; swollen, blood-filled kidneys tinged with yellow; pale muscles with pinpoint-sized bloody spots in muscles and organs; shriveled spleen and cloacal bursa

RESEMBLES — coccidiosis, infectious bursal disease, ulcerative enteritis, poisoning; aflatoxicosis, except that chickens are unlikely to be exposed to high enough doses of aflatoxin to produce these symptoms

DIAGNOSIS — flock history, symptoms (sudden deaths without symptoms), postmortem findings (fatty bone marrow, liver appearance), microscopic examination of liver

CAUSE — unknown, possibly an adenovirus and/or a parvovirus called "chicken anemia agent;" may be related to vitamin K deficiency and/or drug toxicity (especially sulfa drugs); often found in combination with or following infectious bursal disease and/or secondary bacterial or fungal infections

TRANSMISSION — ingesting bacteria from droppings of infected birds; spreads from breeders to chicks through hatching eggs; contaminated litter or equipment (especially hatching-egg cartons)

PREVENTION — healthy birds in clean surroundings develop natural immunity after about 3 weeks of age; do not hatch eggs from breeders whose previous chicks had infectious anemia; vaccinate breeder flock for infectious bursal disease; avoid chilling, vaccinating, or prolonged use of sulfonamides in young birds; thoroughly clean contaminated facilities with disinfectant containing iodine

TREATMENT — none other than supportive therapy (see page 192) including a supplement containing trace minerals and vitamins B and K; avoid coccidiostats, which increase the disease's severity; treatment with antibiotics or sulfa drugs may worsen the disease

HUMAN HEALTH RISK — none known

Infectious Avian Encephalomyelitis. *See* Epidemic Tremor

Infectious Bronchitis

ALSO CALLED — avian infectious bronchitis, IB, mild cold

INCIDENCE — common worldwide

SYSTEM/ORGAN AFFECTED — respiratory

INCUBATION PERIOD — 18 to 36 hours

PROGRESSION — acute, starts suddenly, spreads rapidly, runs through flock in 24 to 48 hours, individuals recover in 2 to 3 weeks

SYMPTOMS — in birds of all ages: gasping, coughing, sneezing, rattling, wet eyes, nasal discharge

— in young and growing birds: watery nasal discharge, huddling near heat, loss of appetite, slow growth; sometimes swollen sinuses

— in maturing birds: sometimes swollen wattles

— in hens: sharp drop in laying to near zero, eggs with soft, thin, misshapen, rough, or ridged shells and watery whites

PERCENTAGE AFFECTED — 100 percent

MORTALITY — limited in older birds; 25 percent in chicks, but can be up to 90 percent, especially in cold weather and/or in the presence of a secondary bacterial infection

POSTMORTEM FINDINGS — in chicks: yellowish cheesy plugs in throat; swollen, pale kidneys

— in growing and mature birds: swollen, pale kidneys; urate crystals in tubes leading from kidneys; fluid yolk or whole eggs in abdominal cavity of hens

RESEMBLES — infectious laryngotracheitis, except that laryngo spreads less rapidly and is more severe; Newcastle, except that Newcastle is more severe, produces a greater drop in egg production, and can cause nervous symptoms; infectious coryza, except that coryza often has a foul odor and produces facial swelling (bronchitis rarely does); egg drop syndrome, except that EDS does not cause runny egg whites; nutritional roup, except that roup does not affect egg whites or shells

DIAGNOSIS — difficult; symptoms, laboratory identification of virus

CAUSE — several strains of coronavirus that survive no more than one week off chickens and are easily destroyed by disinfectants; infects only chickens, which vary in susceptibility among breeds and strains

TRANSMISSION — the most contagious poultry disease; spreads by contact with infected birds or their respiratory discharges; spreads on contaminated equipment; travels over 1,000 yards through air

PREVENTION — defies good management; avoid mixing birds of different ages or from different sources; vaccinate with strain(s) of virus found locally (infectious bronchitis may still occur due to a different or new strain of virus); be prepared to treat with broad-spectrum antibiotic if signs of air-sac disease follow vaccination; hens that have a strong reaction to vaccine may never lay well

TREATMENT — electrolytes in drinking water (see page 193); keep birds warm and well fed; avoid crowding; watch for secondary bacterial infection, particularly air sac disease; survivors are permanently immune but become carriers (hens return to production in 6 to 8 weeks, but may never produce the same egg quality or quantity as before due to permanent ovary damage)

HUMAN HEALTH RISK — none known, a different virus causes bronchitis in humans

Infectious Bursal Disease

ALSO CALLED — Gumboro disease, IBD

INCIDENCE — common worldwide (except in New Zealand), primarily in large flocks

SYSTEM/ORGAN AFFECTED — lymph tissue, especially cloacal bursa

INCUBATION PERIOD — 1 to 3 days

PROGRESSION — acute, appears suddenly, spreads rapidly, runs through flock in 1 to 2 weeks

SYMPTOMS — in young birds 3 to 18 weeks old (most often broilers 3 to 6 weeks old): droopiness, ruffled feathers, vent picking (bird picks at own vent), straining while trying to eliminate, whitish or watery (sometimes blood-tinged) diarrhea staining feathers below vent (making litter sticky), slight trembling, loss of appetite, dehydration, incoordination, fever followed by drop in body temperature to below normal, prostration, death

PERCENTAGE AFFECTED — nearly 100 percent

MORTALITY — 0 to 30 percent, peaking within a week; greater in Leghorns than in heavy breeds, in chicks fed 24 percent protein starter, and in birds infected with bronchitis, Newcastle, or cecal coccidiosis

POSTMORTEM FINDINGS — none significant or dark, shriveled breast muscles flecked with bloody streaks; mucus-filled intestine; cloacal bursa may be yellow, pink, red, or black, swollen, oblong-shaped, filled with creamy or cheesy material, and surrounded by gelatinous film (as the disease progresses, the bursa returns to normal size, then shrinks and shrivels up); swollen spleen covered with gray dots; birds that die from infection have swollen, pale kidneys

RESEMBLES — coccidiosis, except that cocci does not cause bloody flecks in muscles or swelling of cloacal bursa

DIAGNOSIS — flock history (age of birds, rapid onset, number of birds involved), symptoms (white or watery diarrhea, birds picking own vents, deaths peaking within a week, rapid recovery), postmortem findings (swollen or shriveled cloacal bursa)

CAUSE — birnavirus that affects primarily chickens and is common in every major poultry-producing area; survives in feed, water, and droppings for weeks and in housing for at least 4 months after removal of infected birds

Transmission — highly contagious; spread from infected birds through their droppings in contaminated litter and dust in air, and on equipment, feed, shoes, insects, rodents, and wild birds; may be spread by darkling beetle, or lesser mealworm *(Alphitobius diaperinus)* found in litter

Prevention — good sanitation helps but virus defies good management and is difficult to eradicate; vaccinated breeders pass temporary immunity to their chicks; natural immunity develops in chicks exposed to infection before the age of 2 weeks; vaccinate only where disease is prevalent

Treatment — none; keep birds warm and well ventilated and provide plenty of drinking water; recovered chickens are more susceptible to other diseases and may not develop immune response to vaccines, especially Marek's

Human Health Risk — none known

Infectious Catarrh. *See* Infectious Coryza

Infectious Coryza

Also Called — cold, contagious catarrh, coryza, hemophilus infection, infectious catarrh, IC, roup

Incidence — common worldwide, particularly in fall and winter in tropical and temperate climates (southeastern United States and California)

System/Organ Affected — respiratory

Incubation Period — 1 to 3 days

Progression — acute and spreads rapidly or chronic and spreads slowly

Symptoms — in chicks at least 4 weeks old: depression, nasal discharge, facial swelling, one or both eyes closed, death

— in growing and mature birds (most likely group affected): watery eyes with eyelids stuck together, reddish foul-smelling discharge from nose, drop in feed and water consumption, drop in egg production, swollen face, eyes, and sinuses; sometimes diarrhea, rales or wheezing

Percentage Affected — high (more in an acute outbreak than in a chronic outbreak)

Mortality — low

Postmortem Findings — thick, grayish fluid, or yellowish solid material in nasal passages

ARTHUR A. BICKFORD. DVM. U. CAL. DAVIS

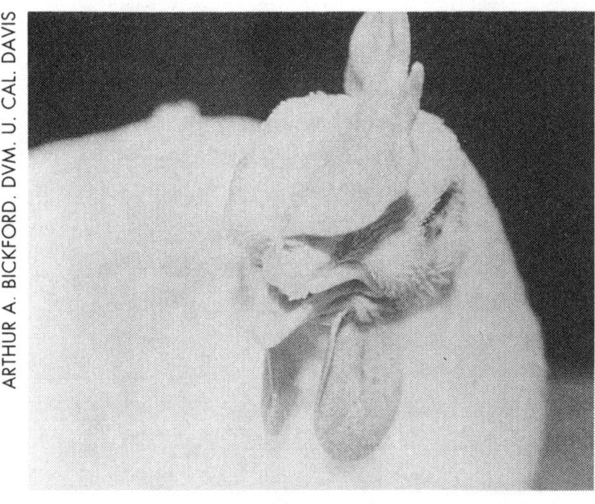

Face swollen with infectious coryza

RESEMBLES — cholera, except that coryza causes facial swelling; chronic respiratory disease, infectious laryngotracheitis, Newcastle, nutritional roup, infectious bronchitis, influenza, except that coryza produces a characteristic odor

DIAGNOSIS — symptoms (facial swelling, characteristic odor), laboratory identification of bacteria

CAUSE — *Haemophilus paragallinarum* bacteria that do not survive long in the environment and are easily destroyed by disinfectants; often found in combination with chronic respiratory disease, cholera, pox, infectious bronchitis, or infectious laryngotracheitis

TRANSMISSION — contagious; contact with infected or carrier birds and their nasal or respiratory discharges in dust, drinking water, or feed

PREVENTION — avoid combining birds from different flocks and of different age groups; remove infected birds, disinfect, and leave housing vacant for 3 weeks before bringing in new birds; vaccinate only if the disease has been positively identified; vaccinated breeders pass temporary immunity to their offspring; after an outbreak, clean and disinfect housing and leave vacant for a few days

TREATMENT — erythromycin (Gallimycin), streptomycin (Vetstrep), sulfadimethoxine; disease may recur after treatment is discontinued; culling is preferable since survivors (including all birds in the flock) may be carriers

HUMAN HEALTH RISK — none known

Infectious Enterohepatitis. *See* Blackhead

Infectious Hepatitis. *See* Campylobacteriosis

Infectious Laryngotracheitis

ALSO CALLED — avian diphtheria, ILT, laryngo, LT

INCIDENCE — common worldwide

SYSTEM/ORGAN AFFECTED — upper respiratory tract

INCUBATION PERIOD — 6 to 12 days

PROGRESSION — acute, spreads slowly, most birds die or recover within 2 weeks, runs through flock in 2 to 6 weeks

SYMPTOMS — in maturing or mature birds (mild infection): watery inflamed eyes, swollen sinuses, nasal discharge, drop in egg production, unthriftiness

— in maturing or mature birds (acute infection): nasal discharge, coughing (sometimes producing bloody mucus that gets on face or feathers), head shaking, breathing through mouth, gasping (neck extended during inhale, head on breast during exhale), choking, gurgling, rattling, whistling, or "cawing," swollen sinuses and wattles, watery eyes, drop in egg production, soft-shelled eggs

PERCENTAGE AFFECTED — 5 percent in mild case, 90 to 100 percent in acute infection

MORTALITY — 10 to 20 percent average, can be up to 70 percent in acute infection; least in young birds during warm weather, greatest in layers during winter

POSTMORTEM FINDINGS — swollen windpipe clogged with bloody mucus or a cheesy plug

RESEMBLES — infectious bronchitis, except that laryngo spreads less rapidly and is more severe; Newcastle, except that laryngo does not cause nervous symptoms; pox (wet), except that laryngo does not produce facial sores; swallowed feed-sack string wrapped around tongue, except that string affects only one bird at a time; gapeworm, except that in laryngo birds die more quickly with no worms in throat

DIAGNOSIS — flock history, symptoms (coughing up blood, high death rate), postmortem findings, confirmed by laboratory procedures

CAUSE — a herpes virus that affects primarily chickens and pheasants and does not live long off the bird

TRANSMISSION — highly contagious; inhaled virus from infected or carrier birds or contaminated litter; can be spread on equipment or the feet of rodents, dogs, and humans

PREVENTION — flock isolation and scrupulous sanitation; do not mix vaccinated or recovered birds with others; vaccinate *if* laryngo is common in your area, you show your chickens in areas where it is common, you regularly bring in new adult birds, or you frequently visit with chicken-keepers from laryngo-prevalent areas

TREATMENT — none, cull; vaccination keeps disease from spreading and survivors are immune, but survivors (and vaccinated birds) are carriers; disinfect housing and leave it empty for 6 weeks; this is a **reportable disease** in many states, see "Reportable Diseases" page 196

HUMAN HEALTH RISK — none known

Infectious Leukemia. *See* Typhoid

Infectious Sinusitis. *See* Chronic Respiratory Disease

Infectious Stunting Syndrome

ALSO CALLED — broiler runting syndrome, ISS, malabsorption syndrome, pale bird syndrome, split-wing syndrome, stunting syndrome, helicopter syndrome

INCIDENCE — increasingly more common in the United States, Europe, and Australia

SYSTEM/ORGAN AFFECTED — digestive

INCUBATION PERIOD — 1 to 13 days

PROGRESSION — chronic

SYMPTOMS — in 1- to 6-week-old birds (primarily intensively raised broilers): uneven or seriously stunted growth (chicks reach only half their normal size by 4 weeks of age), pale skin, slow feather development; sometimes protruding abdomen, undigested feed in droppings, diarrhea, increased thirst; lameness and/or reluctance to walk (when disease occurs in combination with viral arthritis or osteoporosis)

PERCENTAGE AFFECTED — 5 to 20 percent

MORTALITY — less than 6 percent, peaking early

POSTMORTEM FINDINGS — enlarged, sometimes bloody stomach (proventriculus); pale, distended intestines; small intestine filled with poorly digested feed; sometimes thin, white, fibrous pancreas

RESEMBLES — infectious anemia, runting syndrome

DIAGNOSIS — symptoms, postmortem findings

CAUSE — unknown, possibly due to a combination including one or more reoviruses and/or bacteria and/or fungal toxins; may occur in combination with encephalomalacia

TRANSMISSION — unknown; possibly transmitted by inhaling or ingesting virus generated by infected birds; or spread from infected breeders through hatching eggs

PREVENTION — unknown; avoid crowding and practice good sanitation

TREATMENT — unknown; following an outbreak, thoroughly clean and disinfect housing with lye or 0.5 percent organic iodine solution

HUMAN HEALTH RISK — none known

Infectious Synovitis. *See also* Colibacillosis

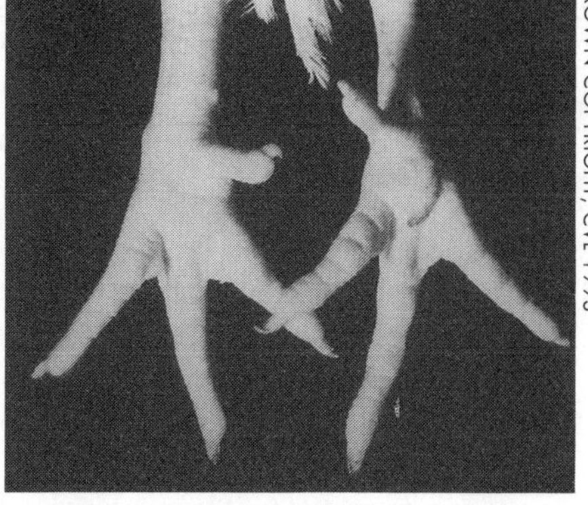
CROWN COPYRIGHT, CVL 1993

Leg swollen with infectious synovitis

ALSO CALLED — enlarged hock disease, *Mycoplasma synoviae* infection, MS (one form of mycoplasmosis)

INCIDENCE — worldwide but not common except in large commercial flocks, especially in cold, damp weather

SYSTEM/ORGAN AFFECTED — joints, sometimes upper respiratory tract

INCUBATION PERIOD — 11 to 21 days

PROGRESSION — usually acute with slow recovery in young birds, chronic in older birds (survivors of acute form become chronic)

SYMPTOMS — in growing broilers, 4 to 12 weeks old: no signs or slow growth, lameness, pale comb, followed by depression, ruffled feathers, shrunken comb, hunkering around feeders and waterers, emaciation; sometimes swollen hocks, shanks, and foot pads (swollen areas feel hot), breast blister from squatting on floor, slight rales, bluish comb, green droppings capped with large amounts of white urate deposits

PERCENT AFFECTED — usually 100 percent, but only 15 to 20 percent have symptoms

MORTALITY — up to 10 percent (usually due to secondary infection)

POSTMORTEM FINDINGS — creamy yellowish or grayish fluid (acute) or thick orange yellow matter (chronic) in joints, keel, and foot pad; swollen, mottled, pale kidneys; enlarged, greenish liver

RESEMBLES — staphylococcic or viral arthritis, except that infectious synovitis more often involves wing joints and produces breast blisters

DIAGNOSIS — flock history, symptoms, postmortem findings, blood tests, laboratory identification of bacteria

CAUSE — *Mycoplasma synoviae* bacteria, often infecting following stress due to Newcastle or infectious bronchitis; may be caused by *Escherichia coli,* in which case some birds recover in about a week, others remain infected and become emaciated

TRANSMISSION — inhaling bacteria from infected or carrier birds; spread by breeders through hatching eggs

PREVENTION — keep litter dry; do not combine birds from different sources; acquire only MS-free stock; hatch eggs only from MS-free breeders; blood test and remove positive reactors; vaccinate where infection is prevalent (expensive)

TREATMENT — none effective; aureomycin or terramycin in water or streptomycin by intramuscular injection may help, but survivors may be carriers

HUMAN HEALTH RISK — none known

Influenza

Also Called — avian influenza, AI, European fowl pest, fowl plague

Incidence — worldwide, but serious outbreaks are rare

System/Organ Affected — primarily respiratory, sometimes involves digestive and nervous systems

Incubation Period — a few hours to 3 days

Progression — acute, spreads rapidly, runs through flock in 1 to 3 days

Symptoms — in birds of all ages: sudden death without signs, or severe depression, droopiness, coughing, sneezing, rattling, watery eyes, huddling, ruffled feathers, loss of appetite, weight loss, reduced fertility, sudden drop in egg production, increased broodiness, eggs with soft or no shells, skin hemorrhages, fever; sometimes bloody nasal discharge, greenish diarrhea, darkened head, comb, wattles, and/or swollen eyes, comb, and wattles; sometimes twisted neck, loss of coordination, paralysis of legs or wings, swollen hock joints, purplish shanks; rapid deaths

Percentage Affected — 100 percent

Mortality — 0 to 100 percent, usually low

Postmortem Findings — none obvious; mild form: cheesy plugs in sinuses, throat, air sacs, oviduct

— severe form: large and small reddish brown spots or blotches (hemorrhages) along the interior of the upper and lower digestive tract, on the ovaries, and over the fat of the abdomen; straw-colored fluid beneath skin of face; enlarged blood vessels; loose gizzard lining

Resembles — mild form: infectious bronchitis, chlamydiosis, chronic respiratory disease, Newcastle

— severe form: acute cholera, exotic Newcastle, infectious laryngotracheitis

Diagnosis — symptoms (high rate of rapid deaths), confirmed by laboratory identification of virus

Cause — several strains of type A influenza orthomyxoviruses, some mild, some lethal, that affect a wide variety of bird species but do not survive long in the environment; often infect in combination with a bacterial or mycoplasmal disease

Transmission — highly contagious; contact with infected birds (either domestic or wild) and their body discharges, especially droppings; spreads through improper disposal of infected birds and their manure, on contaminated equipment and the feet of insects, rodents, and humans

Prevention — do not visit flocks or let people visit your flock if an outbreak occurs in your area; keep chickens away from water frequented by wild waterfowl

Treatment — mild form: antibiotic to prevent secondary bacterial or mycoplasmal infection; survivors are immune for several months but are carriers

— severe form: this is a **reportable disease,** see "Reportable Diseases" page 196

Human Health Risk — type A influenza viruses have the *potential* for causing infection in humans and other mammals, but no case is known of a human getting the flu from a chicken

Iritis. *See* Marek's Disease

- J -

Jittery Chicks. *See* Congenital Tremor

- K -

Keel Bursitis. *See* Breast Blister
Keel Cyst. *See* Breast Blister
Keratoconjunctivitis. *See* Conjunctivitis

Kinky Back

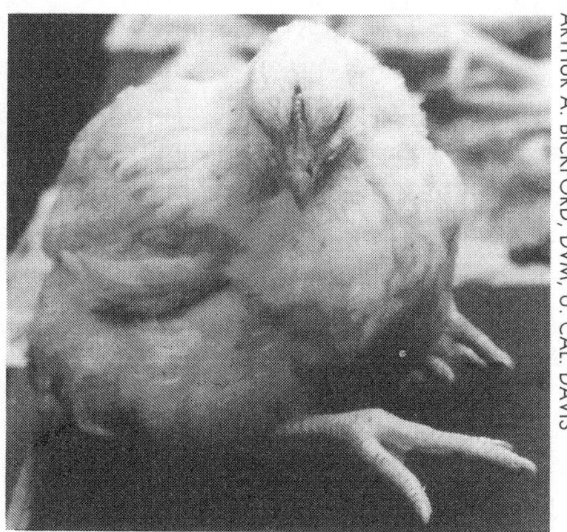

ARTHUR A. BICKFORD, DVM, U. CAL. DAVIS

Broiler with kinky back

ALSO CALLED — spondylolisthesis

INCIDENCE — common in broiler flocks

SYSTEM/ORGAN AFFECTED — joints or vertebrae

SYMPTOMS — in broilers 3 to 6 weeks of age: arched back, extended neck, squatting with weight on hocks and tail, feet off the ground, struggling backward on hocks to move around (backpedaling), sometimes falling over with inability to get up, paralysis

PERCENTAGE AFFECTED — 2 percent

MORTALITY — 100 percent (due to dehydration)

POSTMORTEM FINDINGS — deformed spinal column

RESEMBLES — any crippling condition including infection that causes swelling and pressure to the spinal cord

DIAGNOSIS — symptoms (few birds involved at once)

CAUSE — unknown, possibly hereditary; rapid growth causes vertebrae to twist and pinch the spinal cord

TRANSMISSION — genetic and/or feed related, does not spread from bird to bird

PREVENTION — breed for resistance; do not feed for rapid growth

TREATMENT — none, cull

HUMAN HEALTH RISK — none

- L -

Laryngotracheitis. *See* Infectious Laryngotracheitis

Leucocytozoonosis

ALSO CALLED — *Leucocytozoon* disease

INCIDENCE — only in areas where biting midges *(Culicoides)* and blackflies *(Simuliidae)* are prevalent, especially during summer and fall; in North America occurs in southeastern states, Minnesota, and Wisconsin

SYSTEM/ORGAN AFFECTED — blood

PROGRESSION — sudden onset, spreads rapidly, acute in young birds, chronic in mature birds

SYMPTOMS — in young birds (particularly those carrying heavy loads of internal parasites): droopiness, weakness, lameness, fever, loss of appetite, emaciation, increased thirst, vomiting, increased excitability, rapid labored breathing, sometimes green diarrhea; birds recover or die within 3 days

— in older birds: no symptoms but may remain carriers for months

PERCENTAGE AFFECTED — high

MORTALITY — 10 to 80 percent

POSTMORTEM FINDINGS — enlarged spleen, pale muscles and other tissues; sometimes flabby, yellow flesh; often upper intestine filled with blood

RESEMBLES — malaria

DIAGNOSIS — requires laboratory procedure (blood smear)

CAUSE — *Leucocytozoon* spp protozoan parasites that infect many other kinds of birds more often than chickens

TRANSMISSION — spread by biting midges from infected or carrier birds; does not spread through direct contact with infected birds

PREVENTION — control blackflies and midges (see page 62) or do not raise chickens in areas where they are abundant; isolate brooding chicks from infected adults; dispose of breeder flock each year to eliminate carriers; continuous drug treatment (pyrimethamine in feed plus sulfadimethoxine or sulfaquinoxaline in feed or water) is a preventative but not a cure

TREATMENT — ineffective; recovered birds are carriers, may be stunted, and will never lay well

HUMAN HEALTH RISK — none known

Leukosis/Sarcoma. *See* Lymphoid Leukosis, Osteopetrosis

Limberneck. *See* Botulism

Listeriosis

ALSO CALLED — circling disease

INCIDENCE — worldwide in temperate areas, but rare (chickens are resistant)

SYSTEM/ORGAN AFFECTED — brain and heart (encephalitic) or entire body (septicemic)

INCUBATION PERIOD — 5 to 15 days

PROGRESSION — acute, moves through flock slowly

SYMPTOMS — in young birds: walking in circles with twisted neck (encephalitic form); diarrhea, gradual weight loss, death (septicemic form)

— in mature birds: sudden death (septicemic)

PERCENTAGE AFFECTED — low

MORTALITY — usually low but can reach 40 percent

POSTMORTEM FINDINGS — patchy spots on liver; pale, inflamed heart

RESEMBLES — encephalitic form: encephalomalacia, epidemic tremor, exotic Newcastle

— septicemic form: any acute septicemia

DIAGNOSIS — difficult; laboratory identification of bacteria

CAUSE — *Listeria monocytogenes* bacteria commonly found in soil and the bowels of birds and other animals

TRANSMISSION — inhaling or ingesting bacteria; bacterial contamination of a wound

PREVENTION — good sanitation

TREATMENT — none, cull

Human Health Risk — conjunctivitis and listeric abortion from contact with infected or carrier birds; see "Listeriosis," page 236

Liver Disease. *See* Campylobacteriosis

Long-Bone Distortion. *See* Twisted Leg

Lymphoid Leukosis

Also Called — big liver disease, LL, lymphatic leukosis, visceral lymphoma (one disease in the leukosis/sarcoma group)

Incidence — common worldwide

System/Organ Affected — entire body

Incubation Period — 14 weeks

Progression — usually chronic

Symptoms — in birds 16 weeks or older (especially those nearing maturity): depression, death

— in birds over 6 months old: death without symptoms or pale shriveled comb, loss of appetite, diarrhea, emaciation, weakness; sometimes bluish comb, vent feathers spotted with white (urates) or green (bile); sometimes you can feel enlarged kidney, cloacal bursa, liver, or nodular tumors through skin

— in hens: reduced egg production, enlarged abdomen, loose droppings

Percentage Affected — sporadic

Mortality — up to 25 percent (rapidly following first symptoms)

Postmortem Findings — in birds 16 weeks or older: large and numerous soft, smooth, shiny white or gray tumors in liver, spleen, and cloacal bursa; sometimes swollen grayish crumbly or gritty liver, enlarged joints, tumors in kidney, lungs, heart, bone marrow, testes or ovary

Resembles — Marek's disease (see chart page 128), blackhead, pullorum, tuberculosis

Diagnosis — flock history (birds' age), symptoms (progression and mortality), postmortem findings (especially involvement of cloacal bursa)

Cause — a group of retroviruses that primarily infect chickens and do not live long off a bird's body

Transmission — contact with infected birds; spreads from infected breeders through hatching eggs (main source of transmission) or by infected chicks to non-infected chicks through droppings; mechanically by blood-sucking parasites or unhygienic vaccination method

Prevention — defies good management but can be controlled by: buying and breeding resistant strains (heavier meat breeds are more resistant that lighter laying breeds); identifying and eliminating breeders that produce infected chicks (requires testing for reactors); not reusing chick boxes; raising chicks on wire; not combining chickens of different ages or from different sources; thoroughly cleaning facilities before introducing new birds; thoroughly cleaning and disinfecting incubator and brooder between hatches; controlling blood-sucking parasites; avoiding use of same needle for flockwide injections or vaccinations

Treatment — none, cull; clean up and disinfect

Human Health Risk — none known

- M -

Malabsorption Syndrome. *See* Infectious Stunting Syndrome

Malaria

Also Called — avian plasmodia, *Plasmodium* infection
Incidence — worldwide in temperate climates
System/Organ Affected — blood
Incubation Period — 5 to 7 days
Progression — acute to chronic
Symptoms — in all ages: none to death
Percentage Affected — 5 to 20 percent
Mortality — 0 to 90 percent
Postmortem Findings — anemia
Resembles — leucocytozoonosis
Diagnosis — laboratory testing (blood smear)
Cause — *Plasmodium* spp protozoan parasites
Transmission — mosquito bites
Prevention — control mosquitoes; isolate chickens in mosquito-proof housing
Treatment — none
Human Health Risk — none known

Marble Bone. *See* Osteopetrosis

Marek's Disease

Also Called — MD, neuritis, neurolymphomatosis, range paralysis (eye form: gray eye, iritis, ocular lymphomatosis, uveitis)
Incidence — very common worldwide (more so in large breeds than in bantams)
System/Organ Affected — organs (liver, lungs, and others), nerves, or skin; see page 127 for chart describing forms of Marek's disease
Incubation Period — 2 weeks
Progression — often acute
Symptoms — in chicks over 3 weeks old (most commonly 12 to 30 weeks): growing thin while eating well (most common form), deaths starting at 8 to 10 weeks and persisting until 20 to 25 weeks

— in maturing birds (6 to 9 months old): enlarged, reddened feather follicles or white bumps (tumors) on skin that scab over with a brown crust (skin form); stilted gait or lack of coordination, pale skin, wing or leg paralysis (involves nerve); when both legs are paralyzed, one points forward and the other points back under body; sometimes rapid weight loss, gaping or gasping, transient paralysis lasting 1 to 2 days (pseudo-botulism form), dehydration, emaciation, coma; death due to inability to get to food and water or trampling by other chickens

— in breeds with reddish bay eyes: cloudy grayish, dilated, irregular pupil ("gray eye," involves optic nerve); distorted or blinded eye

— in all ages: sudden death of apparently healthy birds

Percentage Affected — 30 to 50 percent in unvaccinated flocks, less than 5 percent in vaccinated flocks
Mortality — can be nearly 100 percent; gradually increasing for up to 10 weeks, higher in pullets than in cockerels

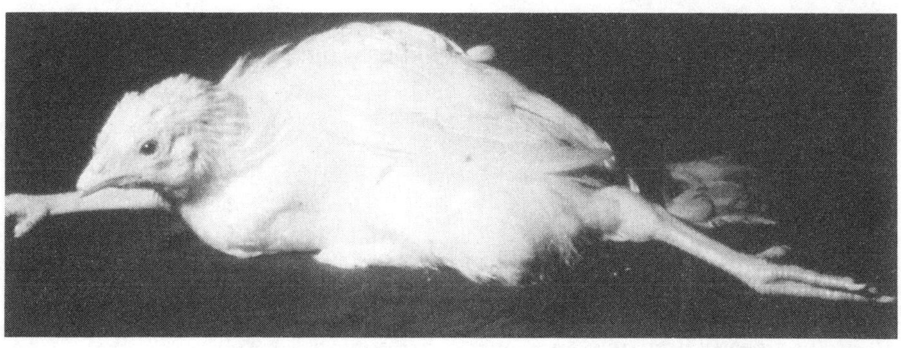
ARTHUR A. BICKFORD, DVM, U. CAL., DAVIS

Chicken paralyzed with Marek's disease

Postmortem Findings — in cases of sudden death, massive tumors, especially along the spinal column; otherwise, enlarged nerves with nodules (usually only on one side — compare same nerve on opposite side of body); tumors in testes or ovary (ovary takes on a "cauliflower" appearance); solidified lungs; extremely enlarged liver, spleen, or kidneys with grayish white, soft areas; sometimes coarse, granular liver

Resembles — primarily lymphoid leukosis (see page 128 for chart on how to tell the two apart); respiratory disease when Marek's affects the lungs; transient paralytic Marek's (called "pseudo-botulism" or "false botulism") resembles botulism, except that in pseudo-botulism birds recover quickly; paralysis and/or internal changes may resemble blackhead, epidemic tremor, joint infection or injury, Newcastle disease, slipped tendon, riboflavin deficiency, tuberculosis, or tick paralysis (see "Soft Ticks," page 73)

Diagnosis — flock history (birds not yet mature), symptoms (especially discolored iris and irregular pupil), postmortem findings (two or more organs affected)

Cause — six different herpes viruses concentrated in feather follicles, shed in dander, survive for years in dust and litter; in pullets, often infect in combination with coccidiosis

Transmission — contagious; contact with carrier or infected birds or their feathers; contact with contaminated litter; inhaled contaminated dust or dander; spread by darkling beetle or lesser mealworm *(Alphitobius diaperinus)* found in litter; not transmitted through hatching eggs or on their shells

Prevention — breed for resistance (some chickens carry a resistance factor, "B21," detected through blood testing); practice good sanitation; provide good ventilation; brood chicks away from adult birds until 5 months of age (by which time they develop resistance); keep turkeys with chickens (turkeys carry a related though harmless virus that keeps Marek's virus from causing tumors); inject vaccine under skin lifted at nape of neck of newly hatched chicks, one-time vaccination confers lifetime immunity; do not expose vaccinated chicks to infection until immunity develops within 7 days; not all vaccines are effective against all six strains of Marek's virus

Treatment — none, cull affected birds (unless you're breeding for resistance); some tumors, particularly those of the feather follicles, clear up and the bird recovers on its own, but survivors are carriers

HUMAN HEALTH RISK — none known from the virus, but handling vaccine may make your eyes itch for a few days

Mesogenic Newcastle. *See* Newcastle Disease

Moniliasis. *See* Thrush

Monocytosis. *See* Bluecomb

Mud Fever. *See* Bluecomb

Muguet. *See* Thrush

Muscular Dystrophy. *See* White Muscle Disease

Mushy Chick Disease. *See* Omphalitis

Mycoplasma gallisepticum. *See* Chronic Respiratory Disease

***Mycoplasma synoviae* Infection.** *See* Infectious Synovitis

Mycoplasmosis. *See* Air-Sac Disease, Chronic Respiratory Disease, Infectious Synovitis

Mycotic Pneumonia. *See* Aspergillosis (acute); Aspergillosis (chronic)

Mycotoxicosis. *See* Aflatoxicosis, Fusariotoxicosis, Ochratoxicosis

- N -

Navel Ill/Infection. *See* Omphalitis

Necrotic Dermatitis

ALSO CALLED — avian malignant edema, clostridial dermatomyositis, gangrenous cellulitis, gangrenous dermatitis, gangrenous dermatomyositis, gas edema disease, wing rot

INCIDENCE — worldwide but rare

SYSTEM/ORGAN AFFECTED — skin

INCUBATION PERIOD — 2 to 3 days

PROGRESSION — acute

SYMPTOMS — in birds 3 to 20 weeks old (commonly 4 to 8 weeks old): sudden deaths (sometimes with small, moist sores between toes) or depression, lameness, incoordination, prostration, loose feathers or skin that easily rubs off; skin that pops or crackles when rubbed (due to gas underneath); reddish black patches of dead, featherless skin on wings, breast, abdomen, or legs; death within 24 hours, body decomposes rapidly, turning green within 1 or 2 hours

PERCENTAGE AFFECTED — low

MORTALITY — 60 to 100 percent

POSTMORTEM FINDINGS — bloody, gelatinous fluid beneath skin; gray or tan breast and thigh muscles that look cooked; usually shriveled cloacal bursa; sometimes enlarged liver and spleen, swollen kidneys, degenerated lungs

RESEMBLES — blister burn or contact dermatitis caused by wet or improperly managed litter; nutritional deficiencies leaving skin unprotected due to slow feathering

DIAGNOSIS — symptoms, postmortem findings

CAUSE — *Clostridium septicum* bacteria commonly found in droppings, soil, dust, litter, feed; often occurs in combination with necrotic enteritis, staphylococcosis, and colibacillosis; usually follows an outbreak of infectious bursal disease, sometimes follows infectious anemia or infectious stunting syndrome

TRANSMISSION — through wounds caused by caponizing, fighting, cannibalism, injury on poorly designed equipment

PREVENTION — good sanitation and nutrition; good management to avoid wounds; ventilation to prevent excessive humidity in housing; breed for resistance to infectious bursal disease

TREATMENT — broad-spectrum antibiotic (penicillin, erythromycin, tetracyclines), proper selection requires laboratory identification of all organisms involved; vitamin-electrolyte supplement hastens recovery

HUMAN HEALTH RISK — none, if good sanitation is practiced after handling infected chicks

Necrotic Enteritis

ALSO CALLED — cauliflower gut, crud, enterotoxemia, NE, rot gut

INCIDENCE — worldwide but rare

SYSTEM/ORGAN AFFECTED — intestines

INCUBATION PERIOD — 3 to 10 days

PROGRESSION — acute, appears suddenly, progresses rapidly, runs through flock in 5 to 10 days

SYMPTOMS — in intensively raised birds, 2 weeks to 6 months old (commonly 2 to 5 weeks old): depression, loss of appetite, ruffled feathers, reluctance to move, diarrhea, death within hours; or sudden death without symptoms

PERCENTAGE AFFECTED — up to 15 percent

MORTALITY — 2 to 50 percent

POSTMORTEM FINDINGS — cauliflower-like yellow or green membrane lining small intestine filled with gas or foul-smelling brown fluid

RESEMBLES — intestinal coccidiosis *(Eimeria brunetti),* except that cocci is usually less severe; ulcerative enteritis, except that necrotic enteritis rarely affects the cecum or liver

DIAGNOSIS — postmortem findings, laboratory identification of bacteria

CAUSE — *Clostridium perfringens* bacteria and their toxins, sometimes following change in feed; often found in conjunction with coccidiosis and occasionally salmonellosis (both of which increase susceptibility)

TRANSMISSION — droppings from infected birds and spores in built-up litter, dust, or feed

PREVENTION — good sanitation management to prevent coccidiosis and other intestinal infections; make feed changes gradually

TREATMENT — bacitracin in drinking water at the rate of ½ gram per gallon for 4 days, combined with amprolium to control coccidia; vitamin supplement following treatment hastens recovery

HUMAN HEALTH RISK — do not slaughter sick birds: toxins in meat contaminated by infected droppings during butchering can cause mild to serious illness; see "Clostridium Poisoning," page 241

Nephrosis. *See* Gout (visceral), Infectious Bursal Disease

Neuritis. *See* Marek's Disease
Neurolymphomatosis. *See* Marek's Disease
Neurotropic Velogenic Newcastle Disease. *See* Newcastle Disease (exotic)

Newcastle Disease

ALSO CALLED — avian distemper, domestic Newcastle, endemic Newcastle, parainfluenza, pneumoencephalitis, pseudofowl pest, mesogenic Newcastle, mild Newcastle, ND

INCIDENCE — common worldwide

SYSTEM/ORGAN AFFECTED — respiratory and nervous systems

INCUBATION PERIOD — 2 to 15 days (5 to 6 average)

PROGRESSION — acute, starts suddenly, spreads rapidly, runs through flock in about a week

SYMPTOMS — in growing birds: wheezing, gasping, coughing, chirping, sometimes followed within 10 to 14 days by nervous disorders (drooping wing, draggy leg, twisted neck), death due to being trampled by other chickens

— in mature birds: slight wheezing, temporary cessation of laying, eggs with soft, rough, or deformed shells; sometimes nasal discharge, cloudy eye

PERCENTAGE AFFECTED — high

MORTALITY — few or none but can be high when nervous symptoms appear

POSTMORTEM FINDINGS — none significant; sometimes mucus in throat and thickened air sacs containing yellowish matter

RESEMBLES — infectious bronchitis and other respiratory diseases, except that Newcastle produces nervous symptoms; a disease known as "fowl plague" that does not occur in North America

DIAGNOSIS — symptoms (chicks with both nervous and respiratory signs), laboratory identification of virus

CAUSE — paramyxovirus that affects many different birds

TRANSMISSION — contagious; spread by inhaling or ingesting the virus from body excretions of infected birds or carriers in air, water, or feed

PREVENTION — defies good management; breed for genetic resistance (tests for antibodies against the virus commonly find healthy reactors, suggesting a high degree of resistance); vaccination not necessary unless virus is common in your area, then vaccinate chicks at 1 day old (or between 7 and 10 days) and repeat every 4 months or as required by risk of exposure; vaccinate all adult birds when chicks are first vaccinated

TREATMENT — keep birds warm and well fed; watch for secondary bacterial infections, particularly air-sac disease and chronic respiratory disease; survivors are immune but will be carriers for up to a month

HUMAN HEALTH RISK — temporary (3 to 7 days) eye infection may result from handling vaccine or infected birds

Newcastle Disease (exotic)

ALSO CALLED — Asiatic Newcastle disease, neurotropic velogenic Newcastle disease, NVND, the plague (in the Philippines), pseudo-poultry plague, velogenic Newcastle, viscerotropic velogenic Newcastle disease, VVND

INCIDENCE — rare but worldwide, especially in young, concentrated, confined flocks

SYSTEM/ORGAN AFFECTED — respiratory and nervous systems, sometimes digestive system

INCUBATION PERIOD — 2 to 15 days (5 to 6 average)

PROGRESSION — acute, spreads rapidly, runs through flock in 3 to 4 days, lasts 3 to 4 weeks

SYMPTOMS — in all ages: sudden, high rate of death without symptoms or

— in chicks: gasping, sneezing, coughing, "chirping" sound, rattle in throat; followed by slow growth, drooping wings, dragging legs; sometimes twisted head and neck, circling, somersaulting, walking backward, paralysis; birds recovering from respiratory symptoms but retaining nervous symptoms

— in mature birds: listlessness, rapid or difficult breathing, progressive weakness, near total cessation of laying within 3 days (sometimes shells have odd shapes or colors with flabby, blood-stained yolks and watery whites); followed by loss of coordination, loss of appetite, muscular tremors, twisted neck, wing and leg paralysis; sometimes watery, greenish (blood-stained) diarrhea, swollen, blackish eyes with straw-colored fluid draining from eyes and nose, bleeding through nose, death within 2 to 3 days

PERCENTAGE AFFECTED — up to 100 percent

MORTALITY — usually 50 percent in adults, 90 percent in young birds, can be 100 percent in all ages

POSTMORTEM FINDINGS — yellow patches on roof of mouth; large and small reddish brown spots or blotches (hemorrhages) in the upper and lower digestive tract, over abdominal fat, and on the ovary; wrinkled or discolored yolks; broken egg in abdominal cavity of hens

RESEMBLES — aflatoxicosis, blackhead, canker, coccidiosis, acute cholera, influenza, infectious laryngotracheitis, mild Newcastle, nutritional roup, thrush

DIAGNOSIS — flock history (human handler's contact with infected chickens or smuggled cage bird), symptoms, postmortem findings, confirmed by laboratory identification of virus

CAUSE — several strains of paramyxovirus that survive for up to 30 days in broken eggs, feathers, drinking water, and droppings in litter, but are sensitive to sunlight

TRANSMISSION — highly contagious; usually introduced by illegally imported cage birds that have not gone through USDA quarantine; spread by contact with infected birds and their body discharges; spreads in feed, water, air, and on equipment and the feet of rodents and humans; eggs laid by infected hens rarely hatch but may break in incubator and spread the virus

PREVENTION — avoid mixing birds of different ages or from different sources; avoid contact with illegally imported birds; do not visit flocks or let people visit your flock if an outbreak occurs in your area; vaccination does not offer 100 percent protection and birds vaccinated with live vaccine become carriers

TREATMENT — none; this is a **reportable disease,** see "Reportable Diseases" page 196; infected flocks are quarantined and destroyed; thoroughly clean up and disinfect equipment and housing with lye, 2 percent quaternary ammonium compound, or 5 to 20 percent chlorine bleach

HUMAN HEALTH RISK — temporary (3 to 7 days) eye infection requiring medical treatment may result from handling vaccine or infected birds

New England Disease. *See* Epidemic Tremor

New Wheat Disease. *See* Bluecomb

Nutritional Myopathy. *See* White Muscle Disease

Nutritional Roup. *See* Roup (nutritional)

- O -

Ochratoxicosis

INCIDENCE — sporadic in North America, Europe, and Asia

SYSTEM/ORGAN AFFECTED — kidney

PROGRESSION — gradual and cumulative

SYMPTOMS — in hens: yellow diarrhea, thin-shelled eggs

PERCENTAGE AFFECTED — 5 to 50 percent, depending on age of birds and level of toxicity

MORTALITY — usually low, depending on amount of toxin ingested

POSTMORTEM FINDINGS — swollen, pale kidneys, sometimes swollen, spotted liver, intestine filled with mucus

RESEMBLES — other mycotoxicoses

DIAGNOSIS — symptoms, postmortem findings, feed analysis

CAUSE — ochratoxins produced by *Aspergillus ochraceous* and *Penicillium viridicatum* fungi in barley, corn, sorghum, and wheat and in pelleted feed made with contaminated grain

TRANSMISSION — poisoning from contaminated rations; does not spread from bird to bird

PREVENTION — avoid moldy feeds

TREATMENT — replace contaminated feed

HUMAN HEALTH RISK — danger of ochratoxin residue in meat is low as most of the toxin is rapidly excreted in droppings; residue rarely appears in eggs

Ocular Lymphomatosis. *See* Marek's Disease

Oidica. *See* Thrush

Oidiomycosis. *See* Thrush

Omphalitis

ALSO CALLED — mushy chick disease, navel ill, navel infection (one form of colibacillosis)

INCIDENCE — common

SYSTEM/ORGAN AFFECTED — navel

INCUBATION PERIOD — 1 to 2 days (present at time of hatch)

PROGRESSION — acute

SYMPTOMS — dead embryos late in incubation; newly hatched chicks feel wet
— in chicks to 4 weeks of age: drooping head, puffed-up down, huddling near heat, lack of uniformity in size, lack of interest in food or water, distended abdomen with unabsorbed yolk sac; unhealed, reddened, swollen, and wet, mushy or scabby navel; sometimes diarrhea; death

PERCENTAGE AFFECTED — usually low unless incubator sanitation is poor

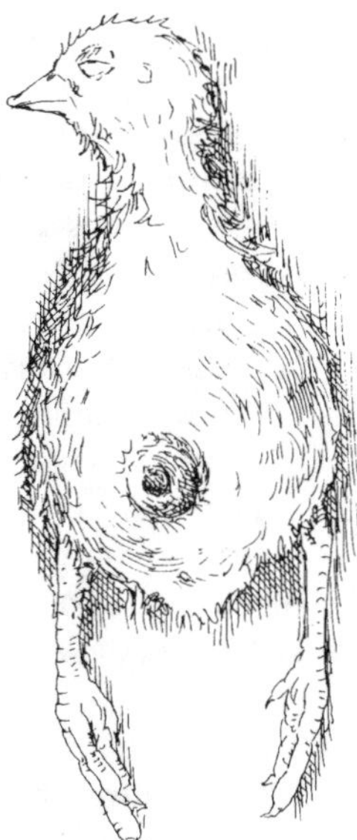
Chick infected with omphalitis

Mortality — up to 15 percent, starting just prior to hatch and continuing for up to 3 weeks; may increase as hatching season progresses

Postmortem Findings — incompletely healed navel, fluid under skin, bluish abdomen, unabsorbed yolk in abdomen (sometimes yellowish green and watery or yellowish brown and cheese-like, often bad smelling)

Diagnosis — symptoms, postmortem findings

Cause — *Escherichia coli* combined with *Staphylococcus aureus, Streptococcus faecalis,* and other bacteria

Transmission — contaminated droppings on hatching eggs; high incubation humidity keeps navel from closing properly, infectious organisms in incubator or brooder (or within egg, having penetrated shell before or during incubation) enter unhealed navel; feed, water, litter contaminated with droppings; not transmitted between growing or mature birds

Prevention — hatch only clean, uncracked eggs; control incubator humidity; clean and disinfect incubator and brooder between hatches

Treatment — none effective, cull; if newly purchased chicks experience a high death rate, notify seller and/or hatchery

Human Health Risk — none, if good sanitation is practiced after handling infected chicks

Ornithosis. *See* Chlamydiosis

Osteomalacia. *See* Rickets

Osteopetrosis

Also Called — marble bone, thick leg disease (one disease in the lymphoid/sarcoma group)

Incidence — common

System/Organ Affected — bones

Incubation Period — 30 days

Progression — usually chronic

Symptoms — in young or mature birds (more often male than female): thickened (sometimes unusually warm) leg bones, puffy looking shanks, lameness or stilted gait, faulty body conformation, stunting

Percentage Affected — low

Mortality — up to 10 percent

Postmortem Findings — thickened, deformed bones

Resembles — rickets, except that osteopetrosis does not cause bones to become porous; cage fatigue, except that in cage fatigue the bones twist but do not thicken

Diagnosis — flock history, symptoms, postmortem findings, laboratory tests

Cause — retrovirus; often occurs in combination with lymphoid leukosis

Transmission — contact with infected birds; spread by infected breeders through hatching eggs or by infected chicks to non-infected chicks through droppings; mechanically by bloodsucking parasites or unhygienic vaccination method

Prevention — defies good management but can be controlled by: buying and breeding resistant strains; identifying and eliminating breeders that produce infected chicks (requires testing for reactors); not reusing chick boxes; raising chicks on wire; not combining chickens of different ages or from different sources; thoroughly cleaning facilities before introducing new birds; thoroughly cleaning and disinfecting incubator and brooder between hatches; controlling bloodsucking parasites; avoiding flockwide injections or vaccinations using one needle

Treatment — none, cull; clean up and disinfect

Human Health Risk — none known

Osteoporosis. *See* Cage Fatigue

- P -

Pale Bird Syndrome. *See* Infectious Stunting Syndrome

Paracolon. *See* Arizonosis

Parainfluenza. *See* Newcastle Disease

Paratyphoid

Also Called — paratyphoid infection, PT (one kind of salmonellosis)

Incidence — very common worldwide

System/Organ Affected — digestive or entire body (septicemic)

Incubation Period — 5 days

Progression — acute or chronic

Symptoms — in embryos at time of hatch: numerous dead in shell, pipped or unpipped

— in chicks up to 5 weeks old: death at time of hatch or depression, weakness, poor growth, drooping wings, decreased appetite, increased thirst, “chirping” or “peeping” sounds, huddling around heat with feathers ruffled, eyes closed, head down, wings drooping; sometimes swollen joints, swelling or blindness in one or both eyes, watery diarrhea with pasting, dehydration

— in adult carriers: no symptoms or reduced egg production; purplish head, comb, and wattles (septicemic form)

Percentage Affected — high

Mortality — 10 to 20 percent, sometimes 100 percent; peaks at 6 to 10 days of age

Postmortem Findings — in chicks: none recognizable, or unabsorbed yolk sac, dehydration, swollen liver with red streaks or white dots, creamy or yellowish cheesy cores in ceca

— in adult birds: none recognizable, or inflamed intestine, swollen liver, spleen, kidneys

Resembles — arizonosis, typhoid, pullorum, septicemia due to colibacillosis (see “Colibacillosis,” page 112), infectious synovitis when joints are swollen

Diagnosis — flock history (birds' age), symptoms, postmortem findings, laboratory identification of bacteria

CAUSE — over 150 different *Salmonella* bacteria (*S. heidelberg* and *S. typhimurium* most commonly affect chickens, *S. enteritidis* also affects humans) that reside in soil and litter and infect a variety of birds and mammals

TRANSMISSION — contaminated soil or litter (persists for up to 7 months); contaminated droppings (persists for up to 28 months); contaminated feathers, dust, hatchery fluff (persists for up to 5 years); feed containing contaminated animal by-products (not including pellets and crumbles) or feed and water containing contaminated droppings; spreads from infected breeders to chicks through hatching eggs (eggs can blow up during incubation, further spreading contamination); spread on dirty equipment, feet of rodents and humans

PREVENTION — difficult, due to bacteria's wide range of animal hosts; collect hatching eggs often; hatch only eggs from paratyphoid-free breeders; replace nesting litter often; clean and disinfect incubator and brooder after each hatch; minimize chilling, overheating, parasitism, withholding of water or feed; keep drinking water free of droppings; control rodents, reptiles, wild birds, cockroaches, beetles, fleas, and flies; avoid mixing chickens of various age groups; keep breeders on wire flooring

TREATMENT — none effective, survivors may be carriers; *Salmonella Enteritidis* infection is **reportable,** see "Reportable Diseases" page 196

HUMAN HEALTH RISK — mild to serious illness from eating raw or undercooked contaminated meat or eggs, see "Salmonellosis," page 239

Parrot Fever. *See* Chlamydiosis

Pasted Vent

ALSO CALLED — cloacitis, vent gleet

INCIDENCE — common in chicks, less common in mature birds

SYSTEM/ORGAN AFFECTED — vent

PROGRESSION — chronic

SYMPTOMS — in chicks up to 10 days old: droopiness, droppings sticking to vent
—in laying hens: offensive odor from droppings sticking to vent feathers

PERCENTAGE AFFECTED — usually limited

MORTALITY — possible, if vent gets sealed shut

POSTMORTEM FINDINGS — distended rectum filled with droppings

RESEMBLES — in chicks: arizonosis and paratyphoid, except that pasted vent involves fewer chicks and they appear otherwise healthy

DIAGNOSIS — symptoms

CAUSE — in chicks: unknown, may be due to improper consistency of droppings caused by rations or chilling
— in hens: loss of muscle tone due to hereditary weakness

TRANSMISSION — does not spread from bird to bird

PREVENTION — keep chicks warm; do not hatch eggs from affected hens to avoid passing on hereditary weakness

TREATMENT — carefully pick away adhering matter; cull chicks that don't recover

HUMAN HEALTH RISK — none

Pasteurellosis. *See* Cholera (acute); Cholera (chronic)

Pediculosis. *See* "Lice," page 63

Pendulous Crop. *See* Crop Impaction
Perosis. *See* Slipped Tendon
Pink Disease. *See* Fatty Liver Syndrome
The Plague. *See* Newcastle Disease (exotic)
Plantar Pododermatitis. *See* Bumblefoot
***Plasmodium* Infection.** *See* Malaria
Pleuropneumonialike Organism (PPLO) Infection. *See* Chronic Respiratory Disease
Pneumoencephalitis. *See* Newcastle Disease
Pneumomycosis. *See* Aspergillosis (acute); Aspergillosis (chronic)
Poisoning. *See* page 139

Pox (dry)

ALSO CALLED — avian pox, chicken pox (has nothing to do with human chicken pox), cutaneous pox, fowl pox, sore head, (sometimes mistakenly called "canker")

INCIDENCE — common in some areas worldwide, especially in confined flocks in cold weather

SYSTEM/ORGAN AFFECTED — skin

INCUBATION PERIOD — 4 to 14 days

PROGRESSION — spreads slowly (except when spread by mosquitoes), lasts 3 to 5 weeks in individual birds

SYMPTOMS — in birds of all ages, except newly hatched chicks: raised clear or whitish wart-like bumps on comb and wattles that grow larger, turn yellowish, and later become reddish brown, gray, or black bleeding scabs appearing singly, in clusters, or clumping together; scabs fall off to form smooth scars; sometimes scabs spread to eyelids, unfeathered areas of head and neck, vent area, feet, or legs; retarded growth or weight loss (sores around eyes inhibit feeding), drop in egg production

PERCENTAGE AFFECTED — low to 100 percent

MORTALITY — 1 to 2 percent

RESEMBLES — comb wounds due to fighting, except that wounds do not spread

DIAGNOSIS — symptoms, confirmed by laboratory identification of virus

CAUSE — pox virus that affects a wide variety of birds and survives for many months on scabs and feathers of infected birds

TRANSMISSION — through skin wounds (due to insect bites, dubbing, fighting, cannibalism, or other injury); spreads by means of feathers and scabs from infected birds; spread mechanically by mites, mosquitoes, and wild birds; *may* spread from infected breeders to chicks through hatching eggs, causing disease when infected birds come under stress

PREVENTION — defies good management; control mites and mosquitoes; vaccinate where pox is prevalent (on day-old chicks, use only vaccine designated *for chicks)*; if large number of vaccination sites do not swell and scab over within 7 to 10 days, revaccinate with new batch of vaccine; since pox spreads slowly, it may be checked by vaccinating while disease is in progress

TREATMENT — none; isolate infected birds in uncrowded housing; remove scabs around mouth and eyes so birds can eat; prevent secondary infection with 300 mg oxytetracycline (Terramycin) per gallon of drinking water for 3 days followed by vitamin supplement in water; infected birds naturally recover in 2 to 4 weeks and are immune (but some remain carriers and may become reinfected during molt and other times of stress); thoroughly clean housing after outbreak to remove all infective scabs

Human Health Risk — none known; "chicken pox" in humans is caused by a different virus that has nothing to do with chickens

Pox (wet)

Also Called — diphtheritic pox, fowl diphtheria

Incidence — worldwide, less common than dry pox

System/Organ Affected — upper respiratory

Incubation Period — 4 to 14 days

Progression — spreads slowly (except when spread by mosquitoes), lasts 3 to 5 weeks in individual birds

Symptoms — in birds of all ages, except newly hatched chicks: transparent whitish wart-like or scabby bumps on face, eyes (can cause blindness), throat, and windpipe (possibly becoming large enough to suffocate bird), growing larger until they join and turn yellow and cheesy; rales or wheezing, nasal or eye discharge, death due to suffocation

Percentage Affected — low to 100 percent

Mortality — up to 50 percent

Postmortem Findings — yellowish or brownish cheesy masses in mouth, upper throat, and windpipe, anchored by cheese-like roots

Resembles — infectious laryngotracheitis, nutritional roup
— in chicks: biotin deficiency, canker

Diagnosis — flock history, symptoms, confirmed by postmortem findings, laboratory identification of virus

Cause — same virus as dry pox invading the upper respiratory tract

Transmission — same as for dry pox

Prevention — same as for dry pox

Treatment — if thick discharge interferes with breathing, clear airways with

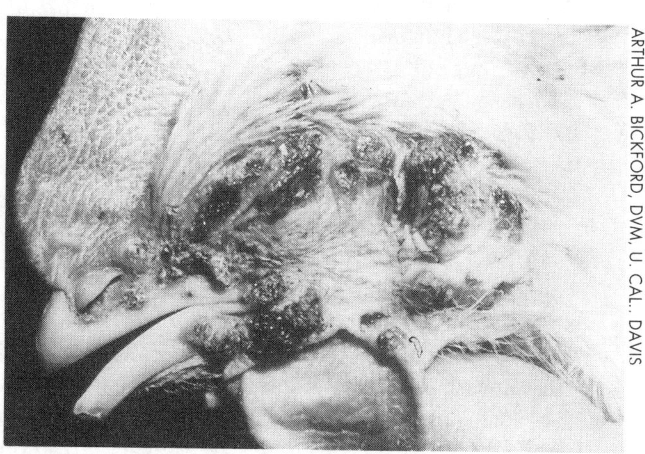

ARTHUR A. BICKFORD, DVM, U. CAL., DAVIS

Head of a chicken with pox

cotton swab coated with iodine; otherwise, treat as for dry pox

HUMAN HEALTH RISK — none known, not related to diphtheria in humans

Pseudo-Botulism. *See* Marek's Disease

Prolapse. *See* "Prolapsed Oviduct," page 53

Pseudofowl Pest. *See* Newcastle Disease

Pseudomonas

INCIDENCE — rare

SYSTEM/ORGAN AFFECTED — entire body

INCUBATION PERIOD — 3 days

PROGRESSION — acute to chronic

SYMPTOMS — in embryos or newly hatched chicks: death

— in older birds: lameness, loss of coordination, swollen head and wattles, swollen hock joints and foot pads, diarrhea, death within 1 to 2 days

PERCENTAGE AFFECTED — up to 10 percent

MORTALITY — usually no more than 10 percent but can be up to 90 percent

POSTMORTEM FINDINGS — swollen, spotty liver, spleen, kidneys

RESEMBLES — septicemic colibacillosis

DIAGNOSIS — characteristic fruity odor, laboratory identification of bacteria

CAUSE — *Pseudomonas aeruginosa* bacteria commonly found in chicken droppings, soil, water, and humid environments; infects birds with reduced resistance due to some other cause

TRANSMISSION — droppings of infected birds in feed, water, litter; infects chicks through shells of hatching eggs; spreads in vaccines and antibiotics handled in an unhygienic manner; infects chickens with reduced susceptibility due to other bacterial or viral diseases

PREVENTION — good incubator and brooder sanitation; hygienic handling of vaccines and antibiotics; avoid mixing birds of different ages; avoid stress

TREATMENT — bacteria are resistant to many antibiotics, but treatment *may* reduce losses *if* started early *and* a suitable antibiotic (such as gentamicin) is determined through laboratory sensitivity testing

HUMAN HEALTH RISK — rare but potentially serious infection due to bacteria entering an open wound or deep puncture

Pseudo-Poultry Plague. *See* Newcastle Disease

Psittacosis. *See* Chlamydiosis

Pullet Disease. *See* Bluecomb

Pullorum

ALSO CALLED — bacillary white diarrhea, BWD, pullorum disease, PD, white diarrhea (one kind of salmonellosis)

INCIDENCE — worldwide, rare in North America

SYSTEM/ORGAN AFFECTED — digestive or septicemic

INCUBATION PERIOD — 7 to 10 days

PROGRESSION — acute or chronic

SYMPTOMS — in chicks up to 4 weeks old: sudden death or loss of appetite, sleepiness, weakness, huddling near heat, swollen hock joints, white (or greenish-brown) pasty diarrhea; sometimes gasping, shrill peeping or chirping while trying to expel droppings; uneven growth among survivors

— in mature birds: no signs or loss of appetite, increased thirst; sometimes pale, shriveled comb, green diarrhea, drop in egg production

PERCENTAGE AFFECTED — up to 100 percent

MORTALITY — up to 90 percent in chicks, increasing on 4th or 5th day and peaking at 2 to 3 weeks of age (100 percent if infected chicks are shipped, chilled, or kept in unsanitary conditions)

POSTMORTEM FINDINGS — in chicks: none recognizable; or unabsorbed yolk; cheesy material in abdominal cavity or ceca; enlarged liver, heart, kidneys, and spleen; small white or gray nodules (pinpoint to pea-size) in liver, heart, gizzard, intestine, and lungs

— in adult birds: none recognizable; or enlarged liver, heart, spleen, and kidneys; swollen ceca or oviduct filled with firm, cheesy material

— in hens: brownish or greenish shriveled yolks, yolk material in abdominal cavity

— in cocks: shriveled testes (testicles)

RESEMBLES — omphalitis, paratyphoid, typhoid; white diarrhea due to simple chilling

DIAGNOSIS — history (birds' age), symptoms (pattern of deaths), laboratory identification of bacteria

CAUSE — *Salmonella pullorum* bacteria, survives for years in dry litter, but is easily destroyed by cleaning and disinfection

TRANSMISSION — from infected breeders to chicks through hatching eggs; spread from chick to chick in incubator or brooder; occasionally transmitted by contaminated litter, shoes, equipment

PREVENTION — purchase certified pullorum-free stock; hatch eggs only from pullorum-free breeders; do not mix certified pullorum-free stock with other birds; control flies, rodents, and wild birds; breed for resistance (heavy breeds such as Rocks and Reds are more susceptible than Leghorns and other light breeds); blood test birds (home kits are available) and eliminate carriers until two tests, no less than 21 days apart, are negative (some states require blood testing of all exhibition birds)

TREATMENT — cull, survivors are carriers; this is a **reportable disease** in most states, see "Reportable Diseases" page 196

HUMAN HEALTH RISK — eating highly contaminated meat can cause acute intestinal infection (characterized by explosive onset, high fever, and prostration); recovery is spontaneous and rapid

Pulmonary Aspergillosis. *See* Aspergillosis (acute), Aspergillosis (chronic)]

- Q -

Quail Disease. *See* Ulcerative Enteritis

- R -

Rachitic Chicks. *See* Rickets

Range Paralysis. *See* Marek's Disease

Renal Failure/Gout. *See* Gout (visceral)

Reovirus Infection. *See* Viral Arthritis

Reticuloendotheliosis. *See* Runting Syndrome

Rickets

Also Called — osteomalacia, rachitic chicks

Incidence — rare, yet the most common nutritional deficiency of growing birds, especially those housed in confinement

System/Organ Affected — bones

Progression — depends on degree of deficiency

Symptoms — in young birds: depression, frequent squatting, stiff-legged gait or inability to stand, slow growth, ruffled feathers, black feather parts in red or buff breeds, easily bendable beak, bowed or twisted legs and wings, enlarged joints, paralysis

— in mature birds: easily broken bones, bent keel dished in near the middle

Percentage Affected — can be high

Mortality — up to 20 percent

Postmortem Findings — soft, rubbery bones, string of round knobs caused by beading of inner surfaces of rib heads where ribs join spine (called "rickety rosary" or "rachitic rosary")

Resembles — cage fatigue, except that birds need not be in cages to get rickets

Diagnosis — flock history (birds' age), symptoms (especially soft beak), postmortem findings (especially rib beading), ration evaluation

Cause — deficiency of vitamin D3; deficiency or imbalance of calcium or phosphorus (too much calcium ties up phosphorus); inability to absorb nutrients due to infectious stunting syndrome

Transmission — nutritional, does not spread from bird to bird

Prevention — feed oyster shell or coarse limestone free choice; use commercially prepared ration fortified with vitamin D3; let birds out into the sunshine; range birds on legume or legume-grass pasture

Treatment — vitamin D3 supplement at three times the normal amount for 3 weeks, then reduce to normal amount (take care, excess vitamin D in feed can

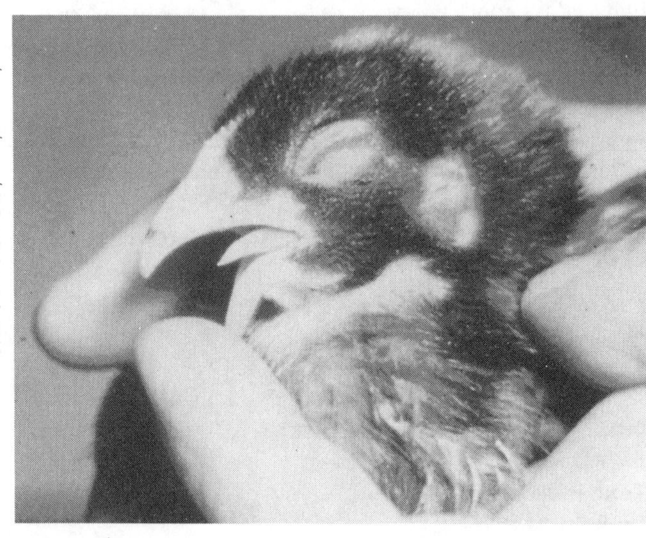

ARTHUR A. BICKFORD, DVM, U. CAL., DAVIS

Bent beak from rickets

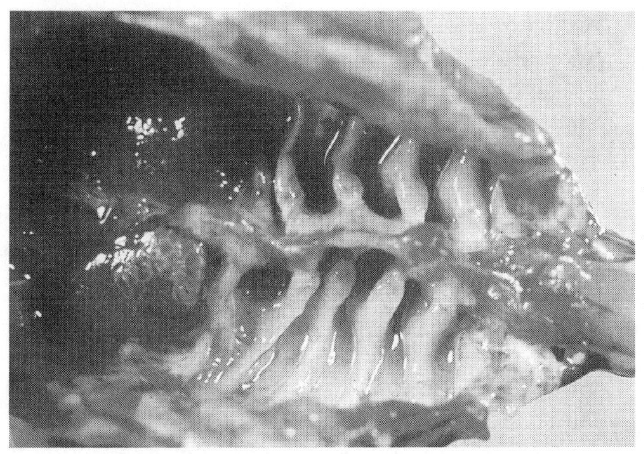

Beaded ribs from rickets

be toxic); for chicks, one-time dose of 15,000 IU vitamin D3; in case of paralysis, give a calcium phosphate supplement

HUMAN HEALTH RISK — none

Rotaviral Enteritis

ALSO CALLED — rotaviral infection, viral enteritis

INCIDENCE — worldwide and increasingly more common

SYSTEM/ORGAN AFFECTED — digestive

INCUBATION PERIOD — 2 to 5 days

PROGRESSION — lasts 5 to 10 days

SYMPTOMS — in young birds: depression, profuse watery diarrhea, inflamed vent, appetite loss, weight loss, dehydration, death

PERCENTAGE AFFECTED — nearly 100 percent

MORTALITY — up to 50 percent

POSTMORTEM FINDINGS — yellowish, watery, gas-filled matter in intestines and ceca

RESEMBLES — any other (enteric) disease causing diarrhea

DIAGNOSIS — laboratory identification of diarrhea's cause

CAUSE — rotavirus common in the poultry environment, but doesn't always cause disease

TRANSMISSION — contact with infected birds and their droppings; spreads on contaminated equipment; *may* be transmitted in or on hatching eggs

PREVENTION — clean and disinfect housing periodically; do not start new chickens on used litter

TREATMENT — none, cull; penicillin and supportive therapy (see page 192) help, but survivors do not grow well; thoroughly clean and disinfect before introducing new flock

HUMAN HEALTH RISK — none known

Rot Gut. *See* Necrotic Enteritis

Round Heart Disease

INCIDENCE — extremely rare and only during winter in birds maintained on deep litter

SYSTEM/ORGAN AFFECTED — heart

PROGRESSION — acute
SYMPTOMS — in birds 4 to 8 months old: sudden death
PERCENTAGE AFFECTED — no illness evident
MORTALITY — up to 50 percent
POSTMORTEM FINDINGS — enlarged, yellowish, soft heart, rounded at the tip
RESEMBLES — sudden death syndrome, except that in SDS birds go into convulsions just prior to death and usually die on their backs
DIAGNOSIS — symptoms, postmortem findings
CAUSE — unknown, possibly related to nutritional deficiency
TRANSMISSION — unknown
PREVENTION — provide proper nutrition
TREATMENT — none
HUMAN HEALTH RISK — none known

Roup. *See* Canker, Cholera (chronic), Infectious Coryza, Roup (nutritional)

Roup (nutritional)

ALSO CALLED — A-avitaminosis
INCIDENCE — rare except when homemade rations are fed
SYSTEM/ORGAN AFFECTED — upper respiratory (eyes, nose, throat)
PROGRESSION — chronic
SYMPTOMS — in chicks 1 to 7 weeks old: droopiness, pale combs, and failure to grow followed by sore, swollen eyelids, sticky or cheesy discharge from eyes and nostrils, swollen sinuses, difficulty breathing
— in hens: unthriftiness and decreased egg production followed by runny eyes and nose, eyelids stuck together, ruffled feathers, whitish-yellow mouth sores in severe cases, weakness, emaciation, increased interval between clutches, increased blood spots
PERCENTAGE AFFECTED — high
MORTALITY — up to 100 percent
POSTMORTEM FINDINGS — dry, dull respiratory lining; excess urates in cloacal bursa
RESEMBLES — cholera (chronic), chronic respiratory disease, infectious bronchitis, infectious coryza, influenza
DIAGNOSIS — symptoms, postmortem findings, microscopic examination of body tissue, ration evaluation
CAUSE — vitamin A deficiency for 2 to 5 months; chicks hatched from deficient breeders will be deficient unless fed fortified starter ration
TRANSMISSION — does not spread from bird to bird
PREVENTION — use only fresh feed (buy small quantities so it won't go stale); allow birds to free range or feed them good sources of vitamin A such as new yellow (not white) corn and alfalfa meal
TREATMENT — water-soluble vitamin A supplement in drinking water; vitamin A injections in severe cases
HUMAN HEALTH RISK — none

Runting Syndrome

ALSO CALLED — runting disease syndrome (a form of reticuloendotheliosis)
INCIDENCE — rare, occurs in Australia, Israel, Japan, and southeastern United States

System/Organ Affected — entire body

Symptoms — in birds 4 to 10 weeks, after receiving contaminated vaccine as day-old chicks: poor growth, abnormal feathering (barbules compress against the shaft for a short distance); sometimes paralysis

— in naturally infected birds of all ages: no symptoms

Postmortem Findings — sometimes enlarged nerves; atrophy of cloacal bursa

Resembles — Marek's disease, except that runting syndrome involves nerves to a lesser extent; infectious anemia, infectious bursal disease, infectious stunting syndrome (a different disease sometimes also called "broiler runting syndrome")

Diagnosis — flock history (use of potentially contaminated vaccine), symptoms, postmortem findings, laboratory identification of virus

Cause — retrovirus that affects a variety of birds accidentally introduced to chickens through vaccines contaminated during manufacture

Transmission — contact with infected birds, their body fluids, or droppings; occasionally spread from breeders (cocks as well as hens) through hatching eggs; possibly spread by mosquitoes and other insects

Prevention — none known; insect control and good sanitation help

Treatment — none known

Human Health Risk — none known

Ruptured Tendon. *See* Viral Arthritis

- S -

Salmonella enteritidis. *See* Paratyphoid

Salmonellosis. *See* Arizonosis, Typhoid, Paratyphoid, Pullorum

Sinusitis. *See* Chronic Respiratory Disease

Slipped Tendon

Also Called — chondrodystrophy, perosis

Incidence — common in heavy, fast-growing breeds

System/Organ Affected — hock

Symptoms — in young birds, starting at 9 days of age: swollen, flat hock joint; hopping on one leg, sometimes one or both legs twist or rotate to the side; death due to inability to obtain food and water

Percentage Affected — 3 to 5 percent

Mortality — low

Postmortem Findings — sometimes shortened, thickened long bones of legs and wings

Resembles — twisted leg, except that in twisted leg the bones are not shortened

Diagnosis — history (birds' age, size, breed), symptoms, postmortem findings, ration evaluation

Cause — deficiency in manganese or one of five B vitamins (biotin, choline, folic acid,

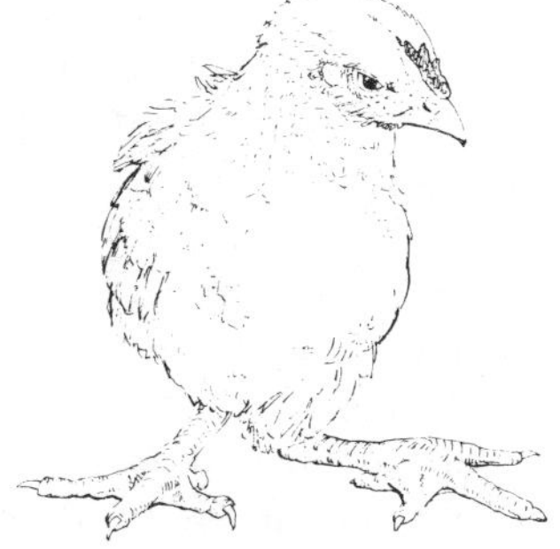

Typical case of slipped tendon

nicotinic acid, pyridoxine)

TRANSMISSION — nutritional, does not spread from bird to bird

PREVENTION — breed for genetic resistance; feed at least 95 percent commercial ration (no more than 5 percent corn or other treats); avoid crowding young birds; brood on litter rather than on slats, wire, or slick floor

TREATMENT — manganese and B-vitamin supplement won't reverse permanent damage but will minimize future damage

HUMAN HEALTH RISK — none

Sod Disease. *See* Ergotism

Sore Head. *See* Pox (dry)

Sour Crop. *See* Thrush

Spirochetosis

ALSO CALLED — fowl spirochetosis

INCIDENCE — common in free-ranged flocks in tropical and temperate climates, rare in North America (although the fowl tick that carries it is found in the southwestern United States)

SYSTEM/ORGAN AFFECTED — entire body (septicemic)

INCUBATION PERIOD — 3 to 12 days

PROGRESSION — acute or chronic

SYMPTOMS — in birds of all ages: droopiness, ruffled feathers, huddling, yellow green diarrhea with large amounts of white urates, increased thirst, loss of appetite, weak legs, pale or purplish comb, incoordination, loss of interest in perching, lying with head on ground, convulsions, fever, paralysis, drop in temperature to below normal just before death

PERCENTAGE AFFECTED — 1 to 2 percent in carrier flocks with immunity due to constant exposure to ticks, up to 100 percent in susceptible birds mingled with immune birds

MORTALITY — usually no more than 75 percent, but can be up to 100 percent

POSTMORTEM FINDINGS — swollen, mottled spleen; sometimes greenish mucus in intestines, enlarged, spotted liver, swollen, pale kidneys and/or enlarged, pale heart

RESEMBLES — influenza or Newcastle, except that spirochetosis does not cause respiratory symptoms and bloody intestines; Marek's disease, except that spirochetosis does not produce tumors; cholera, typhoid, and septicemic colibacillosis, except that in spirochetosis *Salmonella, Pasteurella,* or *E. coli* bacteria cannot be found by laboratory

DIAGNOSIS — flock history (presence of fowl ticks, *Argus persicus),* symptoms, postmortem findings, identification of spirochetes

CAUSE — *Borrelia anserina* bacteria that affect many birds but do not survive long in the environment

TRANSMISSION — contact with moist droppings, blood, tissue, and mucus of infected birds; spread by eating or being bitten by an infective fowl tick, mosquito, or other bloodsucker; spread through cannibalism (including picking carcasses of dead infected birds), contaminated droppings in feed or water, using the same needle for flockwide inoculation, vaccination, or blood testing

PREVENTION — control ticks and other bloodsucking insects; do not combine tick-infested and susceptible birds; do not house clean birds where outbreak has occurred within 3 years; vaccine not available in the United States

TREATMENT — none effective; inject individual birds with 20 mg oxytetracycline (intramuscular) once a day for 2 days or add 1 gram oxytetracycline per gallon of drinking water for 3 days; survivors are immune and are not carriers; treat only under supervision, this is a **reportable disease,** see "Reportable Diseases" page 196

HUMAN HEALTH RISK — none known (little is understood to date about the spread of a related tick-borne spirochete, *B. burgdorferi,* which causes Lyme disease in both birds and humans)

Split-Wing Syndrome. *See* Infectious Stunting Syndrome

Spondylolisthesis. *See* Kinky Back

Staphylococcic Arthritis

ALSO CALLED — arthritis/synovitis, staphylococcic septicemia

INCIDENCE — common worldwide

SYSTEM/ORGAN AFFECTED — joints or entire body (septicemic)

INCUBATION PERIOD — 2 to 3 days (septicemic form)

PROGRESSION — acute (septicemic form) or chronic (arthritic form)

SYMPTOMS — in all ages (most often growing birds): fever, reluctance to move, ruffled feathers, depression, swollen joints (hot to the touch), resting on hocks and keel, lameness (chronic), death (acute)

PERCENTAGE AFFECTED — low

MORTALITY — low

POSTMORTEM FINDINGS — joints (especially hock) and surrounding area are inflamed and contain whitish, fleck-filled pus that appears cheesy in an advanced infection; sometimes swollen, spotted liver and spleen

RESEMBLES — in young birds: joint infections (synovitis) caused by other bacteria; viral arthritis, except that in viral arthritis fluid surrounding joints is yellowish or pinkish

— in mature birds: acute cholera (septicemic form), except that cholera involves a greater number of deaths

DIAGNOSIS — symptoms, laboratory identification of bacteria

CAUSE — *Staphylococcus aureus* bacteria common in the poultry environment

TRANSMISSION — bacteria entering body through wounds

PREVENTION — prevent injuries by providing safe, uncrowded housing

TREATMENT — staph bacteria are resistant to many antibiotics, but treatment *may* be successful *if* a suitable antibiotic is determined through laboratory sensitivity testing

HUMAN HEALTH RISK — unsanitary handling of meat during or following butchering can cause food poisoning in humans; see "Staphylococcal Food Poisoning" page 243

Staphylococcic Septicemia. *See* Staphylococcic Arthritis

Staphylococcosis. *See* Bumblefoot, Omphalitis, Staphylococcic Arthritis

Star-Gazing Syndrome. *See* Epidemic Tremor

Sternal Bursitis. *See* Breast Blister

Stomatitis. *See* Thrush

Streptococcosis. (*See also* Omphalitis)

INCIDENCE — worldwide but not common

SYSTEM/ORGAN AFFECTED — entire body (septicemic)

INCUBATION PERIOD — 5 to 21 days

PROGRESSION — acute (septicemic) or chronic

SYMPTOMS — in mature birds: depression, weight loss; sometimes lameness, head tremors, yellow diarrhea, pale combs and wattles, fever (108-110°F, 42-43°C), eventual or sudden death

PERCENTAGE AFFECTED — up to 50 percent

MORTALITY — up to 50 percent

POSTMORTEM FINDINGS — enlarged, pale heart; light-colored or dark red patchy areas on liver

RESEMBLES — septicemic forms of staphylococcosis, colibacillosis, pasteurellosis, erysipelas, other bacterial diseases

DIAGNOSIS — symptoms and laboratory identification of bacteria

CAUSE — *Streptococcus zooepidemicus* bacteria that normally live in a chicken's intestines; infection is considered secondary, since it occurs only if resistance is reduced by some other disease

TRANSMISSION — inhalation, ingestion, skin wounds; bacteria are extremely susceptible to drying and so cannot be spread on equipment

PREVENTION — practice good sanitation; avoid stress

TREATMENT — bacteria are resistant to many antibiotics, but treatment *may* reduce losses *if* started early *and* suitable antibiotic is determined through laboratory sensitivity testing

HUMAN HEALTH RISK — none known

Stress Disease. *See* Chronic Respiratory Disease

Stunting Syndrome. *See* Infectious Stunting Syndrome

Sudden Death Syndrome

ALSO CALLED — SDS, acute death syndrome, ADS, acute heart failure, fatal syncope, flip-over disease, heart attack ("sudden death syndrome" in maturing broiler breeders in Australia is caused by an unrelated nutritional deficiency)

INCIDENCE — common worldwide, especially in intensively managed broilers

SYSTEM/ORGAN AFFECTED — heart and lungs

INCUBATION PERIOD — days to weeks

PROGRESSION — acute

SYMPTOMS — in apparently healthy broilers, 1 to 12 weeks of age, primarily cocks: extended neck, gasping or squawking, wing beating, leg pumping, flipping onto back, death within 1 minute of first symptoms

— in laying hens: cloacal tissue protrudes through vent, death

PERCENTAGE AFFECTED — up to 5 percent

MORTALITY — 100 percent

POSTMORTEM FINDINGS — feed-filled intestine; bloated, bright red lungs; pools of fluid between ribs and lungs; empty gall bladder; sometimes mottled muscles, liver, and kidneys;

— in hens: numerous blood vessels covering egg yolk cluster, sometimes internal broken-shelled egg

RESEMBLES — round heart disease, except in sudden death syndrome birds go into convulsions before dying

DIAGNOSIS — symptoms, postmortem findings

CAUSE — unknown; may be caused by high carbohydrate feeds and rapid weight gain relative to feed intake

TRANSMISSION — nutritional, does not spread from bird to bird; do not feed for rapid weight gain

PREVENTION — low-intensity lighting; avoid noise and other disturbances

TREATMENT — none

HUMAN HEALTH RISK — none known

Summer Disease. *See* Bluecomb

Swollen Head Syndrome

ALSO CALLED — dikkop, facial cellulitis, SHS, thick head

INCIDENCE — not found in North America; prevalent in Israel, South Africa, and parts of Europe

SYSTEM/ORGAN AFFECTED — head

INCUBATION PERIOD — 36 hours

PROGRESSION — spreads rapidly

SYMPTOMS — in broilers and broiler breeders: sneezing, red swollen eyes, progressive swelling of the head and wattles, scratching of face with feet, drop in egg production; sometimes nervous symptoms; death

PERCENTAGE AFFECTED — less than 4 percent

MORTALITY — 4 to 10 percent

POSTMORTEM FINDINGS — inflamed pus-filled tissue beneath the skin of head

RESEMBLES — infectious bronchitis, infectious coryza, Newcastle

DIAGNOSIS — flock history (contact with infected turkeys), symptoms, laboratory tests

CAUSE — combination of *Escherichia coli* and possibly turkey coryza virus; often follows debeaking or vaccination for Newcastle

TRANSMISSION — contact with turkeys infected with turkey coryza (rhinotracheitis) or drinking water contaminated with the virus

PREVENTION — provide adequate ventilation; avoid crowding; practice good sanitation and litter management; avoid mixing birds of different ages or species

TREATMENT — improve ventilation; keep birds warm and well fed with high protein rations and a vitamin E supplement; treat with broad-spectrum sulfonamides

HUMAN HEALTH RISK — none known

Synovitis. *See* Infectious Synovitis

-T-

Tenosynovitis. *See* Viral Arthritis

Thick Head. *See* Swollen Head Syndrome

Thick Leg Disease. *See* Osteopetrosis

Thrush

Also Called — candidiasis, crop mycosis, moniliasis, muguet, oidica, oidiomycosis, sour crop, stomatitis

Incidence — common

System/Organ Affected — upper digestive tract

Incubation Period — 2 to 4 weeks

Progression — chronic

Symptoms — in growing birds: depression, rough feathers, diarrhea, distended sour crop, slow growth or weight loss

Percentage Affected — up to 20 percent

Mortality — up to 5 percent

Postmortem Findings — grayish white, rough, circular, thickenings that join to create a "Turkish towel" appearance in mouth, esophagus, and crop lining, sometimes in stomach, rarely in the intestine

Resembles — canker, capillary worms, pox (wet)

Diagnosis — flock history (age of birds, outbreak of coccidiosis or use of antibiotics), symptoms (unthrifty birds), postmortem findings

Cause — *Candida albicans* yeast-like fungus commonly living in the bowels of chickens that infect when normal flora are disrupted by coccidiosis or antibiotics, growth promoters, and other drugs; sometimes found in connection with another disease (especially coccidiosis or chlamydiosis)

Transmission — contaminated droppings in drinking water

Prevention — good nutrition and sanitation; avoid parasites; clean feeders and waterers regularly; avoid crowding; avoid prolonged treatment with antibiotics and other drugs

Treatment — isolate infected birds; clean and disinfect feeders and waterers; flush with molasses or Epsom salts (see "Flushes," page 192), followed by ½ teaspoon copper sulfate (powdered bluestone) per gallon drinking water every other day for 5 days served in a nonmetal waterer, repeat monthly; clean mouth sores with an antiseptic such as hydrogen peroxide and treat with nystatin

Human Health Risk — *C. albicans* can cause mouth and genital infection in humans, see "Candidiasis" page 232

Tibial Rotation. *See* Twisted Leg

Toxicoinfection. *See* Botulism

Toxoplasmosis

Also Called — toxoplasma

Incidence — worldwide but sporadic and rare

System/Organ Affected — central nervous system; sometimes reproductive system, muscles, and organs

Incubation Period — 3 to 12 days

Progression — usually acute in young birds, chronic in older birds

Symptoms — primarily in young, stressed birds: loss of appetite, emaciation, pale, shriveled comb, white droppings; sometimes diarrhea, incoordination, walking in circles with head twisted back, muscle spasms, paralysis, blindness;

lasts as long as 3 weeks, often ends in death

PERCENTAGE AFFECTED — high

MORTALITY — up to 50 percent

POSTMORTEM FINDINGS — enlarged, mottled liver; blood-filled lungs

RESEMBLES — Marek's disease, Newcastle, or any other infection involving the nerves

DIAGNOSIS — laboratory identification of protozoa

CAUSE — *Toxoplasma gondii* protozoan parasite

TRANSMISSION — picking in infected droppings of housecats or related animals, picking at infected meat (including infected chickens, dead or live), eating infected earthworms, eating flies or cockroaches carrying toxoplasma on their bodies

PREVENTION — control flies, cockroaches, dung beetles, rodents

TREATMENT — none known

HUMAN HEALTH RISK — eating undercooked meat contaminated with infected droppings can (though rarely does) cause infection in humans, see "Toxoplasmosis" page 235

Trichomoniasis. *See* Canker

Trichothecene Mycotoxicosis. *See* Fusariotoxicosis

Tuberculosis

ALSO CALLED — avian tuberculosis, AT, TB

INCIDENCE — common worldwide, especially in backyard flocks in temperate northern climates (northcentral United States)

SYSTEM/ORGAN AFFECTED — starts in intestinal tract and migrates to other internal organs

INCUBATION PERIOD — years

PROGRESSION — usually chronic, rarely acute, spreads very slowly

SYMPTOMS — in birds 2 years old or older (especially living in contact with soil): dull, ruffled feathers, gradual weight loss despite good appetite, shrunken breast muscles, prominent (often deformed) keel; persistent diarrhea, pale (sometimes bluish) combs and wattles, decrease in laying; sometimes lameness; death

PERCENTAGE AFFECTED — 10 to 50 percent, spread over many months

MORTALITY — 100 percent

POSTMORTEM FINDINGS — hard, knobby grayish to yellowish nodules (tubercles) in liver, spleen, intestine, and bone marrow, increasing in size and number with the length of time the bird is infected

RESEMBLES — blackhead, except that in blackhead organ spots are dished rather than knobby; avian leukosis complex, except that leukosis usually affects younger birds; air-sac mites, which can be detected only by seeing tiny translucent dots moving around in air sacs soon after bird dies (see page 71)

DIAGNOSIS — flock history (bird's age, chronic disease conditions), symptoms (extreme emaciation, continuing deaths), postmortem findings, laboratory identification of bacteria, whole-blood test to identify live positive reactors; live birds may be skin tested by using a 1 ml tuberculin syringe and ½-inch (1.3

cm), 26 gauge needle to inject 0.05 ml avian tuberculin into wattle skin; swelling after 48 hours indicates test is positive, although infected birds occasionally react negatively

CAUSE — *Mycobacterium avium* bacteria that survive for 6 months or more in litter and up to 4 years in soil, affect a wide variety of birds

TRANSMISSION — droppings of infected birds or picking at contaminated carcasses of dead birds; spread on contaminated shoes and equipment

PREVENTION — do not keep chickens over 18 months old; do not mix birds from different age groups; design housing so birds can't pick in droppings; rotate range; remove reactors to wattle test

TREATMENT — none effective, cull; thoroughly clean and disinfect housing with a cresylic compound, remove the top 4 inches of soil in dirt-floor housing and replace it with uncontaminated soil; remove 2 inches of range topsoil or keep new birds off contaminated range for at least 4 years

HUMAN HEALTH RISK — *M. avium* is not the same bacterium that normally causes human TB; human infection is rare but possible in people who have been sensitized to human or bovine TB or who have acquired immune deficiency syndrome

Twisted Leg

ALSO CALLED — crooked legs, long-bone distortion, tibial rotation, valgus leg deformity, valgus or varus deformation, VVD, windswept

INCIDENCE — common in battery-raised broilers

SYSTEM/ORGAN AFFECTED — long bones of leg

PROGRESSION — rapid onset (1 to 2 days)

SYMPTOMS — in broilers 1 week of age and older, primarily cockerels: one or both legs bend outward at hock joints by as much as 90°, sometimes with a pointed protrusion at the hock joint; sometimes birds walk on bruised, swollen hocks

ARTHUR A BICKFORD, DVM, U. CAL., DAVIS

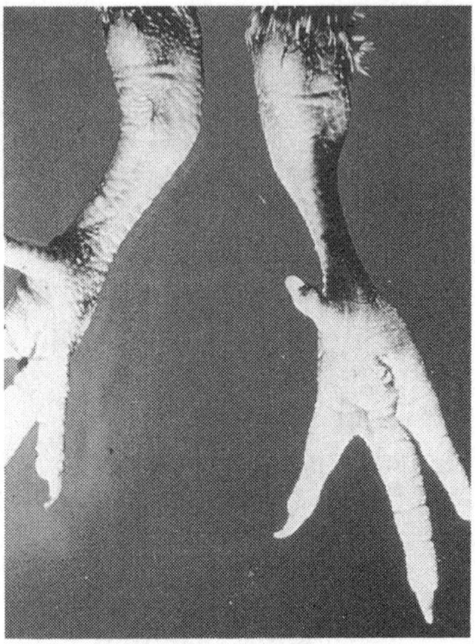

Twisted leg

PERCENTAGE AFFECTED — up to 2 percent in mixed flocks, up to 25 percent in all-cockerel flocks; highest in birds brooded on wire

MORTALITY — none

POSTMORTEM FINDINGS — outward or inward angulation of upper or lower bones

RESEMBLES — slipped tendon, except that twisted leg bones are not widened and shortened

DIAGNOSIS — symptoms

CAUSE — unknown, may be genetic or nutritional; possibly related to slipped tendon

TRANSMISSION — unknown

PREVENTION — raise broilers on litter (rather than on wire) and do not feed for rapid growth

TREATMENT — none, condition is not reversible

HUMAN HEALTH RISK — none known

Typhoid

ALSO CALLED — fowl typhoid, FT, infectious leukemia (one kind of salmonellosis)

INCIDENCE — worldwide, rare in North America

SYSTEM/ORGAN AFFECTED — digestive or system wide (septicemic)

INCUBATION PERIOD — 4 to 5 days

PROGRESSION — usually acute, running through flock in about 5 days, sometimes chronic

SYMPTOMS — in chicks: sudden death soon after hatching or loss of appetite, sleepiness, weakness, droopy wings and head, labored breathing, increased thirst

— in growing birds over 12 weeks old (most common group affected): sudden loss of appetite, droopiness, ruffled feathers, huddling near heat, pale heads, shrunken combs, temperature 1 to 5 °F (1 to 3°C) above normal, diarrhea

— in mature bird: depression, ruffled feathers; sometimes pale heads, increased thirst, dehydration, shrunken combs, greenish or yellowish diarrhea

PERCENTAGE AFFECTED — varies widely

MORTALITY — in chicks: up to 90 percent

—in growing and mature birds: 10 to 50 percent

POSTMORTEM FINDINGS — in young birds: swollen, red liver, spleen, and kidneys

— in older birds: dark, swollen green or bronze liver, sometimes with gray spots; enlarged, sometimes mottled spleen; swollen kidneys; slimy, inflamed intestines; brownish lungs; thin, watery blood

RESEMBLES — paratyphoid and pullorum, except that typhoid often continues for months, usually affects older birds, and causes higher mortality

DIAGNOSIS — flock history, symptoms, postmortem findings, laboratory identification of bacteria

CAUSE — *Salmonella gallinarum* bacteria that affect turkeys as well as chickens and survive for 6 months or more in litter and soil

TRANSMISSION — from infected breeders to chicks through hatching eggs; contaminated litter, equipment, shoes, flies, feet of animals and wild birds

PREVENTION — purchase certified typhoid-free stock; blood test birds and eliminate carriers; clean and disinfect regularly; control flies, rodents, animals, and wild birds; keep chickens away from contaminated ponds and other surface water; rotate range-fed flock; chickens raised in areas where typhoid is prevalent tend to develop resistance

TREATMENT — not recommended, survivors are carriers; this is a **reportable disease** in most states, see "Reportable Diseases" page 196

HUMAN HEALTH RISK — none known, not the same disease as typhoid fever in humans

- U -

Ulcerative Enteritis

ALSO CALLED — quail disease, UE

INCIDENCE — common worldwide

System/Organ Affected — digestive (lower intestine and ceca)
Incubation Period — 1 to 3 days
Progression — acute or chronic, runs its course in 2 to 3 weeks
Symptoms — in young birds, 4 to 12 weeks old (commonly 5 to 7 weeks): sudden death with no symptoms; or listlessness, dull, ruffled feathers, hunched-up posture with head pulled in and eyes closed, diarrhea (sometimes bloody), extreme emaciation, death within 2 to 3 weeks
Percentage Affected — low
Mortality — less than 10 percent, peaking within a week
Postmortem Findings — yellowish button-like dots (ulcerations) throughout intestinal tract, concentrating in lower intestine and cecum; patchy tan or yellow areas on liver; enlarged, mottled spleen; shriveled breast muscle
Resembles — blackhead, except that blackhead does not involve the spleen or lower intestine; coccidiosis, except that cocci often causes bloody droppings (UE rarely does not); necrotic enteritis, except that NE rarely involves the liver or ceca
Diagnosis — symptoms, postmortem findings (buttons in intestine, colorful patchy liver)
Cause — *Clostridium colinum* bacteria that affect game birds more often than chickens, persist under varying conditions (hot, cold, dry, humid), and resist disinfectants; often occurs in combination with coccidiosis, mycoplasmosis, or parasites (internal or external); often follows infectious anemia or infectious bursal disease; outbreak results in permanent contamination of housing
Transmission — contagious; spreads in droppings of infected or carrier birds picked from litter, feed, or water; spread by flies
Prevention — in problem areas, remove and replace litter between flocks or raise birds on wire; avoid crowding; manage flock to avoid coccidiosis, internal and external parasites, and viral diseases (all of which reduce resistance); do not combine birds of different ages or from different sources
Treatment — streptomycin in drinking water at the rate of 15 grams per gallon for 10 days, then 1 gram per gallon for 5 more days; remove old litter; natural survivors are resistant, treated survivors remain susceptible, all survivors may be carriers
Human Health Risk — none known

Urolithiasis. *See* Gout (visceral)
Uveitis. *See* Marek's Disease

- V -

Valgus Leg Deformity. *See* Twisted Leg
Valgus or Varus Deformation (VVD). *See* Twisted Leg
Velogenic Newcastle. *See* Newcastle Disease (exotic)
Vent Gleet. *See* Pasted Vent
Vesicular Dermatitis. *See* Ergotism
Vibrionic Hepatitis. *See* Campylobacteriosis

Viral Arthritis

ALSO CALLED — arthritis/tenosynovitis, reovirus infection, ruptured tendon
INCIDENCE — worldwide but rare
SYSTEM/ORGAN AFFECTED — joints and tendons
INCUBATION PERIOD — 1 to 13 days
PROGRESSION — acute or chronic
SYMPTOMS — in young birds (primarily heavy breeds) 4 to 16 weeks old: lameness, stunted growth, uneven gait, swollen hocks, foot, and other joints
— in mature birds: bowed or spraddled legs (may go undetected)
PERCENTAGE AFFECTED — nearly 100 percent
MORTALITY — 2 to 10 percent, primarily in young birds
POSTMORTEM FINDINGS — hocks and associated tendons sometimes surrounded by yellowish or pinkish sticky fluid
RESEMBLES — staphylococcic arthritis, except that in staph arthritis fluid surrounding joints is whitish and contains flecks; simple leg injury, except that injury involves only individual birds
DIAGNOSIS — flock history (age of birds), symptoms (both shanks swollen), confirmed by laboratory identification of virus
CAUSE — avian reovirus that infects only chickens
TRANSMISSION — contact with infected birds and their droppings or respiratory discharges; spreads from breeders to chicks through hatching eggs
PREVENTION — avoid crowding; do not hatch eggs from infected breeders; vaccinate breeder flock to pass parental immunity to chicks; chicks start developing natural immunity by 2 weeks of age
TREATMENT — none; mildly infected birds recover in 4 to 6 weeks; cull severely affected birds, as they rarely recover; following an outbreak, thoroughly clean and disinfect housing with lye or 0.5 percent organic iodine solution
HUMAN HEALTH RISK — none

Visceral Lymphoma. *See* Lymphoid Leukosis
Visceral Urate Deposition. *See* Gout (visceral)
Viscerotropic Velogenic Newcastle Disease. *See* Newcastle Disease (exotic)
Vitamin A Deficiency. *See* Roup (nutritional)
Vitamin E Deficiency. *See* Encephalomalacia, Exudative Diathesis, White Muscle Disease

- W -

Water Belly. *See* Broiler Ascites
Western Duck Sickness. *See* Botulism
Wet pox. *See* Pox (wet)
White Comb. *See* Favus
White Diarrhea. *See* Pullorum

White Muscle Disease

Also Called — muscular dystrophy, nutritional myopathy
Incidence — not common

SYSTEM/ORGAN AFFECTED — muscles
SYMPTOMS — in chicks 4 weeks old: degeneration of breast and sometimes leg muscles
PERCENTAGE AFFECTED — 10 to 15 percent until diet is corrected
MORTALITY — low
POSTMORTEM FINDINGS — yellow to grayish white streaks (degenerated muscle fibers) in leg or breast muscle
DIAGNOSIS — symptoms, postmortem findings, ration evaluation, absence of infection
CAUSE — deficiency of vitamin E and selenium
TRANSMISSION — nutritional problem, does not spread from bird to bird
PREVENTION — use only fresh commercial rations fortified with Vitamin E and selenium; store feed in cool, dry place and use within 2 weeks of purchase
TREATMENT — vitamin E supplement by injection, in feed, or orally (300 IU per bird); replace old feed; with proper treatment, condition is reversible
HUMAN HEALTH RISK — none

Windpuff. *See* Emphysema
Windswept. *See* Twisted Leg
Wing Rot. *See* Necrotic Dermatitis

- X -

X Disease. *See* Aflatoxicosis, Bluecomb

- Y -

Yolk Sac Infection. *See* Colibacillosis, Omphalitis

Glossary

The following words are defined in the context of chicken health. In another context, some words may have other or broader meanings.

Abscess. Pocket filled with pus.

Acariasis. Mite infestation.

Acute. Having a severe and short development, often measured in hours and ending in death or recovery; opposite of chronic.

Anemia. Deficiency of the blood in quantity or quality due to blood loss or disease, characterized by weakness and pale skin.

Anthelmintic. Wormer.

Antibiotic. A soluble chemical produced by a microorganism or fungus and used to destroy or inhibit the growth of bacteria and other microorganisms.

Antibody. A natural substance in the blood that recognizes and destroys foreign invaders and that causes an immune response to vaccination or infection.

Antigen. A foreign protein that differs from natural body proteins and therefore stimulates the production of antibodies.

Antiseptic. Anything that destroys or inhibits microorganisms responsible for disease, decomposition, or fermentation.

Antitoxin. An antibody that neutralizes toxins produced by bacteria.

Arthritis. Inflammation of the joint and surrounding tissue.

Ascaridiasis. Roundworm infection.

Ascites. Accumulation of fluid in the abdominal cavity.

Atrophy. Shrinking or wasting away of a body part.

Attenuated. Weakened so as not to produce disease but still induce immunity when used as vaccine (said of viruses).

Avian. Pertaining to birds.

Bacteria. Microscopic, single-celled plants that may or may not produce disease (singular: bacterium).

Bactericide. A substance that kills bacteria.

Bacterin. A vaccine produced from bacteria or their products.

Bacteriostat. A substance that inhibits or retards bacterial growth.

Ballooning. Distention of the intestine or ceca due to accumulated blood, mucus, or other materials.

Benign. Not likely to recur or spread.

Biosecurity. Disease-prevention management.

Blow-out. Vent damage due to laying an oversized egg.
Booster. Vaccination other than the first in a series.
Bursa of Fabricius. Cloacal bursa.
Cannibalism. Eating one's own kind.
Cancer. Malignant tumor that tends to spread.
Cankers. Whitish bumps that erupt to form sores, usually on the face or in the mouth.
Capillariasis. Capillary worm infection.
Carrier. An apparently healthy individual that transmits disease-causing organisms to other individuals.
Cauterize. To use a hot iron to burn, sear, or destroy tissue.
Cecum. A blind pouch at the juncture of the small and large intestine that resembles the human appendix (plural: ceca).
Cephalic. Pertaining to the head or skull.
Cestode. Tapeworm.
Cestodiasis. Tapeworm infection.
Chondrodystrophy. Having short bones.
Chromosome. Microscopic cell containing the genes that carry hereditary determination.
Chronic. Having long duration measured in days, months, or even years and being somewhat resistant to treatment; opposite of acute.
Clinical. Having signs or symptoms that can be readily observed.
Cloaca. The lower end of the digestive tract where the digestive, reproductive, and excretory tracts come together.
Clubbed down. Down that fails to emerge in an embryo or newly hatched chick, most commonly around neck and vent.
Coccidiasis. Infection with coccidial protozoa without showing any signs.
Coccidiosis. Infection with coccidial protozoa.
Coccidiostat. A chemical added at low levels to feed or water to prevent coccidiosis.
Cockerel. A male chicken under 1 year of age.
Coliform. Any bacteria resembling *Escherichia coli* bacteria.
Congested. Filled with blood.
Congenital. Existing at birth but not hereditary.
Conjunctiva. Mucous membrane covering the eyeball and inner surface of the eyelid.
Conjunctivitis. Inflammation of the conjunctiva.
Contagious. Readily transmitted from one individual or flock to another.
Crop. To surgically remove wattles; also, the pouch at the base of a bird's neck where feed is temporarily stored.
Cull. To kill a diseased or otherwise unproductive bird.
Culture. To incubate a sample from a diseased bird for several hours (or

days) and look for the presence of bacterial growth.

Cyst. A sack-like structure containing fluid or semi-solid material.

Debeak. To trim back the top beak to prevent cannibalism.

Dehydration. Loss of body water (over 12 percent loss results in death).

Depopulate. Get rid of an entire flock.

Dermatitis. Inflammation of the skin.

Diarrhea. Frequent, runny bowel movements.

Diathesis. Susceptibility to certain diseases.

Disease. Any departure from normal health or impairment of normal body functions.

Disinfection. Killing infectious agents on facilities or equipment but not on a bird's body.

Drench. To give liquid medication orally (by mouth); also the liquid medication itself.

Dub. To surgically remove a bird's comb.

Duodenal Loop. Upper small intestine (same as "duodenum").

Ectoparasite. External parasite.

Edema. Accumulation of excessive fluid in swollen or damaged tissues.

Electrolyte. Natural chemical in the blood needed by body cells to maintain balance; also, mineral solution used to treat dehydration.

Emaciation. Wasting away of the body.

Embryo. A developing chick within an egg.

Embryonation. Development of an embryo into a larva inside an egg without hatching.

Encephalitis. Inflammation of the brain.

Endoparasite. Internal parasite.

Enteric. Affecting the intestines.

Enteritis. Inflammation of the intestine.

Enteropathogens. Microbes that cause enteritis.

Enterotoxin. A substance that poisons cells lining the intestines.

Enzootic. The continuing presence of a disease or infectious agent in a specific area (equivalent to "endemic" human diseases).

Epizootic. Epidemic among chickens or other animals (similar to the word "epidemic" pertaining to humans).

Esophagus. Channel that moves food from the throat to the stomach.

Etiology. The study of causes of diseases.

Eversion. Turned inside out.

Exudate. Fluid associated with inflammation or swelling.

Exudative diathesis. Accumulation of fluid (exudate) under the skin or around the heart.

Fecal. Pertaining to feces.

Feces. Droppings or body waste.

Flaccid. Limp.

Fluke. Trematode flatworm parasite.

Fomites. Inanimate objects such as shipping crates, feed sacks, clothing, and shoe soles that may harbor disease-causing organisms and may be either a vehicle or a reservoir of infection.

Fungus. A plant that does not contain chlorophyll and that reproduces through spores (plural: fungi).

Genes. Parts of chromosomes that carry hereditary factors.

Genetic. Pertaining to genes.

Germs. Disease-causing microbes.

Gangrene. Dead tissue that has no blood supply and no reaction to pain.

Going light. Growing thin while eating ravenously; synonym for anemia.

Gross. Can be seen with the naked eye.

Gross lesions. Easily observable changes in tissues or organs.

Helminth. A category of parasitic worms.

Helminthiasis. Parasitic worm infestation.

Hemorrhage. Heavy or uncontrolled bleeding.

Hepatitis. Inflammation of the liver.

Horizontal transmission. Transmitted from one bird to another.

Host. A bird (or other animal) on or in which an infectious agent lives.

Ileum. Lower small intestine.

Immune. Resistant.

Immunity. Resistance or ability to resist infection.

Immunity, active. Resistance to a disease as a result of having had the disease or having been vaccinated against it.

Immunity, passive. Resistance to a disease as a result of injection with antiserum.

Immunoglobulin. Antigen.

Impaction. Blockage of a body passage or cavity.

Incidence. Number of cases of a particular disease diagnosed during a particular time period.

Incubation period. The time it takes from exposure to a disease-causing agent until the first symptom appears; also, the time it takes for a bird's egg to hatch.

Infection. The entry of an organism into a body and causing of disease by developing or multiplying therein.

Infectious. Capable of invading living tissue and multiplying therein, causing disease.

Infertility. Inability to reproduce.

Inflammation. Reaction of tissue to injury or irritation, whereby it becomes red, hot, swollen, painful, and possibly loses its function.

Ingest. Eat.

Initial vaccination. First vaccination in a series.
Inoculate. To give an injection.
Inoculant. A substance that's injected.
Intramuscular(IM). Placement of an injection into muscle tissue.
Intraocular. In the eye.
Intranasal. In the nose.
Immunosuppressant. Any cause of reduced disease resistance.
Intravenous (IV). Placement of an injection into a vein.
...itis. Suffix indicating inflammation (e.g. sinusitis means inflammation of the sinus cavities).
IU. International Unit, in which some drugs are measured.
Jejunum. Middle small intestine.
Joint ill. Arthritis.
Laceration. Jagged wound.
Lesion. A change in size, shape, color, or structure of an internal organ.
Leukosis. A disease of the blood-forming organs.
Lymphatic system. Circulating system that contains the immune system's white blood cells.
Lymphoma. Cancer of the lymph system.
Malabsorption. Excessive loss of nutrients through the feces.
Malignant. Tending to worsen, recur, or spread; opposite of benign.
Mechanical transmission. Carried on the surface.
Metabolic disease. A disease involving a breakdown in the body's physical or chemical processes.
Metabolism. All the physical and chemical processes that produce and maintain a living body.
Metastasis. The transfer of disease from one organ to another that it isn't directly touching.
Metastasize. Spread to other tissues or organs.
Microscopic. Cannot be seen by the naked eye.
Mite. A small to microscopic jointed-legged creature.
Mold. A type of fungus.
Molt. Natural shedding and renewal of feathers.
Morbid. Having or causing a disease.
Morbidity. Percentage affected by disease.
Morbidity rate. The number of birds in a flock that contract a disease within a given time period.
Moribund. Dying.
Mortality. Death rate.
Mortality rate. The number of birds in a flock that die from a disease within a given time period.
Mucous membrane. The lining of body cavities.

Mucus. Slimy substance produced by mucous membranes.
Mycosis. Any disease caused by a fungus.
Myopathy. Any disease of the muscles.
Necropsy. A postmortem examination (equivalent to a human autopsy).
Necrotic. Pertaining to dead tissue.
Necrotic enteritis. Inflammation and decaying of intestinal tissue.
Nematode. Roundworm.
Neoplasm. A tumor or other abnormal growth.
Nephritis. Inflammation of the kidneys.
Neural. Pertaining to nerves.
Noninfectious disease. A disease that is not caused by a biological organism.
Noxious. Unpleasant.
Ocular. Pertaining to the eye.
Oocyst. The infective fertilized egg of certain one-celled animal parasites.
Opportunistic. A microorganism that is non-infectious to healthy birds; infectious only to birds with reduced resistance from some other cause.
Organism. A living thing.
Osteomyelitis. Inflammation of the bone marrow.
Osteopetrosis. Increased size, density, and brittleness of the bone.
Osteoporosis. Thinning and weakening of the bone.
Oviduct. Channel through which an egg passes after it leaves a hen's ovary.
Parasite. A living organism that survives on another living organism without providing any benefit in return.
Parental immunity. Resistance to disease passed from breeders to their offspring through the egg.
Parenteral. Located outside the intestines, used in referring to drugs introduced by injection rather than by mouth.
Pasting. Loose droppings sticking to the vent area.
Pathogen. Disease-producing organism or agent.
Pathogenic. Capable of causing disease.
Pathogenicity. Degree of ability to cause disease.
Pathology. The study of damage caused by disease.
Pathologist. A medical professional who looks for internal damage caused by disease.
Pediculosis. Louse infestation.
Peracute. Having extremely severe and short duration, measured in minutes or hours.
Perosis. Malformation of the hock joint.
pH. A number that indicates acidity or alkalinity; 7 is neutral, above 7 is alkaline, below 7 is acid.
Pick-out. Vent damage due to cannibalism.
Pneumonia. Any disease of the lungs.

Popeye. Emaciation of chicks (causing eyes to appear large in relation to body).

Post. To conduct a postmortem examination.

Postmortem. Pertaining to or occurring after death.

Predispose. To cause susceptibility to disease.

Prevalence. The number of cases of a disease in a flock during a given time.

Priming vaccination. Vaccination that increases antibody levels before another product is used to induce immunity.

Prolapse. Slipping of a body part from its normal position, often used incorrectly to describe an everted organ.

Progeny test. Evaluation of breeders based on the performance of their offspring.

Protective synergism. Phenomenon by which two vaccines confer greater protection than the sum of their individual effects.

Protozoan. A single-celled microscopic animal that may be either parasitic or beneficial (plural: protozoa).

Proventriculus. A chicken's stomach, lying between the crop and the gizzard.

Pullet. A female chicken under one year of age.

Purulent. Full of pus.

Pus. Liquid, produced by inflammation, containing dead white blood cells.

Rales. Any abnormal sound coming from the airways.

Rattling. Abnormal sound coming from the throat.

Reactor. A bird that reacts positively to a test for an infectious disease.

Renal. Pertaining to the kidneys.

Reportable. A disease that is so serious it must, by law, be reported to a state or federal veterinarian.

Reservoir of infection. Any animate or inanimate object on which an infectious agent survives and multiplies and from which it can be transmitted to a susceptible host.

Resistance. Immunity or ability to resist infection.

Respiration rate. Number of cycles per minute by which air is moved into and out of the lungs.

Rhinitis. Inflammation of the lining of the nasal passages.

Rigor mortis. Stiffness following death.

Roup. Any condition involving chronic infection of skull membranes, characterized by facial swelling.

Salpingitis. Inflammation of the oviduct.

Secondary infection. A disease that invades after a bird's immune defenses have been weakened by some other disease.

Secretion. Fluid coming from a body organ.

Seleniferous. High in selenium.

Self-limiting. Any disease that runs its course in a specific amount of time then stops without treatment.

Septicemia. Blood poisoning or invasion of the bloodstream by a microorganism.

Serological. Pertaining to the testing of blood serum for antibodies against specific diseases.

Serum. The clear liquid portion of the blood left after clotting (plural: sera).

Sign. Objective evidence of disease consisting of symptoms and lesions.

Sinus. A hollow space or cavity.

Sinusitis. Inflammation of the sinus cavities.

Spleen. Organ near the stomach that aids in the proper functioning of blood.

Spore. The seed of fungi or the inactive form of certain bacteria.

spp. (as in *Salmonella* spp.). More than one species.

Starve-out. Failure of chicks to eat.

Sterile. Entirely free of living organisms; also, permanently unable to reproduce.

Sternum. Breastbone or keel.

Stress. Any physical or mental disruption that lowers resistance.

Subclinical. An inapparent infection for which signs or symptoms can be detected only through laboratory analysis.

Subcutaneous. Directly beneath the skin.

Symptom. Detectable evidence of disease.

Syndrome. A group of symptoms that occur in combination in a particular disease, such as runting syndrome.

Synergistic. Working in cooperation (same as "synergetic").

Syringe. Tube with plunger that holds a drug to be injected.

Systemic. Involving the entire body.

Taeniasis. Obsolete word for cestodiasis (tapeworm infection).

Tenosynovitis. Inflammation of the synovial shield of a tendon.

Three-host tick. A tick that spends the three stages of its life on three different hosts.

Torticollis. Twisted or wry neck.

Toxemia. Generalized poisoning resulting from circulation through the body of toxins produced by bacteria.

Toxin. A poison produced by microorganisms.

Toxoid. An agent that confers immunity against toxins produced by bacteria.

Trachea. Windpipe.

Transovarian transmission. Infection of a hen's egg before the shell is formed.

Trauma. Wound or injury that destroys tissue.

Traumatic ventriculitis. Piercing of the gizzard from the inside by a pointed object.

Trematode. A fluke.
Tubercle (as in tuberculosis). A tumor-like mass.
Tumor. A mass of tissue that develops and grows without benefit to surrounding tissue.
Ulcer. A raw, red sore.
Unthrifty. Unhealthy appearing and/or failing to grow at a normal rate.
Urates. Uric acid (salts found in urine), appearing as white crystals or paste.
Uremia. Poisoning caused by accumulated wastes in the Body, usually due to kidney failure.
Urolith. Urinary stone.
Vaccine. Product made from disease-causing organisms and used to induce imunity.
Vascular. Pertaining to blood vessels.
Vector. A living thing that carries disease organisms within its body from one source to another (examples: mosquitoes, ticks, flies).
Vehicle. Anything that mechanically carries disease from one place to another (examples: clothing, equipment, dust).
Vent. The outside opening of the cloaca.
Ventriculus. The gizzard.
Venipuncture. Inserting a needle into the vein for the purpose of withdrawing blood.
Vertebrae. Bones in the spinal column (singular: vertebra).
Vertical transmission. Transmitted from parent to offspring through hatching eggs.
Veterinary ethology. The study of animal behavior as it relates to health.
Viremic. Of or pertaining to a virus in the blood.
Viscera. Internal body organs and glands.
Viscous. Thick and sticky.
Virulence. Pathogenicity or ability to cause disease.
Virus. An ultra-microscopic organism that multiplies only in living cells.
Warfarin. An anti-coagulant used to poison rodents.
Zoonosis. A disease transmissible from a chicken (or other animal) to a human (plural: zoonoses).

Suppliers

American Livestock Supply
Box 8441
Madison, WI 53708
800-356-0700

First State Veterinary Supply
PO Box 190
Parsonburg, MD 21849
800-950-8387

Foster and Smith, Inc.
2253 Air Park Drive
Rhinelander, WI 54501-0100
800-826-7206

G.Q.F. Manufacturing Company
2343 Louisville Road
Savannah, GA 31498
920-236-0651

Hagenow Laboratories, Inc.
1302 Washington Street
Manitowoc, WI 54220
414-683-3339

Jeffers Vet Supply
PO Box 100
Dothan, AL 36302
800-533-3377

Murray McMurray Hatchery, Inc.
Webster City, IA 50595-0458
800-456-3280

Omaha Vaccine Company
PO Box 7228
3030 "L" Street
Omaha, NE 68107
800-367-4444

Paterson Poultry Supplies
210 Meadowbrooke Lane
Martinsville, VA 24112
703-638-2297

PBS Livestock Drugs
2800 Leemont Avenue N.W.
Canton, OH 44701
800-321-0235

Strecker Supply Company
PO Box 190, Dept. S
Parsonburg, MD 21849
800-765-0065

Vineland Laboratories
2285 East Landis Avenue
Vineland, NJ 08360
609-691-2411

State Poultry Pathology Laboratories

ALABAMA

J.B. Taylor Veterinary Diagnostic Laboratory, 495 AL 203, Elba, AL 36323, 334-897-6340

Charles S. Roberts Veterinary Diagnostic Laboratory, PO Box 2209, Auburn, AL 36831-2209, 334-844-4987

ALASKA

Alaska State Federal Laboratory, 500 South Alaska Street, Palmer, AK 99645, 907-745-3236

ARIZONA

Veterinary Diagnostic Laboratory, University of Arizona, 2831 North Freeway, Tucson, AZ 85705, 520-621-2356

ARKANSAS

Arkansas Livestock and Poultry Commission Diagnostic Laboratory, PO Box 8505, Natural Resource Drive, Little Rock, AR 72215, 501-225-5650

Arkansas Livestock and Poultry Commission Diagnostic Laboratory, 3559 N Thompson, Springdale, AR 72764, 501-751-4869

CALIFORNIA

California Veterinary Diagnostic Laboratory System, University of California, PO Box 1770, Davis, CA 95617, 916-752-8700

Fresno Branch Laboratory, 2789 South Orange Avenue, Fresno, CA 93725, 209-498-7740

San Bernardino Branch Laboratory, 105 West Central Avenue, San Bernardino, CA 92408, 909-383-4287

San Diego County Veterinary Laboratory, 555 Overland Avenue, Building 4, San Diego, CA 92123, 619-694-2838

Tulare Branch Laboratory, 18830 Road 112, Tulare, CA 93274, 209-688-7543

Turlock Branch Laboratory, PO Box 1522, Turlock, CA 95381, 209-634-5837

COLORADO

CSU Veterinary Diagnostic Lab, 27847 RD 21, Rocky Ford, CO 81067, 719-254-6382

Veterinary Diagnostic Laboratory, Colorado State University, Fort Collins, CO 80523, 970-491-1281

Western Slope Animal Diagnostic Laboratory, 425-29 Road, Grand Junction, CO 81501, 970-243-0673

CONNECTICUT

Department of Pathobiology, Box U-89 61 North Eagleville Road, University of Connecticut, Storrs, CT 06269-3089, 860-486-3736

DELAWARE

Poultry and Animal Health Section, State Department of Agriculture, PO Drawer D, 2320 S Dupont Highway, Dover, DE 19901, 302-739-4811

FLORIDA

Bureau of Diagnostic Laboratories, 2700 N. Bermuda Road, PO Box 420460, Kissimmee, FL 34742, 407-846-5200

Live Oak Diagnostic Laboratory, Swanee County Branch, 912 Nobles Ferry Road, PO Box O, Live Oak, FL 32064, 904-362-1216

GEORGIA

Georgia Poultry Laboratory, 150 Tom Fryer Drive, Douglas, GA 31533, 912-384-3719

Georgia Poultry Laboratory, PO Box 20, Oakwood, GA 30566, 770-535-5996

HAWAII

Veterinary Laboratory Branch, Hawaii Department of Agriculture, 99-941 Halawa Valley Street, Aiea, HI 96701, 808-483-7100

IDAHO

Division of Animal Industries, PO Box 7249, 2270 Old Penitentiary Road, Boise, ID 83707, 208-885-6639

ILLINOIS

Animal Disease Laboratory, 9732 Shattuc Road, Centralia, IL 62801, 618-532-6701

Animal Disease Laboratory, 2100 South Lake Storey Road, Galesburg, IL 61401, 309-344-2451

INDIANA

Animal Disease Diagnostic Laboratory, Purdue University, 1175 ADDL, West Lafayette, IN 47907-1175, 765-494-7440

Animal Disease Diagnostic Laboratory, SIPAC, 11367 East Purdue Farm Road, Dubois, IN 47527, 812-678-3401

IOWA

Veterinary Diagnostic Laboratory, Iowa State University, Ames, IA 50011, 515-294-1950

KANSAS

Diagnostic Medicine Pathology Laboratories, 1800 Denison Avenue, Manhattan, KS 66506, 913-532-5650

KENTUCKY

Livestock Disease Diagnostic Center, 1429 Newtown Pike, Lexington, KY 40511, 606-253-0571

Murray State University, Breathitt Veterinary Center, PO Box 2000, 715 North Drive, Hopkinsville, KY 42240, 502-886-3959

LOUISIANA

Central Louisiana Livestock Diagnostic Laboratory, 217 Middleton Drive, Lecompte, LA 71346, 318-473-6500

Louisiana Veterinary Medical Diagnostic Laboratory, LSU School of Veterinary Medicine, 1909 South Stadium Drive, Baton Rouge, LA 70803, 504-346-3193

MAINE

Pathology Diagnostic and Research Laboratory, 5735 Hitchner Hall, University of Maine, Orono, ME 04469, 207-581-2775

MARYLAND

Animal Health Department Laboratory, PO Box 376, Oakland, MD 21550, 301-334-2185

Animal Health Laboratory, Maryland Department of Agriculture, 211 Safety Drive, Centreville, MD 21617, 410-758-0846

Animal Health Laboratory, Maryland Department of Agriculture, Rosemont Avenue, Frederick, MD 21702, 301-663-9528

Animal Health Laboratory, Maryland Department of Agriculture, PO Box J, Salisbury, MD 21802, 410-543-6610

Animal Health Laboratory, 8077 Greenmead Drive, College Park, MD 20740, 301-935-6074

MASSACHUSETTS
Tufts University School of Veterinary Medicine, 200 Westboro Road, North Grafton, MA 01536, 508-839-5302

MICHIGAN
Animal Health Diagnostic Laboratory, PO Box 30076, Lansing, MI 48909, 517-353-1683

MINNESOTA
Minnesota Veterinary Diagnostic Laboratories, 1333 Gortoner Avenue, College of Veterinary Medicine, University of Minnesota, St. Paul, MN 55108, 612-625-8787

MISSISSIPPI
Mississippi Veterinary Diagnostic Laboratory, PO Box 4389, Jackson, MS 39216, 601-354-6091

MISSOURI
Veterinary Diagnostic Laboratory, Missouri Department of Agriculture, PO Box 2510, Springfield, MO 65801, 417-895-6861
Veterinary Medical Diagnostic Laboratory, College of Veterinary Medicine, PO Box 6023, University of Missouri, Columbia, MO 65205, 573-882-6811

MONTANA
Veterinary Diagnostic Laboratory Division, Montana Department of Livestock, PO Box 997, Bozeman, MT 59771, 406-994-4885

NEBRASKA
Diagnostic Laboratory, Department of Veterinary Science, University of Nebraska, Lincoln, NE 68583, 402-472-1434
University of Nebraska, WCREC, Route 4 Box 46A, North Platte, NE 69101, 308-532-3611

NEVADA
Animal Disease Laboratory, Nevada Department of Agriculture, 350 Capital Hill Avenue, Reno, NV 89502, 702-688-1180

NEW HAMPSHIRE
Veterinary Diagnostic Laboratory, University of New Hampshire, 319 Kendall Hall, Durham, NH 03824, 603-862-2726

NEW JERSEY
New Jersey Animal Health Diagnostic Laboratory, John Fitch Plaza, PO Box 330, Trenton, NJ 08625, 609-292-3965

NEW MEXICO
Veterinary Diagnostic Services, 700 Camino de Salud Northeast, Albuquerque, NM 87106, 505-841-2576

NEW YORK
Cornell University Duck Research Laboratory, Box 217, Old Country Road, Eastport, NY 11941, 516-325-0600
Department of Microbiology and Immunology, College of Veterinary Medicine, Cornell University, Ithaca, NY 14853, 607-253-3365

NORTH CAROLINA
Rollins Animal Disease Diagnostic Laboratory, PO Box 12223 Cameron Village Station, 272101 Blue Ridge Road, Raleigh, NC 27605, 919-733-3986

NORTH DAKOTA

North Dakota Veterinary Diagnostic Laboratory, North Dakota State University, Fargo, ND 58105, 701-231-8307

OHIO

Animal Disease Diagnostic Laboratory, Ohio Department of Agriculture, 8995 East Main Street, Reynoldsburg, OH 43068, 614-728-6220

OKLAHOMA

Oklahoma Animal Disease Diagnostic Laboratory, College of Veterinary Medicine, Oklahoma State University, Stillwater, OK 74078, 405-744-6623

OREGON

Oregon State Department of Agriculture, Animal Health Laboratory, 635 Capitol Street Northeast, Salem, OR 97310, 503-986-4550

Department of Animal Sciences, 112 Withycombe Hall, Corvallis, OR 97331, 503-737-2301

Veterinary Diagnostic Laboratory, Oregon State University, PO Box 429, Corvallis, OR 97339, 541-737-3261

PENNSYLVANIA

Department of Agriculture, 2305 N. Cameron Street, Harrisburg, PA 17110-9449, 717-787-8808

Animal Diagnostic Laboratory, Veterinary Science Department, Pennsylvania State University, University Park, PA 16802, 814-863-0837

PUERTO RICO

Department of Agriculture, Veterinary Diagnostic Laboratory, PO Box 490, Dorado, PR 00646, 809-796-1650

RHODE ISLAND

Department of Fisheries, Animal, and Veterinary Science, University of Rhode Island, Kingston, RI 02881, 401-874-2477

SOUTH CAROLINA

Clemson Animal Diagnostic Laboratory, PO Box 102406, Columbia, SC 29224-2406, 803-788-2260

SOUTH DAKOTA

Animal Disease Research and Diagnostic Laboratory, South Dakota State University, 105 Veterinary Science, PO Box 2175, Brookings, SD 57007, 605-688-5171

TENNESSEE

C.E. Kord Animal Disease Laboratory, Ellington Agriculture Center, Porter Building, PO Box 40627 Melrose Station, Nashville, TN 37204, 615-837-5125

TEXAS

PBMDL Poultry Laboratory, PO Box 187, Center, TX 75935, 409-598-4451

Department of Pathology and Biology, College of Veterinary Medicine, Texas A and M University, College Station, TX 77843, 409-845-5941

Poultry Disease Laboratory, Texas Veterinary Medical Diagnostic Laboratory System, PO Box 84, Gonzales, TX 78629, 830-672-2834

UTAH

Utah State University-Provo Veterinary Laboratory, Utah Agricultural Experimental Station, 2031 South State, Provo, UT 84606, 801-373-6383

Department of Agriculture, State Chemist Office, 350 North Redwood Road, Salt Lake City, UT 84114, 801-538-7128

Veterinary Diagnostic Laboratory, Utah State University, Logan, UT 84322-5600, 801-750-1895

VIRGINIA

Division of Animal Health, Regulatory Laboratory, 116 Reservoir Street, Harrisonburg, VA 22801, 540-434-3897

Division of Animal Health, Regulatory Laboratory, 34591 General Mahone Blvd., Ivor, VA 23866, 757-859-6221

Division of Animal Health, Regulatory Laboratory, 272 Academy Hill Road, Warrenton, VA 20186, 540-347-6385

Virginia Dept. of Agriculture & Consumer Services, 250 Cassel Road, Wytheville, VA 24382, 540-228-5501

Veterinary Teaching Hospital, VA-MD Regional College of Veterinary Medicine, Virginia Polytechnic Institute and State University, Blacksburg, VA 24061, 540-231-4621

Virginia Department of Agriculture and Consumer Services, Division of Animal Health Regulatory Laboratory, Bureau of Laboratory Services, 4832 Tyreanna, Lynchburg, VA 24504, 804-947-6731

WASHINGTON

Poultry Diagnostic Laboratory, Washington State University, 7612 Pioneer Way East, Puyallup, WA 98371, 206-840-4536

Washington Animal Disease Diagnostic Laboratory, PO Box 2037 College Station, Washington State University, Pullman, WA 99165, 509-335-9696

WEST VIRGINIA

State-Federal Laboratory, West Virginia Department of Agriculture, Capitol Building, Charleston, WV 25305, 304-348-3418

WISCONSIN

Wisconsin Animal Health Laboratory - Barron, 1521 East Guy Avenue, Barron, WI 54812, 715-537-3151

Wisconsin Animal Health Laboratory, 6101 Mineral Point Road, Madison, WI 53705, 608-266-2465

WYOMING

Wyoming State Veterinary Laboratory, 1174 Snowy Range Road, Laramie, WY 82070, 307-742-6638

CANADA

ALBERTA

Poultry Pathology, O.S. Longman Building, 6909-116 Street, Edmonton, AB, T6H 4P2, 403-427-2238

BRITISH COLUMBIA

Animal Health Center, 1767 Angus Campbell Road, Abbottsford, BC, V3G 2M, 604-576-3737

MANITOBA

Animal Health Center, Agricultural Services Complex, University of Manitoba, 545 University Crescent, Winnipeg, MB, R3T 5S6, 204-945-7650

NEW BRUNSWICK

Veterinary Pathology, Department of Agriculture, PO Box 6000, Fredericton, NB, E3B 5H1, 506-453-2210

NOVA SCOTIA
Veterinary Pathology Laboratory, PO Box 550, Truro, NS, B2N 5E3, 902-893-6538

ONTARIO
Veterinary Laboratory, Guelph Agriculture Centre, Ontario Veterinary College, Guelph, ON, N1G 6N1, 519-823-8800

PRINCE EDWARD ISLAND
Atlantic Veterinary College, University of Prince Edward Island, 550 University Avenue, Charlottetown, PE, C1A 4P3 902-566-0882

QUEBEC
Department of Veterinary Pathology, School of Veterinary Medicine, CP 5000, St. Hyacinthe, PQ, J2S 7C6, 514-773-8521

SASKATCHEWAN
Department of Veterinary Pathology, Western College of Veterinary Medicine, University of Saskatchewan, 52 Campus Drive, Saskateoon, SK, S7N 5B4 306-966-7299

Recommended Reading

Some of the following publications are regularly updated as new information and treatments are made available. When requesting a copy, ask for the latest edition.

Avian Disease Manual, The American Association of Avian Pathologists, University of Pennsylvania, New Bolton Center, 382 West Street Road, Kennett Square, PA 19348; easy-to-read handbook designed for avian pathology students.

Chicken Diseases, F. P. Jeffrey, American Bantam Association, PO Box 127, Augusta, NJ 07822; booklet geared toward the backyard enthusiast.

Code of Federal Regulations Title 9 (vaccines), Title 21 (drugs), Title 40 (pesticides), United States Government Printing Office, Superintendent of Documents, Washington, D.C. 20402-9328; U.S. government regulations, including drug use in poultry (available at many libraries).

Color Atlas of Diseases and Disorders of the Domestic Fowl and Turkey, Iowa State University Press, Ames, IA 50010; color photos illustrating internal organs with various disease conditions.

Diseases of Poultry, Iowa State University Press, Ames, IA 50010; comprehensive tome written in fairly technical language.

The Federal Register, United States Government Printing Office, Superintendent of Documents, Washington, D.C. 20402-9328; U.S. government regulations, including drug use in poultry (available at many libraries).

Feed Additives Compendium, Miller Publishing Company, PO Box 2400, Minnetonka, MN 55343; monthly report on current regulations governing livestock feeds (available at agricultural libraries).

Feedstuffs Reference Issue, Miller Publishing Company, PO Box 2400, Minnetonka, MN 55343; annual feed industry report on livestock nutrition and diseases.

A Manual of Poultry Diseases, Department of Agricultural Communications, Reed McDonald Building, Room 101, Texas A&M University, College Station, TX 77843; handbook for small-flock owners.

National Poultry Improvement Plan Directory of Participants Handling Egg-Type and Meat-Type Chickens and Turkeys, USDA, APHIS Veterinary Services, Room 848, FCB #1, Hyattsville, MD 20782; annually updated list of flock owners, dealers, and hatcheries by state.

National Poultry Improvement Plan Directory of Participants Handling Waterfowl, Exhibition Poultry, and Game Birds, USDA, APHIS-VS, NPIP, Room 205 Presidential Building, 6525 Belcrest Road, Hyattsville, MD 20782; annually updated list of flock owners, dealers, and hatcheries by state.

Nutrient Requirements of Poultry, National Research Council, National Academy Press, 2101 Constitution Avenue, NW, Washington, DC 20418; technical discussions and feed charts for formulating rations.

Poultry Health Handbook, L. Dwight Schwartz, Publications Distribution Center, College of Agricultural Science, The Pennsylvania State Publications Distribution Center, College of Agricultural Sciences, The Pennsylvania State University, 112 Agricultural Administration Building, University Park, PA 16802; guide to identifying and preventing diseases of chickens and other fowl.

Solvay Manual of Poultry Diseases, Solvay Animal Health, Inc., Poultry Business Unit, 1201 Northland Drive, Mendota Heights, MN 55120; color manual helpful in conducting home postmortem.

Veterinary Clinical Parasitology, Margaret W. Sloss and Russell L. Kemp, Iowa State University Press, Ames, IA 50010; laboratory manual describing how to conduct a fecal examination, with photos of some of the parasites that infect fowl.

Index

(Illustrations are indicated by page numbers in *italics;* charts and tables are indicated by pages numbers in **bold.**)